## Praise for *Population-Based Public Health Clir* *The Henry Street Model for Nurses*

"*The foundational Henry Street Model continues to inspire and inform in this third edition of* Population-Based Public Health Clinical Manual. *This new edition has welcome updates, with the newest version of Henry Street Consortium Entry-Level Population-Based Public Health Nursing Competencies. Relationships among students, preceptors, and practitioners are reinforced and illustrated with individual and community-based examples. Ethical parameters are reiterated, and there's a renewed emphasis on both national and global health. Revised tables throughout bolster the narrative. The scholarly and reflective updates from the previous edition assure the continuing value of this text to teachers, learners, and patients seeking healthier communities.*"

–Mary W. Byrne, PhD, DNP, MPH, FAAN
Stone Foundation and Elise D. Fish Professor of Clinical Health Care for the Underserved
Columbia University School of Nursing and College of Physicians and Surgeons

"*This book is well-organized, easy to read and understand, and full of critical information for success as a PHN. The elements included in each chapter make it unique among texts on public health nursing, as it is the most relevant to actual practice. The text provides links to other critical documents, such as the Standards of Public Health Nursing, Core Functions, and Sustainable Development Goals. The examples are specific and easy to follow, and the Notebook sections provide excellent summaries at a student's level. I would recommend this book to faculty in any BSN program and to anyone who wishes to pursue a career in public health nursing.*"

–Joy F. Reed, EdD, RN, FAAN
North Carolina Department of Health & Human Services
Division of Public Health

"*In reviewing this text, I absolutely fell in love with the framework and the Henry Street Consortium model. This book showcases the essence of the public health nursing role and the noble history of the discipline. The content's competency structure is perfect for education and clearly identifies experiences for students and teachers. Advocacy for population health is underscored as a public health nursing role and is grounded in the real world. The authors emphasize leadership and political impact and the core of what it means to be a public health nurse. The text portrays the distinct commitment to principles of social justice, which drives advocacy and taking action for what is right.*"

–Pamela N. Clarke, PhD, MPH, RN, FAAN
Professor, Fay W. Whitney School of Nursing
University of Wyoming

"*This third edition of* Population-Based Public Health Clinical Manual: The Henry Street Model for Nurses *supports the learning, knowledge, and professional development of public health nurses committed to making a difference in health worldwide. The book starts with a description of foundational public health nursing concepts, and each of the following chapters describes one core competency and its characteristics. The book's content is based on the practice of public health nurses, making it an excellent resource for the student nurse, for the new public health nurse, for the practicing public health nurse, and for public health nursing faculty.*"

–Kari Glavin, PhD
Professor and Head of Master and Postgraduate Studies
VID Specialized University
Oslo, Norway

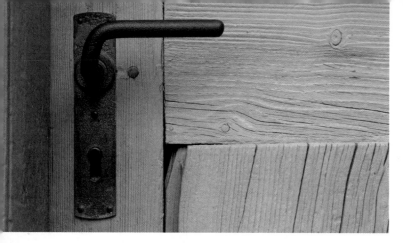
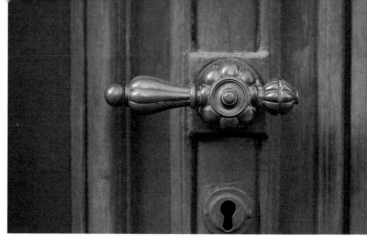
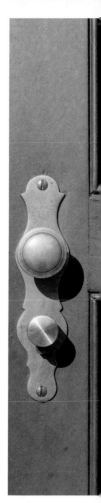

# POPULATION-BASED PUBLIC HEALTH CLINICAL MANUAL

## THE HENRY STREET MODEL FOR NURSES

### THIRD EDITION

**Patricia M. Schoon**, DNP, MPH, RN, PHN
**Carolyn M. Porta**, PhD, MPH, RN, PHN, SANE-A, FAAN
**Marjorie A. Schaffer**, PhD, MS, RN, PHN

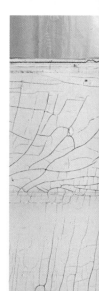

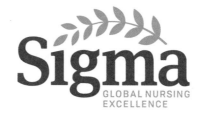

Sigma

GLOBAL NURSING
EXCELLENCE

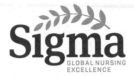

*The Sigma Theta Tau International Honor Society of Nursing (Sigma) is a nonprofit organization whose mission is advancing world health and celebrating nursing excellence in scholarship, leadership, and service. Founded in 1922, Sigma has more than 135,000 active members in over 90 countries and territories. Members include practicing nurses, instructors, researchers, policymakers, entrepreneurs, and others. Sigma's more than 530 chapters are located at more than 700 institutions of higher education throughout Armenia, Australia, Botswana, Brazil, Canada, Colombia, England, Ghana, Hong Kong, Japan, Jordan, Kenya, Lebanon, Malawi, Mexico, the Netherlands, Pakistan, Philippines, Portugal, Singapore, South Africa, South Korea, Swaziland, Sweden, Taiwan, Tanzania, Thailand, the United States, and Wales. Learn more at www.SigmaNursing.org.*

**Sigma Theta Tau International**
**550 West North Street**
**Indianapolis, IN, 46202 USA**

To order additional books, buy in bulk, or order for corporate use, contact Sigma Marketplace at 888.654.4968 (US and Canada) or +1.317.634.8171 (outside US and Canada).

To request a review copy for course adoption, e-mail solutions@sigmamarketplace.org or call 888.654.4968 (US and Canada) or +1.317.634.8171 (outside US and Canada).

To request author information, or for speaker or other media requests, contact Sigma Marketing at 888.634.7575 (US and Canada) or +1.317.634.8171 (outside US and Canada).

| | |
|---|---|
| **ISBN:** | 9781945157752 |
| **EPUB ISBN:** | 9781945157769 |
| **PDF ISBN:** | 9781945157776 |
| **MOBI ISBN:** | 9781945157783 |

---

Library of Congress Cataloging-in-Publication Data

Names: Schaffer, Marjorie, author. | Schoon, Patricia M., author. | Porta, Carolyn M., author. |
Sigma Theta Tau International, issuing body.
Title: Population-based public health clinical manual: the Henry Street model for nurses / Patricia M. Schoon, Carolyn M. Porta, Marjorie A. Schaffer.
Description: Third edition. | Indianapolis, IN: Sigma Theta Tau International, [2018] | Schaffer's name appears first in the first edition. | Includes bibliographical references and index.
Identifiers: LCCN 2018023555 (print) | LCCN 2018024458 (ebook) | ISBN 9781945157769 (epub ebook) | ISBN 9781945157776 (pdf ebook) | ISBN 9781945157783 (mobi ebook) | ISBN 9781945157752 (pbk.) | ISBN 9781945157769 (epub) | ISBN 9781945157776 (pdf) | ISBN 9781945157783 (mobi)
Subjects: | MESH: Henry Street Consortium. | Public Health Nursing | Competency-Based Education | Education, Nursing--standards | Models, Educational | Models, Nursing
Classification: LCC RT97 (ebook) | LCC RT97 (print) | NLM WY 108 | DDC 610.73/4--dc23
LC record available at https://lccn.loc.gov/2018023555

---

**First Printing, 2018**

**Publisher:** Dustin Sullivan
**Acquisitions Editor:** Emily Hatch
**Publications Specialist:** Todd Lothery
**Cover Designer:** Rebecca Batchelor
**Interior Design/Page Layout:** Kim Scott, Bumpy Design
**Illustrator:** Michael Tanamachi

**Principal Book Editor:** Carla Hall
**Development Editor:** Rebecca Senninger
**Copy Editor:** Erin Geile
**Proofreader:** Gill Editorial Services
**Indexer:** Joy Dean Lee

"*We dedicate this third edition to Dr. Linda Olson Keller, DNP, RN, FAAN, whose vision and passion for public health nursing has inspired public health nurses worldwide to improve the health of populations. Her leadership led to the development of the Public Health Intervention Wheel, the Henry Street Consortium, and the Henry Street competencies. Her work has given public health nurses a confident voice in responding to the health needs of people where they grow, live, work, and play.*"

## Acknowledgments

We wish to thank our colleagues in the Henry Street Consortium, who generously shared their knowledge, experiences, and examples of the essence of public health nursing. Linda Olson Keller and Sue Strohschein's vision for developing the public health nursing workforce of the future led to a federal Division of Nursing grant obtained by the Minnesota Department of Health. The Linking Public Health Nursing Practice and Education to Promote Population Health grant provided support for the development of the Henry Street Consortium. As a result of this support, public health nurses and nursing educators collaborated to develop the Henry Street Consortium competencies.

The following Minnesota colleges, universities, health departments, and agencies are represented by Henry Street Consortium members:

### Public Health Agencies

Anoka County Community Health & Environmental Services Department
Carver County Public Health Department
Chisago County Public Health Division of Health and Human Services
City of Bloomington Division of Public Health
Dakota County Public Health Department
Hennepin County Human Services & Public Health Department
Isanti County Public Health
Kanabec County Public Health
Metropolitan Area School Nurses
Minnesota Department of Health
Minnesota Visiting Nurse Agency
Saint Paul-Ramsey County Public Health
Scott County Public Health
Sherburne County Public Health Department
Washington County Department of Public Health & Environment
Wright County Human Services Agency

### Colleges and Universities

Augsburg College
Bethel University
Crown College
Gustavus Adolphus College
Metropolitan State University
Minnesota State University, Mankato
Minnesota State University, Moorhead
St. Catherine University
University of Minnesota

## About the Authors

**Patricia M. Schoon, DNP, MPH, RN, PHN**, is Assistant Professor at Metropolitan State University in St. Paul, Minnesota. She is a founding member of the Henry Street Consortium and has taught nursing and public health for more than 35 years. She was the first geriatric nurse practitioner (GNP) in the United States in 1972. Schoon received the Minnesota Nurses Association Nurse Educator Award in 2005 for her work on Nurses Day on the Hill and an online political advocacy toolkit. She received the Association of Community Nurse Educators 2016 Outstanding Contributions to Community/Public Health Nursing Education Award and March of Dimes 2017 Minnesota Nurse of the Year Education and Research Award. Schoon was President of Chi at-Large Chapter and faculty advisor for Zeta Chapter of Sigma Theta Tau International Honor Society of Nursing (Sigma). She has developed innovative programs in the community, including a foot-care clinic for the homeless and a faith-based program for older adults. She has coauthored articles on the Henry Street Consortium, development of a foot-care clinic in a homeless shelter, and a 2017 article on partnership engagement, an outcome of a Robert Wood Johnson grant to develop best practices in academic-practice collaboration.

**Carolyn M. Porta, PhD, MPH, RN, PHN, SANE-A, FAAN**, is Professor and Director of Global Health in the School of Nursing at the University of Minnesota and holds an adjunct faculty appointment in the School of Public Health. She is engaged in global development projects and the promotion of higher education workforce development. She is active in multiple USAID-funded projects, including One Health Workforce, a large-scale workforce development initiative addressing emerging infectious threats in numerous countries in Africa and Asia. Porta has worked as a public health nurse and sexual assault nurse examiner for more than 20 years, in settings ranging from teen clinics and detention centers to refugee camps in Rwanda and post-9/11 Red Cross disaster relief centers in Washington, DC. She teaches public health nursing courses as well as research and innovative data-collection methods, and advises undergraduate and graduate students in nursing and public health. Porta currently serves on the research committee for the International Association of Forensic Nurses and the editorial review boards for *Public Health Nursing* and the *Journal of Forensic Nursing*, and previously served as president of Zeta Chapter of Sigma.

**Marjorie A. Schaffer, PhD, MS, RN, PHN**, is Professor Emerita of Nursing at Bethel University in St. Paul, Minnesota. A founding member of the Henry Street Consortium, she has taught public health nursing for more than 31 years. She has consulted on nursing education in Norway as a Fulbright Scholar and Fulbright Specialist, and in New Zealand as a Fulbright Specialist. Schaffer has served as President of Chi at-Large Chapter of Sigma and coauthored articles on the Public Health Intervention Wheel and Henry Street Consortium. She has written more than 50 articles and book chapters and coauthored *Being Present: A Nurse's Resource for End-of-Life Communication,* also published by Sigma.

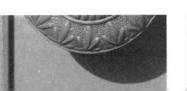
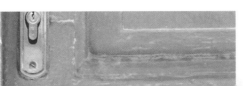
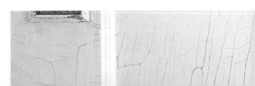

## Contributing Authors

**Linda J. W. Anderson, DNP, MPH, RN, PHN** (Chapters 4, 9) is Professor of Nursing and Director of the Pre-licensure Nursing Program at Bethel University in St. Paul, Minnesota. She teaches public health nursing theory and clinical. Current research interests include investigation of the use of the Public Health Intervention Wheel in school nurse practice. She has served as a Fulbright Specialist to Diakonova University College in Oslo, Norway.

**Christine C. Andres, DNP, RN, PHN, CLC** (Chapters 10, 11, 12) is a nursing faculty member at Anoka-Ramsey Community College in Cambridge, Minnesota. She teaches health promotion and leadership courses in a preprofessional program. She has a passion for supporting the development of the rural nursing workforce. With experience in public health and maternal-child health nursing, she is an advocate for family home visiting and early intervention.

**Bonnie Brueshoff, DNP, MSN, RN, PHN** (Chapters 7, 14) is Public Health Director for the nationally accredited Dakota County Public Health Department in West St. Paul and Apple Valley, Minnesota. She provides leadership for a staff of 100 with a budget of $10 million. Brueshoff has spent the majority of her 38 years in nursing in public health and has a special interest in prevention and early-intervention programs and the development of public health leaders. She is a graduate of the Robert Wood Johnson Executive Nurse Fellows Program and the NACCHO Survive and Thrive Fellowship Program.

**Colleen B. Clark, DNP, MSN, RN, PHN** (Chapter 13) is an adjunct faculty member at Metropolitan State University in the MANE baccalaureate program, St. Paul, Minnesota, and also teaches in the RN-BSN completion programs at Augsburg University, St. Paul, Minnesota, and Mankato State University, Mankato, Minnesota. She currently teaches public health theory and clinical and has previously taught in nursing pre-licensure programs. She has more than 35 years of practice experience in community and school health.

**Desiree Holmquist, BSN, RN, PHN** (Chapter 9) has over 25 years of experience in public health. As the Supervisor for Disease Prevention and Control for Anoka County Community Health in Anoka, Minnesota, she has primary responsibility for communicable disease investigation and management, and immunization services. In her role as coordinator of student nurse clinical experiences, she has championed an agency culture that supports the development of students.

**Melissa L. Horning, PhD, RN, PHN** (Chapter 8) is Assistant Professor at the University of Minnesota School of Nursing. She currently teaches public health nursing and nursing research and theory to pre-licensure nursing students. Grounded in her work in practice as a public health nurse in a wide variety of roles, her research is focused on promoting the health of children, youth, and their families. Her collaborative, community-partnered research is focused on addressing social determinants of health, such as food access, to improve health equity, especially as related to nutrition and obesity.

**Erin Karsten, MSN, RN, PHN** (Chapters 10, 14) is Public Health Supervisor for the Dakota County Public Health Department in Apple Valley, Minnesota. She leads a team of public health nurses and community health workers in the Family Home Visiting Program. Erin also provides mentorship to the public health workforce using a collaborative leadership approach. She has dedicated her entire nursing career to public health and has a special interest in early intervention programs that serve families with a holistic approach.

**Madeleine Kerr, PhD, RN** (Chapter 4) is Associate Professor at the University of Minnesota School of Nursing. She has 10 years of experience as a public health nurse, school nurse, and migrant field nurse and has taught public health nursing for over 30 years. As a health informatics faculty member, she is excited to introduce students to geographic information systems and mapping as a way to explore social and environmental determinants of health.

**Noreen Kleinfehn-Wald, MA, PHN** (Chapters 3, 4, 5, 13) is Public Health Nursing Supervisor for Scott County Public Health in Shakopee, Minnesota. She has 36 years of experience in governmental public health in two Minnesota counties, in inner-city settings, and in East Africa. She has primary responsibility for family home visiting programs, clinic services, and disease prevention and control. She has a passion for data and recently started a community faculty position teaching population-based care at Metropolitan State University in St. Paul, Minnesota.

**Kelly Krumwiede, PhD, MA, RN, PHN** (Chapter 3) is Associate Professor at Minnesota State University, Mankato. She teaches public health theory and clinical in the pre-licensure and RN baccalaureate completion programs. She is Co-chair of the Madelia Community Based Collaborative, which uses the Community-Based Collaborative Action Research framework to address societal health issues.

**Renee Kumpula, EdD, RN, PHN** (Chapters 11, 12) is Clinical Assistant Professor at the University of Minnesota School of Nursing and has taught students of diversity in two previous universities. She has taught theory, public health nursing, care across the life continuum, elder care, and holistic care topics for bachelor to doctoral programs. A former public health nurse in the metropolitan area, she completed her dissertation with honors on spiritual care and how nurses establish patterns in providing care for spiritual needs in practice.

**Raney Linck, DNP, MSN, RN** (Chapters 7, 9) is Clinical Assistant Professor at the University of Minnesota School of Nursing and is part of the VA Nursing Academic Partnership with the Minneapolis VA Health Care System. He has taught public health nursing theory and worked in hospice case management, home health, and substance abuse treatment in addition to critical care and informatics.

**Karen S. Martin, MSN, RN, FAAN** (Chapter 3) is based in Omaha, Nebraska, and has been a healthcare consultant in private practice since 1993. She works with diverse providers, educators, and computer software companies nationally and globally. While employed at the Visiting Nurse Association of Omaha (1978–1993), she was the Principal Investigator of Omaha System research. She has been a visiting scholar and speaker in 24 countries, has served as the chair of numerous conferences, and is the author of more than 100 articles, chapters, and books and 70 editorials.

**Stacie O'Leary, MA, PHN, LSN** (Chapter 5) is Coordinator of School District 197 for West St. Paul, Mendota Heights, Eagan Area Schools in Minnesota. She has over 35 years of nursing experience in various settings: acute, long-term, and school. O'Leary has emphasized the importance of public health in a school setting with various projects and grants and the importance of a strong infrastructure with the School Health Advisory Council (SHAC) to provide the support for the school district and community at large. She implemented the "Whole School, Whole Community, Whole Child" model in the school district as part of the School Health Advisory Council incentive.

**Stephanie Rivery, DNP, RN, PHN** (Chapter 2) recently completed her DNP at the University of Minnesota and is Family Health Program Coordinator at Dakota County Public Health in West St. Paul, Minnesota. She is dedicated to using the holistic scope of public health nursing practice to coordinate care for individuals, communities, and systems and has worked in various nursing roles to increase capacity for well-being with underserved communities in urban and rural areas across the United States. She has a particular interest in the bonding and nutritive aspects that breastfeeding contributes to lifelong well-being. She is a Bentson Scholar and George Fellow.

**Carol J. Roth, MS, RN, PHN, CNE** (Chapters 8, 9, 12) is Assistant Professor at Minnesota State University Moorhead in Moorhead, Minnesota. After 28 years of public health nursing practice, she now teaches public health nursing and nursing leadership. She is a post-master's DNP student with an emphasis in practice and leadership innovations at Winona State University and is completing a research project on provider education and mental health in a nurse-managed homeless clinic using a behavioral health model. She is serving the Xi Kappa Chapter of Sigma in a leadership role on the board.

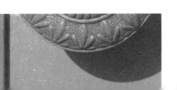
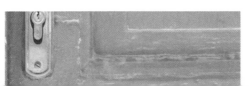
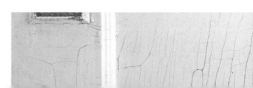

**Jill Timm, JD, RN, PHN** (Chapters 1, 6) is Senior Program Manager with the Washington County Department of Public Health & Environment in Stillwater, Minnesota. She provides nursing direction and leadership to supervisors and staff in family health nursing; disease prevention, control, and outreach; correctional health nursing; and the WIC supplemental nutrition programs. Timm has been in public health nursing for 20 years and appreciates the value public health places on relationships as the primary intervention for moving individual and community goals forward.

**Kelly Zaiser**, **RN, PHN** (Chapter 12) is a public health nurse working for Kanabec County Community Health in Mora, Minnesota. She is working under the evidence-based home visiting program Nurse-Family Partnership, with a focus on improving pregnancy outcomes, child health and development, and self-sufficiency. She has a passion for establishing a therapeutic relationship with the public and those she services in hopes to build trust and facilitate positive change.

## Reviewers

# Table of Contents

## List of Evidence Examples

## List of Figures

## List of Tables and Boxes

*(continues)*

## List of Tables and Boxes (continued)

*(continues)*

## List of Tables and Boxes (continued)

# Foreword

More than a decade ago, I was pleased to lead a group of public health nurses in Wisconsin in designing a project that aimed to connect nurse educators and practitioners to improve public health nursing practice and education in our state. For inspiration and best practices, we needed to journey no farther than our neighboring state of Minnesota. We purposefully took a "follow-the-leader" approach in adopting or adapting many collaborative education and practice improvement strategies pioneered in Minnesota for our Linking Education and Practice for Excellence in Public Health Nursing (LEAP Project). Throughout the 6 years of the LEAP Project, we often looked to public health nursing leaders in Minnesota for guidance because they clearly understood the processes and challenges of academic-practice collaboration and of contemporary public health nursing practice and education. I clearly recall the "Minnesota-nice" generosity of the outstanding faculty and public health nurse members of the Henry Street Consortium in sharing their wisdom on academic-practice collaboration when we consulted with them during a groundbreaking international public health nursing conference held in St. Paul in 2011. In many ways, the Henry Street Consortium epitomizes the best of the best practices for academic-practice partnership and sustainable efforts toward improving public health education and practice.

Publication of the first edition of *Population-Based Public Health Clinical Manual* (2011), authored by members of the Henry Street Consortium, was an important milestone. Its creation demonstrated that magic happens when public health nurses in academic and practice settings work collaboratively. The first and second editions of this book offered a refined set of competencies for entry into contemporary, population-based public health nursing practice. The authors provided clear, practical, evidence-driven content and activities for teaching and learning the knowledge, skills, and values required for becoming a public health nurse in the 21st century. This book was truly a gift to public health nursing faculty, students, and preceptors across the United States and beyond because of its accessible format, applicability to contemporary practice, and clarity of language. It clearly fulfilled the need for a practical guidebook to public health nursing practice for students and novice nurses.

The legacy of excellence continues with the third edition, but in an entirely redesigned format in full color, making it easier to read and more engaging for students and other users. As a former public health nurse and a current public health professor, I think it offers exactly what is needed for readers seeking to teach or learn population-based public health practice. I am impressed with the use of a scaffolding approach that leads students to compare and contrast new information and experiences about public health with what they have already encountered as students in acute care. I am enthused by the many opportunities for readers to apply and develop critical thinking skills, the essence of all knowledge professions. The highly regarded Public Health Intervention Wheel remains central as a core component of the population-based approach. It is refreshing and important that the authors do not expect that students and novice nurses will only be able or asked to work with individuals or families but also provide case examples, stories, and learning activities that support public health nursing interventions provided at the community and systems levels. The case examples and stories included are representative of contemporary practice, while the suggested active learning strategies align with contemporary pedagogy. Past users of this manual will be pleased with the new material in this edition, including a new competency on using principles and science of environmental health to promote safe and sustainable environments, theory applications showing how PHNs use frameworks to further public health, and the inclusion of the United Nations Sustainable Development Goals throughout the text.

While it is a great textbook for student nurses and nurses new to public health practice, this book could also be used in additional ways. First, faculty at the graduate level should find it useful in guiding curricular design for advanced practice public health nurses. Second, the examples that demonstrate the role of nurses as members of interprofessional teams practicing in public health settings make good interprofessional health education activities to help teach collaborative practice and leadership.

Collaboration between academia and practice, although increasingly common, remains challenging. The Henry Street Consortium is one of the finest examples of linking education and practice to improve public health nursing education and practice. The *Population-Based Public Health Clinical Manual*, Third Edition, is one of the best products I have seen that illustrates a successful and sustained academic-practice partnership. Although many community health textbooks are good, none is as clear, organized, practical, and relevant to population-based public health nursing clinical experiences as this one.

Students, teachers, and preceptors will find it the best guidebook for the journey toward becoming a public health nurse.

–*Susan J. Zahner, DrPH, MPH, RN, FAAN*
*Associate Dean for Faculty Affairs*
*Vilas Distinguished Achievement Professor*
*University of Wisconsin-Madison School of Nursing*

# Introduction

Up to this point in your nursing education, you have probably been immersed in learning how to provide nursing care to individuals and families with health concerns in institutional settings such as acute care and long-term care, and possibly in home care. This is what most of you envision as nursing and what you are passionate about. Now we are asking you to spread your wings and think about the community as your client and to use the word *client* instead of *patient*. You might be thinking, "This is not what I was planning to do in my nursing career—why am I here?" or "How can I provide nursing care to an entire community?" As you read this book, you will learn the answers to these questions. You will gain both knowledge and entry-level competencies in providing nursing care for an entire community, an at-risk population group in the community, or at-risk individuals and families in their homes or other community settings.

In today's world, baccalaureate-prepared nurses are expected to be able to manage care for populations, whether in an institutional setting or a community setting. This book will help you learn how to do this in community settings. You are going to learn about and develop skills in entry-level competencies in population-based public health nursing practice. Whether you practice in the community during your nursing career is for you to decide. However, what you learn from reading this book and completing learning activities in your public health/community health nursing clinical will provide you with knowledge about the vast array of resources available in your community that provide support for the patients you see in the emergency department or clinic or discharge from the hospital or nursing home. It is a journey into the unknown, with many challenges and benefits.

Developing competencies (skills, abilities, knowledge) that will help you become a great public health nurse takes more than mere access to or internalization of information and experiences from other people. The tools and resources presented in this manual are important; however, it is the individual—the hands, heart, and mind—who must use the tools to care and positively influence. Lillian Wald used the tools that were available to her, and when something wasn't readily available, she fought to gain access. She was driven by something deep and profound. She was grounded in the lived experiences of those she was working to serve. She acted with purpose that might have begun with caring but was fueled by the relationships she established with the sick, the impoverished, and the needy.

Nursing, especially public health nursing, can be overwhelming. The needs of individuals, families, and communities can appear insurmountable. The idea for this book originated from a shared recognition by public health nursing faculty, agency staff, and preceptors that public health nursing courses and clinical experiences are difficult for students and faculty alike. It has been well established that clinical faculty struggle with finding enough enriching experiences for students. Often, one student is placed in a school-based experience, another student is placed with a local public health agency, and yet another might be placed in a correctional setting. On the one hand, this diversity in settings and opportunities facilitates chances for students to learn from one another as they share and reflect. On the other hand, this diversity also challenges faculty to ensure that all students are learning about and growing in all the core competencies. It can also be confusing for students who have difficulty adapting clinical learning expectations to diverse settings and who might not have a nursing instructor or public health nursing preceptor with them during their clinical experiences.

The Henry Street Consortium (HSC), a group of public health nursing faculty from diverse schools of nursing and public health nurses employed in health departments, schools, and nonprofit community agencies, has been meeting regularly since 2001 to support rich, positive learning experiences for public health nursing students. The HSC developed a set of entry-level public health nursing competencies that all participants agreed to use in developing curriculum and clinical learning experiences. These HSC competencies have been informed by key public health nursing standards and guidelines, including the Quad Council core competencies (Quad Council of Public Health Nursing Organizations, 2011), the scope and standards of public health nursing (American Nurses Association, 2013; American Public Health Association, Public Health Nursing Section, 2013), and the core functions and essential services of public health (Essential Public Health Services Work Group of the Core Public Health Functions Steering Committee

Membership, 1994). Companion documents have included clinical guidelines and a menu of potential learning activities based on the competencies and recognized public health nursing interventions (Minnesota Department of Health, Division of Community Health Services, Public Health Nursing Section, 2001). What had been missing, however, was a manual or guide for students and faculty to develop the skills necessary for effective entry-level public health nursing practice. We wanted to create a manual that would speak to students in an understandable, meaningful way and that would also address student concerns about practicing nursing in the complex and often disorganized community environment. We needed to prepare future public health nurses for population-based practice. We hoped to motivate students to excel in their public health nursing clinical experiences and to engage in activities that facilitate learning and, in direct care, the health promotion of diverse individuals, families, communities, and populations. We sought to encourage students to think, think, think—to use their minds to grapple with moral and ethical dilemmas and complex health needs, disparities, and inequities.

This third edition is guided by an updated set of the HSC *entry-level, population-based public health nursing competencies,* which include a new environmental health competency (HSC, 2017). The third edition retains the strengths of the original manual, including chapter narratives, case studies, evidence-based examples of the competencies in action, and numerous suggestions for reflection, application, and hands-on learning in your own clinical setting. Evidence examples have been updated with recent publications that demonstrate the growth of public health nursing evidence in the US and globally. Theory application examples, a new feature, are found in most chapters. We have given attention to strengthening the global relevance of the manual, with inclusion of examples of the United Nations Sustainable Development Goals. Some chapters have undergone significant revisions to fit the needs of the student learner and the practicing nurse. Some interactive and online content was purposely moved from the manual to the Instructor's Guide to facilitate use of the materials.

### For the Student Nurse:

- You have chosen a career as a nurse, and some of you might become public health nurses. This clinical manual has been developed to serve as a tool you can use as you develop competencies and experience what it means to be a public health nurse.

- The knowledge and skills you acquire in your public health nursing course will enhance your effectiveness as a nurse, regardless of your employment setting. This manual helps you identify the public health principles that guide care for individuals, families, communities, populations, and systems. You will recognize and gain appreciation for public health's promotion of health and well-being and the prevention of disease and illness. You will also become aware of public health nursing's overarching commitment to addressing health disparities and inequities with strategies that improve the well-being of individuals, families, communities, and systems.

- This manual will help you learn who public health nurses are, what they do, and what makes a public health nurse effective. It leads you through the critical, or core, competencies that you need to develop.

### For the New Public Health Nurse:

- This manual provides an opportunity to orient yourself to the core competencies you are expected to demonstrate as a new public health nurse.

- As part of an orientation process, this manual offers opportunities for reflection on a range of issues, challenges, and ethical dilemmas that you will likely experience in one way or another during your initial months of employment.

- Such competencies as assessment, collaboration, communication, and leadership are abilities that all new public health nurses should possess; this manual offers you the opportunity to work through some of these broader competencies using public health nursing case studies and evidence from the literature.

- Additional competencies focus on developing critical relational nursing abilities such as establishing caring relationships; demonstrating nonjudgmental acceptance of others; committing to social justice principles; and holistically undertaking the nursing process of assessment, planning, intervention development, implementation, and evaluation.

- The collaboration of practicing public health nurses and public health nursing faculty to develop this manual has contributed to the high relevance of examples, practical applications, and discussion of each competency contained therein.

### For Public Health Nursing Faculty/Preceptors:

- This manual is a tool to help ensure that your students are equally exposed to core entry-level competencies and a foundational level of knowledge with respect to public health nursing. To ensure that all students receive the same foundational knowledge and skill development, regardless of clinical setting, clinical faculty might choose to assign a particular competency chapter to all students to ensure common ground. Other faculty might decide instead to assign different competencies to different students, depending on the scope of their individual clinical experience.

## Organization of the Manual

This manual begins with a description of foundational public health nursing concepts followed by a chapter on evidence-based public health nursing interventions. The next 12 chapters are each devoted to one core competency. The elements found in each competency chapter are outlined in the following table. A final chapter summarizes the practice of public health nursing and how this practice is consistent with expectations that baccalaureate degree nurses practice population-focused care.

In summary, this manual appreciates public health nursing tradition and encourages adoption of innovative, future-thinking practice. Lillian Wald, the founder of public health nursing, was not bound by the traditions or limitations of nursing practice in her era. She challenged, questioned, and acted. She perpetuated change and demanded that attention be given to the public health needs of children, families, and communities. She used every available asset and resource to combat poverty and disease, and when a resource didn't exist, she created one. She used evidence of the realities and challenges she saw to inform her solutions and strategies.

Today's public health nurse should do no less and has a growing base of evidence upon which to advocate for the health of those being served—evidence that ranges from a child's story to the results of a randomized controlled trial. We hope this manual promotes greater appreciation of what is expected from public health nurses and what makes them effective. We hope the manual's emphasis on evidence-based practice facilitates greater efforts by public health nurses to document effectiveness while continuing to appreciate, not minimize, the value of diverse sources of evidence. The path toward becoming an effective nurse starts with you—with your interest and determination to embrace what it means to be a nurse and, for some of you, a public health nurse. A commitment to figuring out nursing, or public health nursing, will take you on a journey that teaches, models, informs, changes, and challenges. Finally, we hope this book finds its way into your open hands, open heart, and open mind.

| Chapter Element | Description of the Element |
|---|---|
| Chapter Narrative | A new case study is included in each chapter to provide the reader with real-life scenarios experienced by student nurses or new public health nurses that address principles, the public health nursing process, and challenges that are relevant to the core competency. |
| Notebook | A table at the start of each competency chapter lists the competency, its components, and useful definitions of key chapter concepts. |
| Evidence Examples | These examples provide the reader with summaries of research studies and other evidence-based practice sources that are relevant to the competency. These also offer a sense of the level of evidence available for each competency. |
| Theory Application | These theory examples provide students with opportunities to understand how mid-range theories may be applied to clinical practice. |
| Healthy People 2020 | Online Healthy People 2020 activities are integrated into chapters. |
| United Nations Sustainable Development Goals | Examples of the Sustainable Development Goals provide students with examples of how these global goals are implemented in global, national, and local settings. |
| Activities | Learning activities interwoven throughout the text offer opportunities for readers to reflect on and engage with key ideas. |
| Ethical Considerations | This section of each competency chapter applies ethical principles to a common dilemma that public health nurses might face. Three ethical frameworks are used: rule ethics (principles), virtue ethics (character), and feminist ethics (reducing oppression). |
| Key Points | This section summarizes the main ideas of each chapter. |
| Reflective Practice | This section often provides a conclusion to the case study or additional questions for the reader to consider. |
| Application of Evidence | This section poses questions for students to consider that reflect major concepts and competencies presented in the book. |
| References | All references cited in each chapter are listed at the end of each chapter. |

# References

American Nurses Association. (2013). *Public health nursing: Scope and standards of practice.* Silver Spring, MD: Author.

American Public Health Association, Public Health Nursing Section. (2013). *The definition and practice of public health nursing.* Washington, DC: Author. Retrieved from https://www.apha.org/~/media/files/pdf/membergroups/phn/nursingdefinition.ashx

Essential Public Health Services Work Group of the Core Public Health Functions Steering Committee Membership. (1994). *The public health system & the 10 essential public health services.* Retrieved from https://www.cdc.gov/stltpublichealth/publichealthservices/essentialhealthservices.html

Henry Street Consortium. (2017). *Entry-level, population-based public health nursing competencies.* St. Paul, MN: Author. Retrieved from www.henrystreetconsortium.org

Minnesota Department of Health, Division of Community Health Services, Public Health Nursing Section. (2001). *Public health interventions: Applications for public health nursing practice.* St. Paul, MN: Author. Retrieved from http://www.health.state.mn.us/divs/opi/cd/phn/docs/0301wheel_manual.pdf

Quad Council of Public Health Nursing Organizations. (2011). *The Quad Council competencies for public health nurses.* Retrieved from http://www.achne.org/files/Quad%20Council/QuadCouncilCompetenciesforPublicHealthNurses.pdf

# PART I

# Foundational Concepts for Public Health Nursing Practice

# Introduction to Public Health Nursing Practice

■ **Patricia M. Schoon**
*with Marjorie A. Schaffer and Jill Timm*

> *Abby will soon be starting her public health nursing clinical and is struggling with the idea of practicing nursing outside the hospital. She is talking about public health clinicals with Alberto and Sia at lunch. "I can't imagine myself out in someone's home, or in a school, or in a community center or public health agency. I'm not sure I know what I'm supposed to do. I also wonder how I will be respected without scrubs or my uniform. Is it really true that one of the most important skills in public health is listening and that ___ all that you do? I feel like I should be doing something more."*
>
> *___ ds, "My friend, Zack, had public health last semester. He said that it was interesting to ___ as its own intervention. It was hard to not jump in and 'teach' immediately. He often ___. After a while, he started to get comfortable and also started to understand the benefits ___ understand the perspectives of clients in the community."*
>
> *"I worry about all of this too. I was talking with Jen, a friend of mine who took public ___ he said that on her first home visit, she went with her public health nursing preceptor. ___ ance to get a sense for the family's needs and possible interventions."*
>
> *___ m really worried about being out alone. I wonder what the neighborhood where my ___ like and whether I will be safe."*
>
> *___ also curious about the various public health nursing roles that we may be able to ___ ems like the field is so broad and there are so many things to consider."*

**___ OOK**

**___ NS**

___ atient) is the individual/family, community, population or subpopulation, or system that is ___ e's focus of care.

___ unity can refer to (a) a group of people or a population group, (b) a physical place and time ___ n lives and works, or (c) a cultural group that has shared beliefs, values, institutions, and ___ r, Shapiro, & Asselin, 2006, p. 23).

**Health Determinants:** Health determinants are factors that influence the health of individuals, families, and populations. Health determinants can potentially have a positive (protective factors) or negative (risk factors) influence on health.

**Health Status:** Health status refers to the level of health or illness and is the outcome of the interaction of the multiple health determinants. Health status indicators, also called global measures of population health, include birth, longevity, and death rates (mortality); illness (morbidity) patterns; perception of wellness and life satisfaction; level of independence; and functional ability.

*(continues)*

## ABBY'S NOTEBOOK

**USEFUL DEFINITIONS** *(continued)*

**Holistic Nursing:** Holistic nursing is defined as "all nursing practice that has healing the whole person as its goal and honors relation-centered care and the interconnectedness of self, others, nature, and spirituality; focuses on protecting, promoting health and wellness..." (Dossey & Keegan, 2016, p. 3).

**Levels of Prevention:** The levels of prevention comprise a health-intervention framework applied to the stages of health and disease for individuals and groups (Leavell & Clark, 1958; Stanhope & Lancaster, 2008). The levels of prevention are (a) primary—the prevention of disease and promotion of health; (b) secondary—early diagnosis and treatment; and (c) tertiary—limiting of negative effects of disease and restoring of function.

**Population:** A population is defined as the "total number of people living in a specific geographic area." A subpopulation (syn. group or aggregate) "consist[s] of people experiencing a specific health condition; engaging in behaviors that have potential to negatively affect health; or sharing a common risk factor or risk exposure, or experiencing an emerging health threat or risk" (American Nurses Association [ANA], 2013, p. 3).

**Population-Based Practice:** Population-based practice focuses on the population as a whole to determine its priority needs (Minnesota Department of Health [MDH], 2001).

**Public Health:** Public health refers to all organized measures (whether public or private) to prevent disease, promote health, and prolong life among the population as a whole (World Health Organization [WHO], n.d.).

**Public Health Nursing:** Public health nursing is the practice of promoting and protecting the health of populations using knowledge from nursing, social, and public health sciences. Public health nursing is a specialty practice within nursing and public health. It focuses on improving population health by emphasizing prevention and attending to multiple determinants of health. Often used interchangeably with community health nursing, this nursing practice includes advocacy, policy development, and planning, which addresses issues of social justice (American Public Health Association [APHA], Public Health Nursing Section, 2013, p. 1).

**Social Determinants of Health:** The social determinants of health are the conditions in which people are born, grow, live, work, and age. The distribution of money, power, and resources at the global, national, and local levels shape these circumstances. The social determinants of health are mostly responsible for health inequities— the unfair and avoidable differences in health status seen within and between countries (Modified from WHO, 2013).

**System:** A system is an institution or organization that exists within one or multiple communities.

## Practicing Nursing Where We All Live

Public health nursing care is provided to individuals, families, communities, and populations through a population-based lens that enables nurses to view their clients within the context of the community in which they and their clients live. All aspects of the client's life are considered as public health nurses (PHNs) carry out the nursing process. PHNs practice in their communities, where they can make a difference in the lives of their families, the people they serve, and their communities on a daily basis.

As you practice nursing in a variety of clinical settings, you will become aware that the health of people in your families, neighborhoods, and communities affects everyone in the community both socially and economically. As you read this chapter, consider the concepts presented from both your personal and professional perspectives. As nurses, you are all citizens of the world and have civic and

professional responsibilities to promote health and provide for a safe environment.

In the case study at the beginning of the chapter, Abby and her friends are concerned about providing nursing care in the community. It is difficult for nursing students to think about practicing nursing outside the acute and long-term care settings. Many of the skills that nursing students learn in the acute or long-term care setting (e.g., IV therapy, medication administration, tube care) are part of the delegated medical functions of nursing practice, which, by necessity, are priorities when caring for acutely ill, frail, and elderly individuals. In the community setting, most of what PHNs do is part of the independent practice of nursing (e.g., teaching, counseling, coordinating care), as the focus of public health nursing practice is primary prevention. Components of public health nursing can be practiced in any setting, although they are most often practiced in the community. Not all nursing practiced in the community can be described as public health nursing. For example, home care and hospice care, both very important areas of nursing, are practiced in the community and exhibit components of public health nursing but are not traditionally categorized as public health nursing. As you work through this book and engage in nursing activities, think about how you are integrating the components of public health nursing into your nursing practice. Also, think about how you practice nursing where you live and what your civic and professional responsibilities are to promote the health of your community.

## Public Health

The practice of public health nursing includes components of public health and is a part of the broader field of public health. It is important to understand the nature and scope of public health practice. Public health practice focuses on protecting and promoting the health of entire populations. This practice includes the prevention of disease and injury and the promotion of the social conditions and lifestyles that maintain health and prolong life.

Public health professionals monitor and diagnose the health concerns of entire communities and promote healthy practices and behaviors to ensure that populations stay healthy. The World Health Organization uses the term "global public health" to recognize that, as a result of globalization, forces that affect public health can and do come from outside state boundaries. Responding to public health issues now requires paying attention to cross-border health risks, including access to dangerous products and environmental change (WHO, n.d.). PHNs need to take a global perspective about the nature of population health threats and issues when practicing in the community.

## Public Health Nursing

Public health nursing combines the theory and practice of nursing and public health. Public health nursing, like nursing practice everywhere, involves the interaction of the nurse and client; the health of the client; the influence of the home, healthcare, and community environment; and the nursing care provided. One of the unique features of public health nursing is that the client can be an individual or family, a group of people, or a whole community. The client could also be a system within the community (e.g., a school, church, or community health or social service agency). PHNs work to improve population health at the local, state, national, and international levels (ANA, 2013; APHA, 2013). Public health nursing goals are to promote and preserve the health of populations and the public, prevent disease and disability, and protect the health of the community as a whole.

Public health nursing practice is considered population-based because it starts by focusing on the population as a whole to determine the community's priority health needs (Minnesota Department of Health [MDH], Public Health Nursing Section, 2000, 2001; MDH, Center for Public Health Nursing, 2003). PHNs in a variety of work settings can carry out population-based practice. To be population based, public health nursing practice should meet five criteria:

1. Focus on entire populations possessing similar health concerns or characteristics
2. Be guided by an assessment of population health status that is determined through a community health assessment process
3. Consider the broad determinants of health
4. Consider all levels of prevention, with a preference for primary prevention
5. Consider all levels of practice (individual/family, community, system) (MDH, 2001, pp. 2–3; MDH, 2003)

PHNs work in homes, clinics, schools, jails, businesses, religious organizations, homeless shelters, camps, hospitals, visiting nurse associations, health departments, and Indian reservations. Public health nursing is defined by its goals, not by its setting. Although public health nursing is considered a specialty area of practice, its standards include expectations for entry-level baccalaureate nursing graduates. Even at the entry level, PHNs are expected to function as change agents and to help shape the healthcare system to meet the public health needs of the 21st century. This leadership expectation for public health nursing practice is implicit in the American Nurses Association's *Public Health Nursing: Scope and Standards of Practice* (ANA, 2013). The American Public Health Association (APHA) definition of public health nursing, "the practice of promoting and protecting the health of populations using knowledge from nursing, social, and public health sciences" (APHA, 2013, p. 2), implies the importance of the scientific knowledge base for PHN practice.

### Definition of Public Health Nursing Practice

Up to this point in your nursing education, you have focused on nursing care of individuals and families. Public health nursing is population based and focuses on population health. "Public health nursing is the practice of promoting and protecting the health of populations using knowledge from nursing, social, and public health sciences. Public health nursing is a specialty practice within nursing and public health. It focuses on improving population health by emphasizing prevention, and attending to multiple determinants of health" (APHA, 2013, p. 1). While public health nursing practices include primary, secondary, and tertiary prevention, the focus is on primary prevention.

As students, you have already learned about nursing core concepts that also shape public health nursing, which include (Keller, Strohschein, & Schaffer, 2011):

- Care and compassion
- Holistic and relationship-centered practice
- Sensitivity to vulnerable populations
- Independent nursing practice

This book also introduces you to additional public health core concepts that shape public health nursing, which include (Keller et al., 2011):

- Social justice
- Population focus
- Reliance on epidemiology
- Health promotion and prevention
- The greater good
- Long-term commitment to community

## Evolution of Public Health Nursing

In this chapter, you will read about how nurses practice public health nursing in the community, and you will consider how important nurses are to the health of communities at the local, national, and international levels. It is important to mention two key founders of public health nursing. Since the time of Florence Nightingale, the first public health nurse, nurses have always been essential participants in improving and maintaining the health of individuals, families, and communities. Nightingale, who started her nursing career in 1850, provided leadership for the health of vulnerable populations by advocating for changes in the organizations and communities that were responsible for providing healthcare (Selanders & Crane, 2012). Nightingale focused on managing the environment of those who needed care, whether it was on the Crimean War battlefields or working with the London poor. Her concerns about the impact environmental conditions had on health and her work to advocate for healthful environments is as relevant today as it was in the 1800s (Davies, 2012). Lillian Wald, the founder of modern-day public health nursing, founded the Henry Street Settlement in 1893 to provide nursing services to the indigent citizens of New York. In 1903, Wald, in collaboration with Metropolitan Life, started the first insurance reimbursement for nurse home visiting and demonstrated its effectiveness (Abrams, 2008; Buhler-Wilkerson, 1993). The Henry Street Settlement House continues to provide health and social services today.

Public health nursing in the United States developed out of a need to provide nursing services to individuals and families who had unmet health needs, and started with Clara Barton, who founded the American Red Cross as a response to the needs of injured and ill Civil War soldiers

in 1881 (Kulbok, Thatcher, Park, & Meszaros, 2012; Kub, Kulbok, & Glick, 2015; see Figure 1.1). PHNs saw themselves not only as caregivers but also as advocates for those living in unhealthy conditions and experiencing unmet healthcare needs. Care of the ill soon expanded to care of those at risk for poor health and to populations and entire communities. Disease prevention and health promotion for vulnerable or at-risk populations in diverse settings became a second focus.

Until the late 1960s, PHNs working for governmental public health agencies generally provided services to two at-risk populations: mothers and children, and adults living at home with chronic diseases and disabilities. When Medicare legislation was enacted in 1966, home care became a covered service, and private agencies began to offer home care services (see Chapter 7). Many public health agencies renewed their commitment to the goals of health promotion, disease prevention, and protection and risk reduction, and they stopped providing home care to adults with chronic diseases and disabilities. PHNs increased their efforts to address the social determinants of health, which are discussed later in this chapter. Today, public health nurses often work with community groups as well as individuals and families. Community engagement, population-based advocacy, collaboration with other community agencies and groups, and community organizing are all part of the scope of practice of public health nurses (see Chapters 2, 5, and 10). At the same time, nurses practicing in a variety of non-traditional public health settings (e.g., home care, hospice, faith-based nursing, institutional and insurance care coordination and care management, etc.) use public health nursing principles and public health interventions in their practice.

Emerging threats to public health require a dramatic shift in the focus of healthcare, public health, and public health nursing. ANA (2013, p. 2) has identified six 21st-century threats that form a context for the current and future directions of public health nursing practice:

1. Reemergence of communicable disease and increasing incidence of drug-resistant organisms
2. Environmental hazards
3. Physical or civic barriers to healthy lifestyles (e.g., food "deserts")
4. Overall concern about the structure and function of the healthcare system
5. Challenges imposed by the presence of modern public health epidemics, such as pandemic influenza, obesity, and tobacco-related diseases and deaths
6. Global and emerging crises with increased opportunities for exposure to multiple health threats

Nursing continues to expand its leadership role in healthcare in all settings, but in public health nursing, that leadership role often takes place in the community, including in the public policy–making arena (ANA, 2003, 2013).

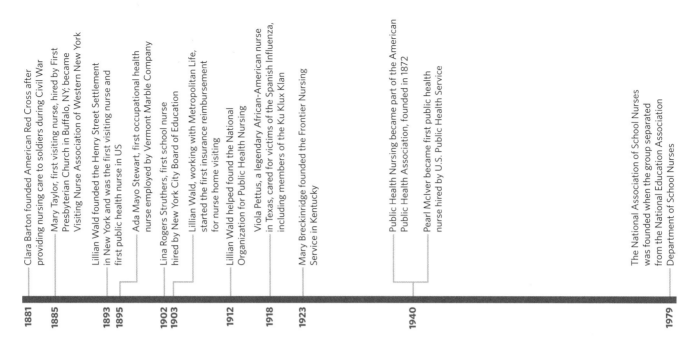

**FIGURE 1.1** Public Health Nursing in the United States

*Sources:* Abrams, 2008; Buhler-Wilkerson, 1993; Kub, Kulbok, & Glick, 2015;
Visiting Nurses Association of Western New York, n.d.

A key principle to keep in mind is that PHNs must place more importance on goals related to the public good than goals for the benefit of individuals in the social and economic systems (see Chapter 13 for a discussion of social justice and Chapter 14 for a discussion of public health nursing leadership).

> *"I still don't really understand how we are going to factor in community or environmental needs when we are working with individuals." Albert sighs.*
>
> *Sia responds, "What I remember from our public health theory class this morning is that even though we are meeting people in their homes, we have to take into account the home environment and the community. Our instructor also talked about public health nurses having a responsibility to improve the health of the public at the local, national, and international levels. She mentioned that this idea can be overwhelming for nursing students and suggested that we focus on what we could do to improve the health of individuals and families as a way to help improve the health of our community. She used the term 'glocal,' which means to think global, but act local."*
>
> *Abby adds, "Maybe we should read more about this in our textbook and look at some of the websites suggested."*
>
> *"Good idea," says Sia.*

## Cornerstones of Public Health Nursing

The Cornerstones of Public Health Nursing (Minnesota Department of Health [MDH], Center for Public Health Nursing, 2007) provide the foundation for population-based nursing practice (Keller et al., 2011). The Cornerstones reflect the values and beliefs that guide public health nursing practice, and they are also closely related to the ANA Principles of Public Health Nursing Practice (ANA, 2013), as represented in Table 1.1.

These Cornerstones are reflected in PHNs' daily practice when they:

- Organize their workload and schedule based on priority health needs of clients and community

- Take time to establish trust when visiting families in their homes

- Carry out holistic assessments of individuals and families within the context of culture, ethnicity, and communities

- Use evidence-based practice from nursing and public health sciences to select appropriate and effective interventions

- Collaborate with other members of the healthcare team

- Make critical decisions about the needs of their clients and the selection, implementation, and evaluation of interventions based on their professional knowledge and professional licensure

**TABLE 1.1  Cornerstones of Public Health Nursing and Related ANA Principles of PHN Practice**

| Cornerstones of Public Health Nursing | ANA Principles of Public Health Nursing Practice |
|---|---|
| Focuses on the health of entire populations | The client or unit of care is the population. |
| Reflects community priorities and needs | The primary obligation is to achieve the greatest good for the greatest number of people or the population as a whole (also related to the social justice cornerstone). |
| Establishes caring relationships with communities, systems, individuals, and families | NA |
| Is grounded in social justice, compassion, sensitivity to diversity, and respect for the worth of all people, especially the vulnerable | A public health nurse is obligated to actively identify and reach out to all who might benefit from a specific activity or service. |
| Encompasses mental, physical, emotional, social, spiritual, and environmental aspects of health | Public health nursing focuses on strategies that create healthy environmental, social, and economic conditions in which populations may thrive. |
| Promotes health through strategies driven by epidemiological evidence | Optimal use of available resources and creation of new evidence-based strategies is necessary to ensure the best overall improvement in the health of the population.<br><br>Primary prevention is the priority in selecting appropriate activities. |
| Collaborates with community resources to achieve those strategies but can and will work alone if necessary | Public health nurses collaborate with the client as an equal partner.<br><br>Collaboration with other professions, populations, organizations, and stakeholder groups is the most effective way to promote and protect the health of the people. |
| Derives its authority for independent action from the Nurse Practice Act | NA |

*Sources for Cornerstones:* Keller et al., 2011; MDH, Center for Public Health Nursing, 2007
*Source for ANA Principles:* ANA, 2013, pp. 8–9

## Activity

Keep a log of your nursing activities. Reflect on how you have demonstrated the cornerstones of public health nursing in your clinical activities.

*Abby is spending the day with her PHN preceptor. Her preceptor receives a referral to visit a family who just moved into the community and is homeless. The PHN knows that a health priority for her community and agency is to improve the health of homeless populations, particularly those in the population with young children. Recent data on the health needs of her county demonstrate that young children in homeless families have higher rates of malnutrition and developmental delays. Abby's PHN preceptor modifies her home-visiting plan for the day so that she can make an initial visit to this family at the local family homeless shelter. The family speaks Spanish but the PHN does not, so she arranges for an interpreter to accompany them on the visit to this family. The PHN has Abby gather information about local homeless shelters and food banks to take to the visit and has her get some bus passes for the family to use when they go to different agencies to apply for assistance. The PHN also brings along important phone numbers so that she can assist the family with follow-up regarding their application for cash assistance. After her busy day with her PHN preceptor, Abby discusses her visit to the homeless family with Alberto and Sia that evening. Their instructor has challenged them to identify the Cornerstones of Public Health Nursing found in their clinical visits that day.*

## Holistic Foundations of Public Health Nursing

Public health nursing and holistic nursing practice have common roots. Florence Nightingale, who believed in care that focused on unity, wellness, and the interrelationship of human beings and their environment, is considered to be one of the first holistic nurses. She is known for her global vision, leadership, and advocacy (Beck, 2010; Dossey & Keegan, 2016; Selanders & Crane, 2012). Lillian Wald was as concerned about the health of the indigent of New York as she was about their social welfare, the tenement environment in which they lived, and the cultural and political environment that needed to change in order to improve the health of her clients and her community (Buhler-Wilkerson, 1993). Both Nightingale's and Ward's nursing practices have informed contemporary holistic public health nursing practice.

A contemporary nursing theory that reflects the synthesis of nursing and public health and reflects holistic public health nursing practice is Watson's Theory of Human Caring, in which the nurse and the client exist within a caring-healing environment. Watson was greatly influenced by the practice of Florence Nightingale and built upon Nightingale's work in emphasizing the "curative factors" of disease and illness, embracing the wholeness of the individual. The Theory of Human Caring reflects an expansive sharing process that changes the self, others, the culture, and the environment; respects the beliefs of others; and recognizes and is open to unexpected life events (Parker & Smith, 2010; Watson, 2008, p. 34, 2010). Some of the public health nursing theoretical perspectives that you will find in later chapters reflect this synthesis of public health nursing and holistic nursing into holistic public health nursing practice.

## Scope and Standards of Public Health Nursing Practice

All professional nurses, regardless of their clinical areas of practice, have a scope of practice. A *scope of practice* refers to the boundaries of safe and ethical practice (see Chapter 6 for a discussion of the scope of practice of public health nursing) and depends on four components: educational preparation, credentials, state licensure law, and clinical or employer role description. A PHN's job description is a good measure of the nurse's scope of practice.

Professional nurses are also guided by standards of practice developed by their professional nursing organizations. One nationally accepted set of standards for public health nursing is the American Nurses Association (ANA) publication *Public Health Nursing: Scope and Standards of Practice* (2013); Table 1.2 lists these standards. Specific criteria for operationalizing these standards and measuring performance are included in the publication.

**TABLE 1.2  Standards of Public Health Nursing Practice and Professional Performance**

**Standards of Public Health Nursing Practice**

*Standard 1. Assessment:* The public health nurse collects comprehensive data pertinent to the health status of populations.

*Standard 2. Population Diagnosis and Priorities:* The public health nurse analyzes the assessment data to determine the diagnosis or issues.

*Standard 3. Outcomes Identification:* The public health nurse identifies expected outcomes for a plan specific to the population or issues.

*Standard 4. Planning:* The public health nurse develops a plan that prescribes strategies and alternatives to attain expected outcomes.

*Standard 5. Implementation:* The public health nurse implements the identified plan.

*Standard 5A. Coordination of Care:* The public health nurse coordinates care delivery.

*Standard 5B. Health Teaching and Health Promotion:* The public health nurse employs multiple strategies to promote health and a safe environment.

*Standard 5C. Consultation:* The public health nurse provides consultation to influence the identified plan, enhance the abilities of others, and effect change.

*Standard 5D. Prescriptive Authority:* Not applicable.

*Standard 5E. Regulatory Activities:* The public health nurse participates in the application of public health laws, regulations, and policies.

*Standard 6. Evaluation:* The public health nurse evaluates progress toward the attainment of outcomes.

*Standard 7. Ethics:* The public health nurse practices ethically.

*(continues)*

**TABLE 1.2  Standards of Public Health Nursing Practice and Professional Performance** *(continued)*

**Standards of Professional Performance**

*Standard 8: Education:* The public health nurse attains knowledge and competence that reflect current nursing practice.

*Standard 9. Evidence-based Practice & Research:* The public health nurse integrates evidence and research findings into practice.

*Standard 10. Quality of Practice:* The public health nurse contributes to quality nursing practice.

*Standard 11. Communication:* The public health nurse communicates effectively in a variety of formats in all areas of practice.

*Standard 12. Leadership:* The public health nurse demonstrates leadership in the professional practice setting and the profession.

*Standard 13. Collaboration:* The public health nurse collaborates with the population and others in the conduct of nursing practice.

*Standard 14. Professional Practice Evaluation:* The public health nurse evaluates her or his own nursing practice in relation to professional practice standards and guidelines, relevant statutes, rules, and regulations.

*Standard 15. Resource Utilization:* The public health nurse utilizes appropriate resources to plan and provide nursing and public health services that are safe, effective, and financially responsible.

*Standard 16. Environmental Health:* The public health nurse practices in an environmentally safe, fair, and just manner.

*Standard 17. Advocacy:* The public health nurse advocates for the protection of the health, safety, and rights of the population.

*Source:* American Nurses Association, 2013, pp. 28–64

## Activity

■ Review your preceptor's job description with your preceptor.

■ Share the list of the ANA practice standards for public health nursing.

■ Discuss how your preceptor's job description and nursing practice incorporate specific ANA standards.

## Global Nature of Public Health Nursing

Public health nurses are citizens of the world as well as their own communities. Travel, communication technology, immigration patterns, the global spread of disease, and the universality of the social determinants of health in all geographic areas and cultures have changed the nature of public health nursing practice.

In 2015, the United Nations (UN) General Assembly adopted resolution *70/1. Transforming Our World: The 2030 Agenda for Sustainable Development* (2015). This resolution addresses the social determinants of health at a global level and sets out an action plan for people, the planet, prosperity, peace, and partnership. This action plan identifies 17 Sustainable Development Goals (SDGs). These goals, represented by the following set of icons (see Figure 1.2), provide a framework for the public health nursing practice wherever PHNs practice. Examples of how SDGs are addressed will be highlighted throughout the chapters of this book.

## EVIDENCE EXAMPLE 1.1

### Health in All Policies

In 2017, an International Health in All Policies Conference was convened in Adelaide, Australia to strategize over how to make progress in achieving the SDGs. A major outcome of the conference was *Health in All Policies: Governance, Partnerships and the Sustainable Development Agenda, Adelaide Statement II on Health in All Policies 2017.*

The statement stresses that:

■ "Health is a political choice, and as such any political, economic, social and ecological decision has health and equity impacts. Mayors play a critical role in agenda 2030 and health.

■ The SDGs are indivisible and universal and should not be addressed in silos but rather through taking into consideration their interconnectedness.

■ The transformative strategies for implementing the SDGs require joint action and policy coherence through the various levels of the government. Thus, health literacy is critical to good governance" (WHO, 2017).

As nurses who care about the social environment in which you and the populations you serve live, you need to consider how your nursing practice fits into both the SDGs and the *Health in All Policies* approach within your local, national, and global communities.

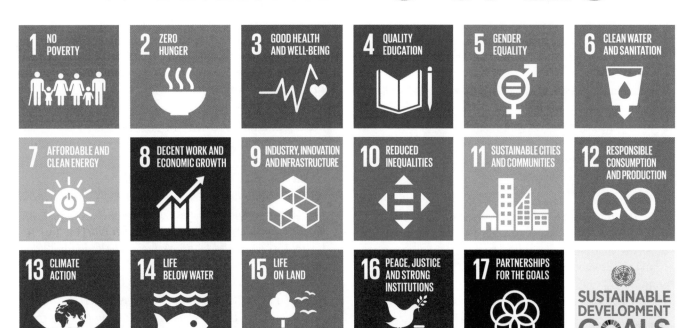

**FIGURE 1.2** UN Sustainable Development Goals With Icons
*Source:* United Nations General Assembly, 2015

## Ethical Framework for Public Health Nursing

The ever-changing healthcare environment, complex healthcare systems, and technological changes require a dual approach according to Ivanov and Oden (2013). They recommend that PHNs employ a rights-based approach consistent with the Universal Declaration of Human Rights passed by the United Nations (UN) in 1948 (United Nations, 1948) and an ethical approach based on ethical standards for nursing practice published by the American Nurses Association. The International Council of Nurses (ICN), in its position statement on *Nurses and Human Rights* (2011; p. 1), states that "all human rights are interdependent and indivisible and that individuals' health and wellbeing can be harmed when their human rights in any category are violated."

Other authors propose a complementary ethical framework that addresses the diversity of client populations and settings. PHNs might experience ethical problems when they have to consider the impact or benefits and burdens of their decisions on multiple clients, population groups, and communities (Racher, 2007). Culturally diverse societies and communities might have moral standards different from each other's and from those of the PHNs, which could lead to conflicts between the PHNs and clients.

Ethnic diversity in the community requires a complex ethical framework that includes the complementary approaches of rule ethics, virtue ethics, and feminist ethics (Racher, 2007; Volbrecht, 2002).

*Rule ethics* uses a framework of guiding principles for decision-making (Racher, 2007). Examples of rules or principles include autonomy, beneficence (promoting good), nonmaleficence (preventing harm), justice, loyalty, truth-telling, and respect (Aiken, 2004; Beauchamp & Childress, 1979; Purtilo, 2005; Scoville Walker, 2004). Rule ethics is based on a biomedical model of decision-making.

In contrast, *virtue ethics* is based on good character (Racher, 2007). One's actions are evaluated in the context of one's community. Examples of nursing virtues include compassion, honesty, courage, justice, self-confidence, resilience, practical reasoning, and integrity (Volbrecht, 2002).

*Feminist ethics* focuses on building relationships and reducing oppression in society (Volbrecht, 2002). Key values in a feminist ethics approach are inclusion, diversity, participation, empowerment, social justice, advocacy, and interdependence (Racher, 2007). Table 1.3 provides additional explanations about these three ethical approaches.

This three-pronged ethical approach is used throughout the book to highlight ethical concerns and principles related to specific public health nursing competencies.

**TABLE 1.3  Ethical Framework for Public Health Nursing Practice**

**Rule Ethics**

■ Rule ethics defines rules or principles that are based on perceptions of fairness.

■ Ethical principles are standards of conduct that guide behavior and specify moral duties and obligations (Racher, 2007).

■ Community rights might be given priority over individual rights in some situations.

■ Resources are given based on need and thus might be distributed unequally (distributive justice).

■ Those who have been unfairly burdened or harmed are compensated (compensatory justice).

**Virtue Ethics**

■ Virtue ethics identifies characteristics of the individual (moral agent) and that person's intentions and behaviors.

■ An individual is responsible for developing good character and good community (Volbrecht, 2002).

■ This type of ethics provides the foundation for professional ethics, which specifies professional values and virtues.

**Feminist Ethics**

■ A core ideal is achieving social justice; feminist ethics applies social justice and distributive justice to social structures and context.

■ This ethical approach focuses on characteristics of relationships, strengthens relationships and connectedness, eliminates oppression, and realigns power imbalances.

■ Feminist ethics is committed to restructuring relationships, social practices, and institutions so that people can live freer and fuller lives (Volbrecht, 2002).

## Key Components of Public Health Nursing

The key components of public health nursing practice discussed in this book include:

■ Cornerstones of Public Health Nursing (MDH, 2007)

■ Core public health functions and essential services of public health (IOM, 1988)

■ The standards of public health nursing practice (ANA, 2013)

■ Health determinants framework (U.S. Department of Health and Human Services [U.S. DHHS], n.d.-b)

■ Levels of prevention (Leavell & Clark, 1958; Stanhope & Lancaster, 2008)

■ Public health nursing process (ANA, 2013; MDH, 2001)

■ Public Health Intervention Wheel (MDH, 2001)

The Cornerstones, health determinants framework, and levels of prevention are included in this chapter. The public health nursing process and Public Health Intervention Wheel are discussed in Chapter 2. In the United States, PHNs and other public health professionals who work for governmental public health agencies have a scope of practice that is based on identified *core public health functions* and the *essential services of public health* (IOM, 1988). Chapter 7 discusses the responsibility and accountability of PHNs who work in governmental agencies.

" *Well, this is all very interesting. But I still don't have a clue how I am actually going to practice public health nursing,"* Albert sighs.

Sia responds, *"I'm realizing that there are a variety of roles in public health nursing. Some PHNs might spend their time working with individual families, but they still have to consider global impacts on health. Our instructor told us we would be practicing at the individual/family level of practice during most of our clinical time. But, I know we still need to consider how basic human rights are impacted by public health nursing work. There are a lot of good internet videos on human rights. I suppose we could look at them. And there is additional information in the textbook itself."*

Abby states, *"Great! But I think I want to spend more time actually doing something. I am going to spend a day with my preceptor tomorrow. Maybe I can apply some of what I have read and watched on the web."*

## Practicing Public Health Nursing

As a student, you will probably be spending most of your clinical hours working with individuals and families. However, the role of the PHN is broader; PHNs also spend time working with community groups and other members of the community team. Public health nursing is carried out at different levels of practice within society: individual/family, community, and systems (MDH, 2001, pp. 4–5).

### Individual/Family Level of Practice

PHNs work with individuals and families to promote health and reduce risks. The family is the essential unit of all communities and societies. A *family* is defined as a social unit of two or more people who identify themselves as a family, share emotional bonds, and carry out the functions of a family, including managing healthcare (Clark, 2008; Friedman, Bowden, & Jones, 2003; Martin, 2005).

PHNs work with individuals and families in many different community settings (see Chapter 3 for information on home visiting and family assessment). Working with families in the community helps you understand the diverse socioeconomic, cultural, and environmental factors that influence the health, wellness, and disease of individuals and families. If you are working with an individual or family to help them adapt or change their values, health beliefs, or behaviors to improve their health status, then you are working at the individual/family level of practice.

## Community Level of Practice

We tend to think of a community as a geographic place, but a *community* may refer to any group of people who share common values, culture, characteristics, and goals, whether they live in a specific geographical locale or are separated by distance (Skemp, Dreher, & Lehmann, 2016). Communities are composed of people, organizations, and social patterns of behavior. If you are working with members of the community to help the community adapt or change its values, health beliefs, or behaviors to improve the members' health status, then you are working at the community level of practice.

PHNs work with two types of populations in the community: populations of interest and populations at risk (MDH, 2001, p. 2). Table 1.4 defines and provides examples of these populations.

## Systems Level of Practice

A *system* is an institution or organization that exists within one or multiple communities. Key systems include healthcare systems, public health systems, schools, churches, government agencies, nonprofit organizations, and businesses.

### TABLE 1.4  Populations Served by Public Health Nurses

| Population | Examples |
|---|---|
| **Population of Interest:** Population who is essentially healthy but could improve factors that promote or protect health (MDH, 2001) | ■ Families who live in urban areas with little opportunity for exercise because of lack of parks, playgrounds, or bike paths<br>■ College students who have increased stress because of study needs and college debts and are looking for ways to reduce their stress level |
| **Population at Risk:** Population with a common identified risk factor or risk exposure that poses a threat to health (MDH, 2001) | ■ Children who are not immunized for major childhood illnesses, such as measles and chickenpox<br>■ Older members of a church congregation who live alone and are at risk for falls |

PHNs practice at the systems level when they work with providers and professionals like teachers, social workers, nurses, doctors, government officials, and members of the business community working for different agencies. If you are working with members of systems to help these systems adapt or change their values, health beliefs, or the way they conduct their business (behaviors) so that they can improve their capacity to meet the health needs of those they serve, then you are working at the systems level of practice.

## The Relationships Between Individuals/Families, Communities, and Systems

Individuals, families, and systems are best understood within the context of the community in which you live. Individuals and families interact with, and are influenced by, their social and physical environments and the systems that influence their health. For example, families living in an inner-city neighborhood might not have access to a grocery store with fresh fruits and vegetables or transportation to the store. The neighborhood's characteristics influence family access to quality food and their nutritional well-being. Figure 1.3 shows an example of the interrelationships among families, communities, and systems.

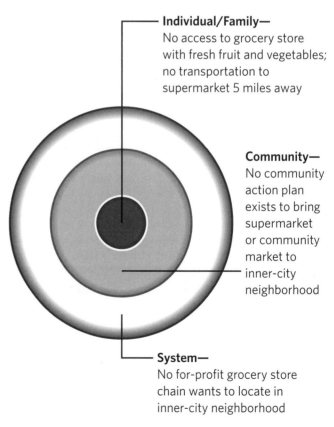

**Individual/Family—** No access to grocery store with fresh fruit and vegetables; no transportation to supermarket 5 miles away

**Community—** No community action plan exists to bring supermarket or community market to inner-city neighborhood

**System—** No for-profit grocery store chain wants to locate in inner-city neighborhood

**FIGURE 1.3** Interrelationships of Families, Communities, and Systems

To make a difference for these families and others in their inner-city neighborhood, PHNs might carry out the following interventions:

■ Refer families who are eligible for food benefits and nutrition services to Women, Infants, and Children (WIC)—individual/family level of practice.

■ Work with a community action council to make its members aware of problems in their inner-city neighborhood and assist them with taking action to obtain bus service from the neighborhood to a shopping center or supermarket—community level of practice.

■ Help form a coalition of nonprofit organizations and businesses to bring a cooperative store or other full-service grocery store to the neighborhood—systems level of practice.

Table 1.5 summarizes the three levels of PHN practice and provides examples of how public health nursing is carried out at these levels. These are all actions that you as a student or a newly practicing public health nurse can also take.

## Health Determinants

Public health nurses consider the multiple factors that determine the health of their clients. *Health determinants* are factors that influence the health of individuals, families, and populations. Health determinants can have a positive or negative influence on health. Table 1.6 presents examples of protective and risk factors at all three levels of practice for communicable disease in childhood:

■ *Protective factors* are health determinants that protect a person from illness or assist in improving the person's health.

■ *Risk factors* are health determinants that contribute to the potential for illness to occur or to a decrease in health or well-being.

Just as holistic nursing practice focuses on the whole, public health nursing focuses on the whole by identifying all of the factors that influence the health of individuals, families, and communities. To ignore this wholeness of the living condition is to ignore many factors that impact health and the ability of public health nurses to promote health. Biological, behavioral, and environmental factors interact

## TABLE 1.5  Levels of Public Health Nursing Practice

| Individual/Family Level | Examples |
|---|---|
| "Population-based, individual-focused practice changes knowledge, attitudes, beliefs, practices, and behaviors of individuals. This practice level is directed at individuals, alone or as part of a family, class, or group. Individuals receive services because they are identified as belonging to a population at-risk" (MDH, 2001, p. 5). | ■ Make home visits to newborns and their parents.<br>■ Teach hand-washing to a first-grade class.<br>■ Assess for the presence of lead-based paint in a home with preschool children.<br>■ Develop a fall-prevention plan for an elderly person living alone. |
| **Community Level** | **Examples** |
| "Population-based, community-focused practice changes community norms, community attitudes, community awareness, community practices, and community behaviors. They [PHNs] are directed toward entire populations within the community or occasionally toward target groups within those populations. Community-focused practice is measured in terms of what proportion of the population actually changes" (MDH, 2001, p. 4). | ■ Write a letter to the editor of a local paper to stress the value of home visits to parents of newborns.<br>■ Create a billboard about the hazards of lead-based paint.<br>■ Participate in a community "town hall" meeting to make the community aware of safety hazards for elderly people living alone. |
| **Systems Level** | **Examples** |
| "Population-based, systems-focused practice changes organizations, policies, laws, and power structures. The focus is not directly on individuals and communities but on the systems that impact health. Changing systems is often a more effective and long-lasting way to impact population health than requiring change from every single individual in a community" (MDH, 2001, pp. 4–5). | ■ Meet with legislators to advocate for reimbursement for home visits with families of newborns.<br>■ Develop a hand-washing program at an elementary school.<br>■ Teach real-estate agents how to recognize lead-based paint in a home.<br>■ Develop a fall-prevention protocol for nurses working with the elderly in the community. |

and contribute to the health and illness of individuals, families, and populations (ANA, 2013; Marmot & Wilkinson, 1999; Zahner & Block, 2006). Individuals and families are able to influence or control some of their biological and many of their behavioral health determinants but are not able to control many of the physical and social environmental determinants of health that occur at the community and systems levels. Health determinants shaped by social, economic, and political forces, including systems put in place to deal with illness, are called the *social determinants of health*. (See Chapter 13 for further discussion on the social determinants of health.) These social determinants of health affect population health in all nations of the world.

The *social determinants of health* are the conditions in which people are born, grow, live, work, and age. These circumstances are shaped by the distribution of money, power, and resources at global, national, and local levels. The social determinants of health are mostly responsible for *health inequities*—the unfair and avoidable differences in health status seen within and between countries (WHO, 2013).

## Health Status

PHNs use the community assessment process and public health nursing process (see Chapter 3) to determine the health statuses of individuals, families, communities, and populations. *Health status* refers to the level of health or illness and is the outcome of the interaction of the multiple health determinants. Health status indicators are frequently represented by statistical measures, such as rates and percentages. Some common examples of population health status indicators are teen pregnancy rates, percentage of low-birthweight babies, neonatal mortality rates, percentage of malnutrition in a group, and obesity rates. Rates and percentages of various population groups can be compared to determine similarities or differences in the health status of those groups. Health status comparisons can also be applied at an individual level, such as identifying a child with malnutrition as having a lower level of health than a child who is not malnourished. Health status comparisons allow PHNs to determine their priorities for actions with specific individuals, families, communities, and populations. Figure 1.4 illustrates a health determinants model.

All of the Healthy People 2020 health determinants, including access to healthcare, are represented in Figure 1.4 (U.S. DHHS, n.d.-b). This model represents a holistic approach to assessment of the protective and risk factors that determine health status in individuals, families, and communities. Health determinants, including protective and risk factors, exist at individual/family, community, and systems levels, so nursing interventions should address health determinants at all levels as needed. PHNs can use this holistic approach to organize and identify the complex contributors to the health status of specific individuals,

## TABLE 1.6 Protective and Risk Factors for Childhood Communicable Diseases

### Protective Factors by Level of Practice

| Individual/Family Level | Community Level | Systems |
|---|---|---|
| ■ Family has insurance that covers immunizations. | ■ 95% of children in the community are immunized (herd immunity). | ■ Immunizations are available at public health clinics, pharmacies, and medical clinics. |
| ■ Children are up to date on immunizations. | ■ Community billboards urge parents to immunize their children. | ■ Free or low-cost immunizations are available to the uninsured. |
| ■ Parents teach children proper hand-washing and the benefits of covering their mouths when coughing. | ■ Low-density housing or single-dwelling homes reduce contact between infected and noninfected children. | ■ Childcare center has effective infection prevention and control practices. |

### Risk Factors by Level of Practice

| Individual/Family Level | Community Level | Systems |
|---|---|---|
| ■ Family is uninsured. | ■ 45% of children in the community are immunized (no herd immunity). | ■ Immunizations are not available at the public health clinic. |
| ■ Family members are not aware of the need for immunizations. | ■ Some community groups oppose childhood immunizations. | ■ Funding for low-cost immunizations for the uninsured is lacking. |
| ■ Parents are not aware of how to prevent the spread of infectious diseases. | ■ Many high-density housing and apartment complexes in the community place people living close together at greater risk. | ■ School district does not track students' immunization records. |

families, and populations and to develop interventions to improve health. PHNs collaborate with their clients by building and strengthening their protective factors and helping them reduce their risk factors. The social determinants of health that play a significant role in health disparities are discussed in Chapter 13.

## Activity

Review the following Health Determinants Analysis Case Study:

■ Identify the health status indicators for this community.

■ Identify health determinants, including protective and risk factors that contribute to the health status of this community.

■ Determine how you would work with community members to build on their protective factors and reduce their risk factors.

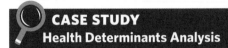

### CASE STUDY
### Health Determinants Analysis

A community assessment in a small rural community determines that more than one-third of the adult residents are overweight or obese. The assessment reveals that 40% of the adults in this community report that they have high cholesterol, and 30% report that they have high blood pressure. The majority of adults admit to eating out at fast-food restaurants at least five times a week. This community contains many fast-food restaurants, and the most common foods sold in them are high in fat, sodium, sugar, and calories. This community has few outdoor recreational sites, such as bike and walking paths, and the county board has voted against increasing tax levies to provide those paths. The local hospital does provide evening and weekend health education classes on modifying diet and exercise to lead a healthier life. A coalition of healthcare clinics, the public health agency, and local businesses is working on a plan to increase healthy living resources in the community.

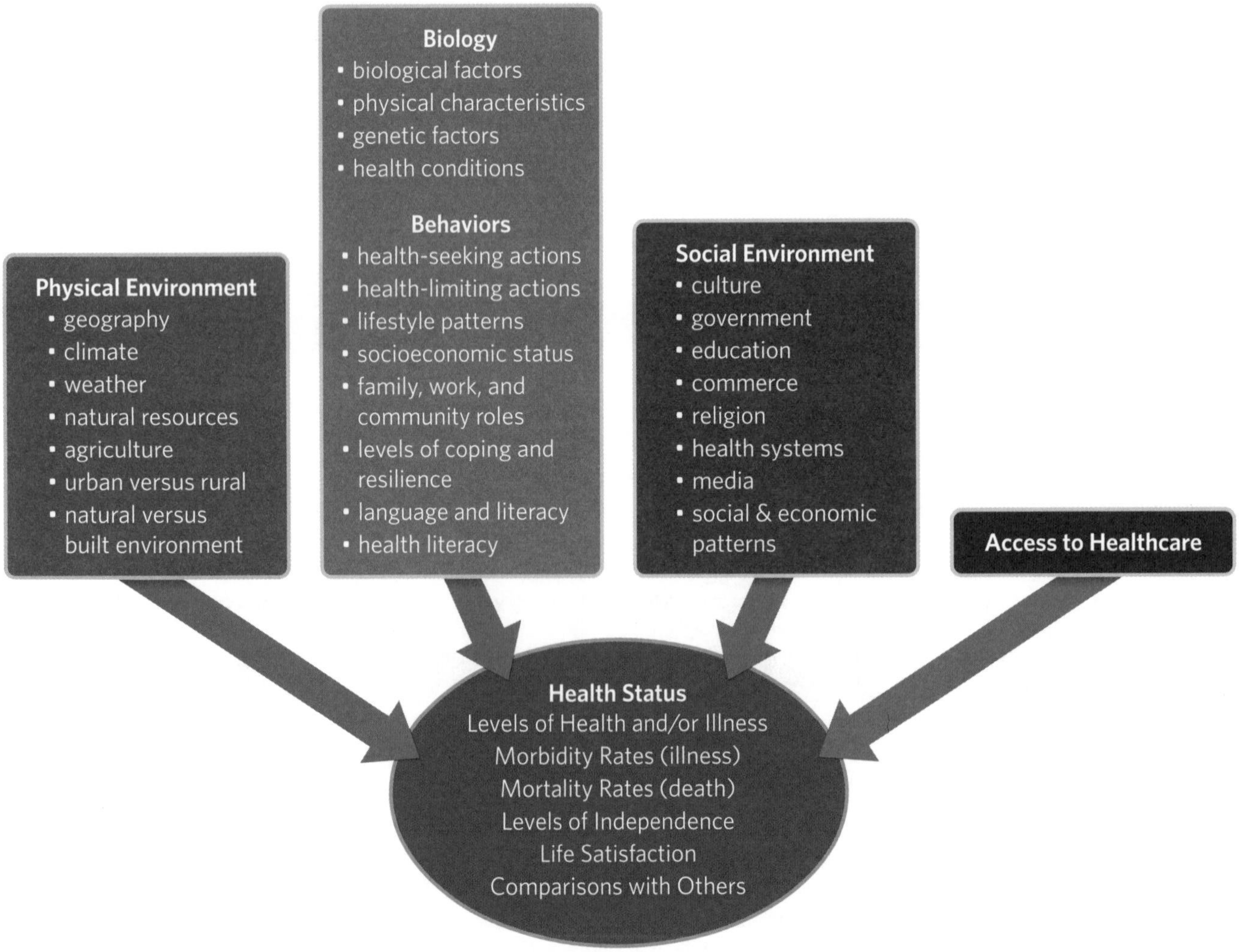

**Biology**
- biological factors
- physical characteristics
- genetic factors
- health conditions

**Behaviors**
- health-seeking actions
- health-limiting actions
- lifestyle patterns
- socioeconomic status
- family, work, and community roles
- levels of coping and resilience
- language and literacy
- health literacy

**Physical Environment**
- geography
- climate
- weather
- natural resources
- agriculture
- urban versus rural
- natural versus built environment

**Social Environment**
- culture
- government
- education
- commerce
- religion
- health systems
- media
- social & economic patterns

**Access to Healthcare**

**Health Status**
Levels of Health and/or Illness
Morbidity Rates (illness)
Mortality Rates (death)
Levels of Independence
Life Satisfaction
Comparisons with Others

**FIGURE 1.4** A Health Determinants Model for Individuals/Families, Communities, and Populations

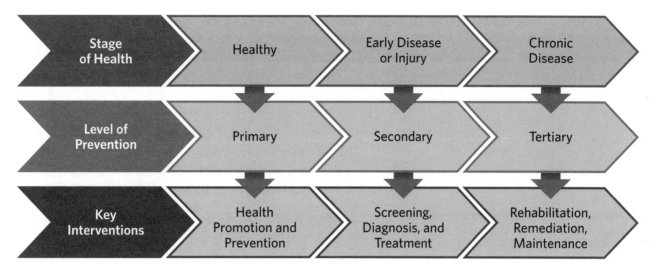

**FIGURE 1.5** Stages of Health and Disease and Levels of Prevention

## Levels of Prevention

The levels of prevention (primary, secondary, and tertiary) provide a framework for health-promotion and disease-prevention efforts in the stages of the natural history of disease (Leavell & Clark, 1958; Stanhope & Lancaster, 2008). The health-promotion progression from primary to secondary to tertiary prevention provides a framework for population-based public health nursing interventions at all levels of public health nursing practice (MDH, 2001; Skemp et al., 2016). It is important to determine the health status of individuals/families, communities, and populations and to determine the level of prevention for specific health concerns to implement the appropriate interventions. Figure 1.5 provides an overview of the stages of health, the levels of prevention, and intervention approaches.

Although the focus of public health nursing is primary prevention, public health nursing practice encompasses all three levels. In contrast, within the hospital setting, the focus of most nursing care is on ill patients and their family members, and nurses more often provide secondary and tertiary prevention but may also provide some primary prevention. Table 1.7 shows the definition of each level with examples.

**Healthy People**
**2020**
**healthypeople.gov**

Healthy People, a program of the U.S. Department of Health and Human Services, has established science-based benchmarks and 10-year national objectives for improving the health of all Americans. Healthy People 2020 is the third set of national health priorities identified over the last 3 decades. Its vision is "a society in which all people live long healthy lives" (U.S. DHHS, n.d.-b, p. 1). The mission and goals are displayed in Table 1.8. This national program seeks to involve all Americans by encouraging community and organizational collaboration, empowering individuals to make informed health decisions, and measuring the outcomes of prevention activities (U.S. DHHS, n.d.-b).

*"Okay! Now I understand why public health nurses do what they do, but I am still not clear about what I am supposed to do!" Albert states in an exasperated tone of voice.*

*Sia responds, "I guess we have to assess our clients' health status, identify their health determinants, and develop a plan of care that builds on their protective factors and reduces their risk factors. Now it makes sense that we would be mostly listening, teaching, and counseling. Did you know that the words* listen *and* silent *have the same letters? I guess we need to use silence to listen to our clients!"*

*Abby states, "I really like all the secondary and tertiary prevention interventions that I do in the hospital setting, so I am afraid I am going to get bored working in the community. I can only sit and listen for so long. I like action!"*

*Albert reflects, "Primary prevention doesn't have to mean you are not doing anything. Just because there isn't already an illness or disease doesn't mean there isn't work to do. Primary prevention is the way that we can identify health determinants and make an impact. Our instructor says we can apply public health nursing in any nursing practice setting. Maybe I will think about how I can use everything I learn in my community clinical in my hospital practice. But, who knows, maybe I will decide to become a public health nurse!"*

*Sia asks, "I understand what we are supposed to focus on when we work with individuals and families, but I am not sure how identifying their health statuses and health needs fits in with the concept of population-based practice. I guess I need to talk to my preceptor about how our home visits fit in with the priority health needs of our community. How do I know whether what we are doing reflects what the community really wants public health nurses to do?"*

**TABLE 1.7  Prevention Continuum With Public Health Nursing Examples**

| Definitions | Examples |
|---|---|
| *Primary prevention* promotes health and protects against threats to it. It is designed to keep problems from occurring in the first place. It promotes resiliency and protective factors or reduces susceptibility and exposure to risk factors. Primary prevention occurs before a problem develops. It targets populations that are essentially well. | PHN Antepartal home visit:<br>■ Teaching parents the importance of taking a newborn home from the hospital in an approved car seat<br>■ Providing parents with information about approved car seats<br><br>PHN Postpartum home visit:<br>■ Checking the car seat to determine that it is correctly installed<br>■ Monitoring the parents' use of car seat |
| *Secondary prevention* detects and treats problems in their early stages. It keeps problems from causing serious or long-term effects or from affecting others. It identifies risks or hazards and modifies, removes, or treats them before a problem becomes more serious. Secondary prevention is implemented after a problem has begun, possibly before signs and symptoms appear. It targets populations that share common risk factors. | PHN at WIC Clinic:<br>■ Using a growth chart to plot children's heights and weights<br>■ Identifying children who are outside established norms<br>■ Referring parents and children who are above 95th percentile or below 5th percentile to a primary care provider for assessment and to a nutritionist for nutritional education and counseling |
| *Tertiary prevention* limits further negative effects from a problem and aims to keep existing problems from getting worse. Tertiary prevention is implemented after a disease or injury has occurred. It alleviates the effects of disease and injury and restores individuals to their optimal levels of functioning. It targets populations that have experienced disease or injury. | School Nurse<br>Beginning of the school year:<br>■ Identifying students with asthma and obtaining asthma plans<br>■ Working with teaching staff to reduce environmental asthma triggers in the school building<br><br>During the school year:<br>■ Monitoring students with asthma for adherence to their asthma plans and their health status<br>■ Providing nebulizer treatments in the health office |

*Source:* Modified from MDH, 2001, p. 4

**TABLE 1.8  Healthy People 2020 Mission and Goals**

| Mission—Healthy People 2020 strives to: | Overarching Goals |
|---|---|
| ■ Identify nationwide health-improvement priorities<br>■ Increase public awareness and understanding of the determinants of health, disease, and disability and opportunities for progress<br>■ Provide measurable objectives and goals that are applicable at the national, state, and local levels<br>■ Engage multiple sectors to take action to strengthen policies and improve practices that are driven by the best available evidence and knowledge<br>■ Identify critical research, evaluation, and data-collection needs | ■ Attain high-quality, longer lives free of preventable disease, disability, injury, and premature death<br>■ Achieve health equity, eliminate disparities, and improve the health of groups<br>■ Create social and physical environments that promote good health for all<br>■ Promote quality of life, healthy development, and healthy behaviors across all life stages |

*Source:* U.S. DHHS, n.d.-b

A set of national health priorities titled Leading Health Indicators (LHIs) is included in Healthy People 2020 (U.S. DHHS, n.d. -a). They include 42 health outcomes organized into 12 health topics. These priorities reflect the greatest unmet national health needs based on an analysis of Healthy People 2010 health outcome data. The 12 health topics are listed in the following "Leading Health Indicators" box. A mid-course review of progress toward achieving the 42 health indicators shows that 21% of the targets have been achieved and 19% are improving while 11% are getting worse (U.S. DHHS, 2017).

### 🌐 OnlineActivity

Go to the Healthy People webpage (http://www.healthypeople.gov) and search for the LHIs.

▪ Read about one of the LHI health outcomes that interests you.

▪ Find the Healthy People 2010 statistical data that measured the achievement of that outcome.

▪ What is the goal for the Healthy People 2020 outcome? Which statistic would demonstrate improvement of that outcome?

## Activity

▪ Explore the community health priorities of your state or local health department. Compare them with the LHIs.

▪ Identify programs or activities in your clinical agency that are related to the LHIs.

▪ Discuss with your preceptor how nurses are involved in these programs or activities.

▪ Consider how you might become involved as a citizen or as a nurse in working on one of the LHI priorities in your community.

---

### Leading Health Indicators, Healthy People 2020

▪ Access to Health Services
▪ Clinical Preventive Services
▪ Environmental Quality
▪ Injury and Violence
▪ Maternal, Infant, and Child Health
▪ Mental Health
▪ Nutrition, Physical Activity, and Obesity
▪ Oral Health
▪ Reproductive and Sexual Health
▪ Social Determinants
▪ Substance Abuse
▪ Tobacco

*Sources:* National Center for Health Statistics, 2012; U.S. DHHS, n.d.-a

## BSN Preparation

The need for nurses to be prepared to both work in the community and have the ability to practice entry-level public health nursing has become more urgent as healthcare moves from the acute care setting to the community and new models of healthcare and nursing practice emerge. The challenge of practicing in the community is influenced by the persistence of health disparities among all age groups and diverse populations, the aging of the population, and the continuous increase in healthcare costs. In addition, healthcare needs and diseases are not isolated by geographic boundaries but evolve within a global environment. Recognition of the need for nurses to have the ability to improve the health of populations by taking leadership roles within the healthcare system and in their communities and by partnering with other health professionals and community leaders has resulted in a renewed commitment to increase the proportion of nurses with baccalaureate degrees and to enrich the baccalaureate nursing curriculum to prepare nurses for the challenges that face them (Education Committee of the Association of Community Health Nurse Educators [ACHNE], 2010; Institute of Medicine [IOM], 2011; Robert Wood Johnson Foundation, 2013). ACHNE has identified 15 basic core knowledge competencies for baccalaureate nursing graduates that should be included in the baccalaureate nursing curriculum (2010):

▪ Communication
▪ Epidemiology and biostatistics
▪ Community/population assessment
▪ Community/population planning
▪ Policy development
▪ Assurance
▪ Health promotion and risk reduction
▪ Illness and disease management
▪ Information and healthcare technology
▪ Environmental health
▪ Global health
▪ Human diversity
▪ Ethics and social justice
▪ Coordination and care management
▪ Emergency preparedness, response, and recovery

## Activity

▪ Which knowledge areas have you already studied?

▪ What are your knowledge and competency goals for your public health nursing clinical?

# Entry-Level Population-Based Public Health Nursing Competencies

This chapter has given you a lot to think about. Now it is time to focus on the entry-level public health nursing competencies that you can work to develop in your community clinical. This book is going to help you focus on the entry-level competencies expected of baccalaureate nursing graduates and novice nurses entering public health nursing.

## Henry Street Entry-Level PHN Competencies

The Henry Street Consortium (HSC) entry-level population-based public health nursing competencies, initially published in 2003 and updated in 2017, are intended for baccalaureate nursing graduates and novice public health nurses (Henry Street Consortium, 2017; Schaffer et al., 2011). These 12 competencies are consistent with national benchmark standards for entry-level public health nursing (ANA, 2013; Quad Council of Public Health Nursing Organizations, 2011). (See Table 1.9.) A consortium of practicing public health nurses and educators developed these simplified entry-level standards to facilitate the teaching and learning of public health nursing knowledge and skills in the clinical setting (Schaffer et al., 2011).

This list presents each competency in broad statements that are not measurable by themselves. A more complete outline of each of the HSC competencies, which provides measures of how to evaluate PHN achievement of each competency, is found in Appendix A. Chapters 3 to 14 each cover one of the 12 competencies and provide specific evidence about best practices for each competency. As you read this book, you will learn how you might meet these entry-level competencies in your public health clinical learning activities.

## Activity

▪ Review the competencies and their related activities in Appendix A. Make a list of activities within each competency that you would like to practice during your community clinical.

▪ Talk with your preceptor about how you might practice these public health nursing activities.

## TABLE 1.9  Henry Street Consortium Entry-Level Population-Based Public Health Nursing Competencies

**Entry-Level Population-Based Public Health Nursing Competencies**

*For the New Graduate or Novice Public Health Nurse*

1. Applies the public health nursing process to communities, systems, individuals, and families

2. Utilizes basic epidemiological (the incidence, distribution, and control of disease in a population) principles in public health nursing practice

3. Utilizes the principles and science of environmental health to promote safe and sustainable environments for individuals/families, systems, and communities

4. Practices within the auspices of the Nurse Practice Act

5. Works within the responsibility and authority of the governmental public health system

6. Utilizes collaboration to achieve public health goals

7. Effectively communicates with communities, systems, individuals, families, and colleagues

8. Establishes and maintains caring relationships with communities, systems, individuals, and families

9. Incorporates mental, physical, emotional, social, and spiritual aspects of health into assessment, planning, implementation, and evaluation

10. Demonstrates nonjudgmental/unconditional acceptance of people different from self

11. Shows evidence of commitment to social justice, the greater good, and the public health principles

12. Demonstrates leadership in public health nursing with communities, systems, individuals, and families

*Source:* Henry Street Consortium, 2017

## ! KEY POINTS

- Public health nursing combines the theory and practice of nursing and public health. It is a required component of baccalaureate nursing education.

- Public health nursing practice is guided by the national scope of practice standards.

- The goal of public health and public health nursing is to improve the health of the public at the local, national, and international levels.

- The Cornerstones of Public Health explain the beliefs and values of the clinical specialty of public health nursing practice.

- Public health nursing practice is population-based, focusing on the priority health needs of populations.

- Primary prevention is the focus of public health nursing, but PHNs also provide secondary and tertiary prevention interventions.

- PHNs work at all three levels of practice: individual/family, community, and systems.

- Emerging threats and challenges in health and healthcare require changes in and leadership from public health nursing.

- The HSC Entry-Level Public Health Nursing competencies, based on accepted national standards, provide a guide for baccalaureate nursing students to achieve the expected outcomes of baccalaureate nursing education.

## REFLECTIVE PRACTICE

*Alberto takes a deep breath, closes his eyes as if in deep thought, and says to Abby and Sia, "Let's see if I have this straight. Public health nursing is part of my professional nursing practice. It can be practiced anywhere, because public health nursing is shaped by its goal, not by its setting, but it is most often practiced in the community. The goal of public health nursing is to improve the health of the public, the health of the communities in which we live. The client in public health nursing may be an individual, a family, the community, or a population within the community. To improve and protect the public's health, I need to assess the health status and identify the health determinants that affect the health status of individuals, families, communities, and populations. Then I need to intervene by helping my clients build on their protective factors and reduce their risk factors. The interventions I will use most often are teaching and counseling, but we will learn about more interventions as we read this book and complete our community clinical. When I practice in the community, I will probably*
*be partnering with other members of the healthcare team as well as community members. I need to demonstrate a set of entry-level public health nursing competencies to successfully complete my baccalaureate nursing education. The Henry Street Consortium Population-Based Public Health Nursing Competencies focus on what I should be learning and practicing in my public health clinical activities. Whew! Do I have that right?"*

*Abby and Sia respond, "Yes. You've got it! You get an 'A' for the course!"*

1. Think about what Alberto, Abby, and Sia have learned about public health nursing from their observations and discussions with their preceptors.

2. How will you analyze what you observe about public health nursing during your clinical experience?

3. How would you describe public health nursing practices you observe in your clinical to your classmates?

# References

Abrams, S. E. (2008). The best of public health nursing, circa 1941. *Public Health Nursing, 25*(3), 285–291. doi:10.1111/j.1525-1446.2008.00706.x

Aiken, T. (2004). *Legal, ethical, and political issues in nursing.* Philadelphia, PA: F. A. Davis.

American Nurses Association. (2003). *Nursing's social policy statement* (2nd ed.). Silver Spring, MD: Author.

American Nurses Association. (2013). *Public health nursing: Scope and standards of practice.* Silver Spring, MD: Author.

American Public Health Association, Public Health Nursing Section. (2013). *The definition and practice of public health nursing.* Washington, DC: Author. Retrieved from https://www.apha.org/~/media/files/pdf/membergroups/phn/nursingdefinition.ashx

Beauchamp, T., & Childress, J. (1979). *Principles of biomedical ethics.* New York, NY: Oxford University Press.

Beck, D-M. (2010). Expanding our Nightingale horizon: Seven recommendations for 21st-century nursing practice. *Journal of Holistic Nursing, 28*(4), 317–326. doi:10.1177/0898010110387780

Buhler-Wilkerson, K. (1993). Bringing care to the people: Lillian Wald's legacy to public health nursing. *American Journal of Public Health, 83*(12), 1778–1786.

Clark, M. J. (2008). *Community health nursing.* Upper Saddle River, NJ: Pearson.

Davies, R. (2012). 'Notes on nursing: What it is and what it is not' (1860), by Florence Nightingale. *Nurse Education Today, 32*(2012), 624–626. Retrieved from http://www.nurseeducationtoday.com/article/S0260-6917(12)00132-3/fulltext

Dossey, B. M., & Keegan, L. (2016). *Holistic nursing—A handbook for practice* (7th ed.). Burlington, MA: Jones & Bartlett Learning.

Dreher, M., Shapiro, D., & Asselin, M. (2006). *Healthy places, healthy people: A handbook for culturally competent community nursing practice.* Indianapolis, IN.: Sigma Theta Tau International.

Education Committee of the Association of Community Health Nurse Educators. (2010). Essentials of baccalaureate nursing education for entry-level community/public health nursing. *Public Health Nursing, 27*(4), 371–382. doi:10.1111/j.1525-1446.2010.00867.x

Friedman, M., Bowden, V., & Jones, E. (2003). *Family nursing: Research, theory, and practice* (5th ed.). Hoboken, NJ: Pearson Education, Inc.

Henry Street Consortium. (2017). *Entry-level, population-based public health nursing competencies.* St. Paul, MN: Author. Retrieved from www.henrystreetconsortium.org

Institute of Medicine. (1988). *The future of public health.* Washington, DC: National Academies Press.

Institute of Medicine. (2011). *The future of nursing—Leading change, advancing health.* Washington, DC: National Academies Press.

International Council of Nurses. (2011). *Nurses and human rights* [Position statement]. Retrieved from http://www.icn.ch/images/stories/documents/publications/position_statements/E10_Nurses_Human_Rights.pdf

Ivanov, L. L., & Oden, T. F. (2013). Public health nursing, ethics and human rights. *Public Health Nursing, 30*(3), 231–238. doi:10.1111/phn.12022

Keller, L. O., Strohschein, S., & Schaffer, M. A. (2011). Cornerstones of public health nursing. *Public Health Nursing, 28*(3), 249–260. doi:10.1111/j.1525-1446.2010.00923.x

Kub, J., Kulbok, P. A., & Glick, D. (2015). Cornerstone documents, milestones, and policies: Shaping the direction of public health nursing 1890–1950. *Online Journal of Issues in Nursing, 20*(2), 3.

Kulbok, P. A., Thatcher, E., Park, E., & Meszaros, P. S. (2012). Evolving public health nursing roles: Focus on community participatory health promotion and prevention. *Online Journal of Issues in Nursing, 17*(2), 1. doi:10.3912/OJIN.Vol17No02Man01

Leavell, H., & Clark, E. (1958). *Preventive medicine for the doctor in his community: An epidemiologic approach.* New York, NY: McGraw-Hill.

Marmot, M., & Wilkinson, R. G. (1999). *Social determinants of health.* Oxford, UK: Oxford University Press.

Martin, K. S. (2005). *The Omaha System: A key to practice, documentation, and information management* (2nd ed.). Omaha, NE: Health Connections Press.

Minnesota Department of Health, Center for Public Health Nursing. (2003). Definition of population-based practice. Retrieved from http://www.health.state.mn.us/divs/opi/cd/phn/docs/0303phn_popbasedpractice.pdf

Minnesota Department of Health, Center for Public Health Nursing. (2007). *Cornerstones of public health nursing.* Adapted from original by Center for Public Health Nursing, 2004. St. Paul, MN: Author. Retrieved from http://www.health.state.mn.us/divs/opi/cd/phn/docs/0710phn_cornerstones.pdf

Minnesota Department of Health, Division of Community Health Services, Public Health Nursing Section. (2001). *Public health interventions: Applications for public health nursing practice.* St. Paul, MN: Author. Retrieved from http://www.health.state.mn.us/divs/opi/cd/phn/docs/0301wheel_manual.pdf

Minnesota Department of Health, Public Health Nursing Section. (2000). *Public health nursing practice for the 21st century: Competency development in population-based practice.* National Satellite Learning Conference. St. Paul, MN: Author. Retrieved from http://www.health.state.mn.us/divs/opi/cd/phn/docs/0001phnpractice_learningguide.pdf

National Center for Health Statistics. (2012). *Healthy People 2010, final review.* Hyattsville, NY: U.S. Department of Health and Human Services. Retrieved from http://www.cdc.gov/nchs/data/hpdata2010/hp2010_final_review.pdf

Parker, M. E., & Smith, M. C. (2010). *Nursing theories and nursing practice* (3rd ed.). Philadelphia, PA: F. A. Davis.

Purtilo, R. (2005). *Ethical dimensions in the health professions* (4th ed.). Philadelphia, PA: Elsevier Saunders.

Quad Council of Public Health Nursing Organizations. (2011). *The Quad Council competencies for public health nurses.* Retrieved from http://www.achne.org/files/Quad%20Council/QuadCouncilCompetenciesforPublicHealthNurses.pdf

Racher, F. E. (2007). The evolution of ethics for community practice. *Journal of Community Health Nursing, 24*(1), 65–76.

Robert Wood Johnson Foundation. (2013). *Forum on the future of public health nursing, February 8, 2012—Proceedings and feedback: Summary report.* Retrieved from http://www.rwjf.org/content/dam/farm/reports/reports/2012/rwjf404144

Schaffer, M. A., Cross, S., Olson, L. O., Nelson, P., Schoon, P. M., & Henton, P. (2011). The Henry Street Consortium population-based competencies for educating public health nursing students. *Public Health Nursing, 28*(1), 78–90. doi:10.1111/j.1525-1446.2010.00900.x

Scoville Walker, S. (2004). Ethical quandaries in community health nursing. In E. Anderson & J. McFarlane (Eds.), *Community as partner: Theory and practice in nursing* (4th ed., pp. 83–113). Philadelphia, PA: Lippincott, Williams & Wilkins.

Selanders, L. C., & Crane, P. C. (2012). The voice of Florence Nightingale on advocacy. *Online Journal of Issues in Nursing, 17*(1), 1.

Skemp, L. E., Dreher, M. C., & Lehmann, S. P. (2016). *Healthy places, healthy people* (3rd ed.). Indianapolis, IN: Sigma Theta Tau International.

Stanhope, M., & Lancaster, J. (2008). *Public health nursing: Population-centered health care in the community* (7th ed.). St. Louis, MO: Mosby.

United Nations. (1948). *Universal declaration of human rights.* New York, NY: Author. Retrieved from http://www.ohchr.org/EN/UDHR/Documents/UDHR_Translations/eng.pdf

United Nations General Assembly. (2015). *Transforming our world: The 2030 agenda for sustainable development.* New York, NY: Author. Retrieved from https://sustainabledevelopment.un.org/content/documents/21252030%20Agenda%20for%20Sustainable%20Development%20web.pdf

U.S. Department of Health and Human Services. (n.d.-a). *Healthy People 2020: About Healthy People 2020: Leading health indicators.* Retrieved from https://www.healthypeople.gov/2020/Leading-Health-Indicators

U.S. Department of Health and Human Services. (n.d.-b). *Healthy People 2020 framework.* Retrieved from https://www.healthypeople.gov/sites/default/files/HP2020Framework.pdf

U.S. Department of Health and Human Services. (2017). *Healthy People 2020: Chapter 3–Overview of midcourse progress and health disparities.* Retrieved from https://www.cdc.gov/nchs/data/hpdata2020/HP2020MCR-B03-Overview.pdf

Visiting Nurses Association of Western New York. (n.d.). Our history. Retrieved from https://www.vnawny.org/about/history.asp

Volbrecht, R. M. (2002). *Nursing ethics: Communities in dialogue.* Upper Saddle River, NJ: Pearson Prentice Hall.

Watson, J. (2008). *Nursing: The philosophy and science of caring* (Rev. ed.). Boulder, CO: University Press of Colorado. In Watson Caring Science Institute and International Caritas Consortium. (2010). *Core concepts of Jean Watson's theory of human caring/caring science.* Retrieved from http://watsoncaringscience.org/files/Cohort%206/watsons-theory-of-human-caring-core-concepts-and-evolution-to-caritas-processes-handout.pdf

Watson, J. (2010). Florence Nightingale and the enduring legacy of transpersonal human caring-healing. *Journal of Holistic Nursing, 28*(1), 107–108.

World Health Organization. (n.d.). Public health. Retrieved from http://www.euro.who.int/en/health-topics/Health-systems/public-health-services

World Health Organization. (2013). About social determinants of health. Retrieved from http://www.who.int/social_determinants/sdh_definition/en/index.html

World Health Organization. (2017). Health in all policies: Progressing the sustainable development goals. Retrieved from http://www.who.int/phe/events/HiAP-conference-March2017/en/

Zahner, S. J., & Block, D. E. (2006). The road to population health: Using Healthy People 2010 in nursing education. *Journal of Nursing Education, 45*(3), 105–108.

# Evidence-Based Public Health Nursing Practice

■ **Patricia M. Schoon and Marjorie A. Schaffer**

*with Stephanie Rivery*

*Abby is talking with Jaime, an RN who has returned to school to get his baccalaureate nursing degree. She is struggling to understand the three levels of public health nursing practice. Abby asks, "How do you use the nursing process in your hospital work? Did you ever think you could use it for more than the patients you are caring for?"*

*Jaime replies, "It still seems kind of strange to me. But I am a member of the Quality Improvement Team. We just finished an audit to look at the incidence of patient falls to find out whether our unit is meeting the goals set by the hospital to reduce the patient fall rate. Our patient fall rate is still higher than the goal set by the hospital, so we decided that we need to hold an in-service on assessing patients for their fall risk and the different protocols we can use to reduce the number of patient falls. So, I guess if we think of my unit as a community, we are using the nursing process at more than one level."*

*Abby ponders, "I guess I can kind of see that you are using the nursing process to assess the fall rate. The idea of using the nursing process at the systems level still seems very strange to me."*

*Jaime thinks about the idea of nursing at the systems level and finally says, "Maybe if I think of the nursing staff on my unit as part of the hospital system, then Quality Improvement Team members can assess what they know about fall risk and prevention and design a program just for our staff members to improve their skills in that area. What do you think?"*

*Abby sighs, "I kind of understand how I can use nursing process to assess the health needs of individuals, families, and communities, but I can't think how I would assess the health status of a system. Do systems have a health status?" Abby muses, "If a system, like a public health agency, doesn't have enough money to provide the health services that the community needs, then I guess it wouldn't be very healthy."*

*Jaime says thoughtfully, "Maybe we need to look at a community's health needs and determine whether specific community systems, such as hospitals, schools, educational systems, and public health agencies, have the resources to meet the priority needs of their community. If they don't have the resources, then maybe we can plan interventions to help them get the resources or services they need."*

Several years ago, a nursing student about to graduate reflected on what she had learned. She said, "I get it. Nursing is about critical thinking!" Nursing is a knowledge profession. That means nurses think before they do (assessment and planning), while they do (modifying interventions), and after they do (evaluation). This chapter explains how to apply the nursing process to public health nursing practice and to identify and use interventions that support public health practice goals. You will learn how to apply what you already know about evidence-based nursing practice to your public health nursing practice. PHNs are accountable to their clients and to the public for practicing effectively and efficiently to achieve the best outcomes using the least amount of resources. This chapter discusses how PHNs use best practice information to improve their clients' health.

## The Public Health Nursing Process

The public health nursing process integrates concepts of nursing and public health. The steps of the nursing process are the same: assessment, diagnosis, planning, implementation, and evaluation. However, the public health nursing process expands the nursing process in that PHNs focus their assessment and interventions on three different levels of practice: individuals and families, communities, and systems (MDH, 2001). Refer to Chapter 1 for a description of the three levels of PHN practice. Critical thinking throughout the PHN process is essential in identifying and modifying the complex determinants of health that influence the health status of individuals, families, and communities. This application of the nursing process is reflected in the American Nurses Association's (ANA's) *Public Health Nursing: Scope and Standards of Practice* (2013), as illustrated in Figure 2.1.

The application of the nursing process to all three levels of practice is discussed in Chapter 3.

An easy way to remember the level of practice is to ask yourself, "Whose knowledge, beliefs, behaviors, and values am I trying to modify?" For example, if you are teaching a group of first grade students how to wash their hands, even though they are in a group, your intention is to modify the handwashing behaviors of the individual students. So, you are intervening at the individual/family level of practice. If you taught the first-grade teachers how to monitor the handwashing behaviors of their students, you would be intervening at the systems level of practice. If you handed out a flyer on the reasons for handwashing and the correct handwashing procedure at a county fair, you would be intervening with the community level, hoping to change community norms for handwashing, not the behaviors of specific individuals.

*Abby comments, "My PHN preceptor told me that we are going to make a joint visit with the social worker to a family where a baby has failure to thrive. My preceptor is going to focus on assessing the health status of the baby, and the social worker is going to focus on the family support system and resources in the community for the mother. It will be interesting to see how they work together."*

*Jaime responds, "I am going to an interdisciplinary child protection team meeting with my preceptor. It is a county-wide team made up of police, social workers, lawyers, and public health nurses. It seems like my preceptor is always working with other people."*

*Abby concurs, "It really does seem that PHNs work with lots of other disciplines. My preceptor says that is the best way to deal with community-wide health problems."*

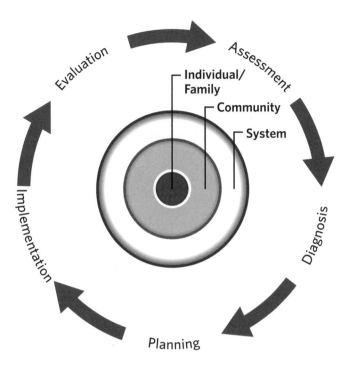

**FIGURE 2.1** Nursing Process at Three Levels of Public Health Nursing Practice

PHNs often work with people in other professions as well as community members to achieve public health goals. (See Chapter 8 for a discussion of interprofessional collaboration.) Many of the interventions that PHNs use are also used by other professionals in the community.

## Public Health Intervention Wheel

The Public Health Intervention Wheel is a major conceptual model in public health nursing (Keller, Strohschein, Lia-Hoagberg, & Schaffer, 1998, 2004; Bigbee & Issel, 2012). Concepts in the Public Health Intervention Wheel include: population-focus, three levels of practice, three levels of prevention, and 17 interventions that define the shared practice of public health nursing. Research supporting the use and effectiveness of many of the interventions in this model are found in this book. This model is supported by evidence from literature and validated by more than 200 public health nurses from a variety of practice settings.

*Public health interventions* are actions that PHNs take on behalf of individuals, families, systems, and communities to improve or protect their health status (MDH, 2001). The Public Health Intervention Wheel identifies 17 population-based interventions specific to public health practice that are found at three levels: individual/family, community, and systems (Keller et al., 1998, 2004; MDH, 2001). Because PHN practice occurs at three levels, interventions must also be implemented at all three levels.

These interventions are organized in the Public Health Intervention Wheel illustrated in Figure 2.2. The Public Health Intervention Wheel is evidence-based and represents what PHNs do (Keller et al., 2004). PHNs often use more than one intervention at more than one level of practice (individual and family, community, or system) to influence the multiple health risks affecting individuals, families, and populations.

The 17 interventions are divided into five wedges with three or four interventions in each wedge. Each group of wedges reflects a cluster of interventions. The cluster of interventions within each wedge often occurs either concurrently or consecutively. The five wedges (also depicted in specific colors) include the following interventions:

- **Wedge 1 (pink):** Surveillance, disease and health event investigation, outreach, and screening (case finding is the individual level for this wedge)
- **Wedge 2 (green):** Referral and follow-up, case management, and delegation
- **Wedge 3 (blue):** Health teaching, counseling, and consultation
- **Wedge 4 (orange):** Collaboration, coalition building, and community organizing (no individual level for coalition building and community organizing)
- **Wedge 5 (yellow):** Advocacy, social marketing, policy development, and enforcement

The three inner circles, called *segments*, represent the three levels of public health nursing practice (individual/family, community, and systems). All but three interventions are carried out at all three levels of practice. Case finding is only carried out at the individual/family level of practice, so it is placed inside the individual/family circle in the wheel diagram. Community organizing and coalition formation are practiced at the community and systems levels but not at the individual/family level. Sixteen of the interventions are independent nursing actions that can be practiced under your state's Nurse Practice Act without medical orders. The seventeenth intervention, delegated functions, can include medical functions delegated by a medical professional, such as immunizations. Nursing activities that the PHN delegates to another health team member, such as vision and hearing screening, are part of the independent practice of nursing and usually reflect one of the other PHN interventions.

Definitions and examples of the 17 population-based public health interventions are outlined in Table 2.1. Interventions are organized within the five wedges on the Public Health Intervention Wheel. Nursing students could do all the intervention examples in the table.

The Public Health Intervention Wheel has been disseminated to public health nursing students, PHNs, other public health professionals, and health departments nationally and internationally. The Wheel is used as a framework for teaching; a guide for planning, documentation, and evaluation in public health practice; and a model for research on intervention use and effectiveness.

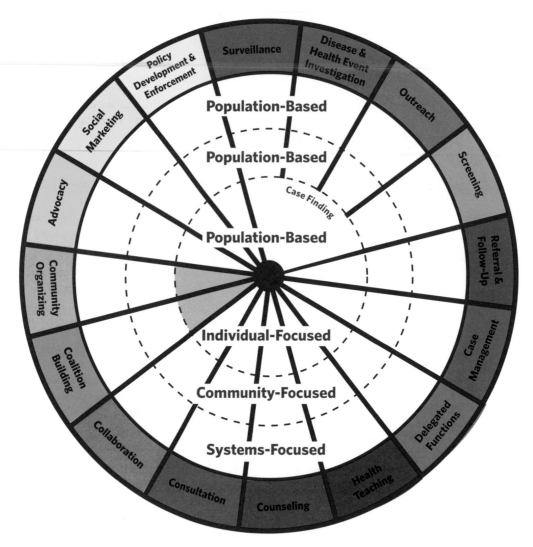

**FIGURE 2.2** Public Health Intervention Wheel
*Source:* MDH, Center for Public Health Nursing (2001)

## TABLE 2.1  Public Health Nursing Interventions at All Three Levels of Practice

| PHN Intervention Definition | PHN Intervention Examples |
| --- | --- |
| **Surveillance (Wedge 1 – Pink)**<br>Surveillance describes and monitors health events through ongoing and systematic collection, analysis, and interpretation of health data for the purpose of planning, implementing, and evaluating public health interventions (MDH, 2001, p. 13). | ■ Investigate and report the incidence and prevalence of sexually transmitted infections in the local teen population (community level).<br>■ Work with a school nurse at an elementary school to develop a tracking program to identify the incidence and prevalence of student-on-student bullying before and after the implementation of an anti-bullying curriculum (systems level). |
| **Disease & Health Event Investigation (Wedge 1 – Pink)**<br>Disease and other health event investigation systematically gathers and analyzes data regarding threats to the health of populations, ascertains the source of the threat, identifies cases and others at-risk, and determines control measures (p. 29). | ■ Identify and follow up on cases of sexually transmitted infection in a high school population to identify sources of infection and provide treatment (individual/family level).<br>■ Gather information about radon levels in your community and determine high-risk geographical areas (community level). |

| PHN Intervention Definition | PHN Intervention Examples |
|---|---|
| **Outreach (Wedge 1 – Pink)**<br>Outreach locates populations of interest or populations at risk and provides information about the nature of the concern, what can be done about it, and how services can be obtained (p. 41). | ■ Interview people at a family homeless shelter to determine who needs information about the location of local food shelves and WIC clinics (individual/family level).<br>■ Develop brochures for local grocery stores to hand out about nutritional needs for children and the location of local food shelves and WIC clinics (systems level). |
| **Case Finding (Wedge 1 – Pink)**<br>Case finding locates individuals and families with identified risk factors and connects them to resources (p. 55). | ■ Identify new immigrants from southeast Asia who might be at risk for tuberculosis (TB) (individual/family level).<br>■ Give at-risk immigrants information on where to receive TB screening (individual/family level). |
| **Screening (Wedge 1 – Pink)**<br>Screening identifies individuals with unrecognized health risk factors or asymptomatic disease conditions in populations (p. 63). | ■ Conduct blood pressure screening for African-American males (community level)<br>■ Organize a blood pressure screening clinic at a community center (systems level) |
| **Referral & Follow-up (Wedge 2 – Green)**<br>Referral and follow-up assists individuals, families, groups, organizations, and communities to utilize necessary resources to prevent or resolve problems or concerns (p. 79). | ■ Give an elderly person who is homebound information about how to contact a local Meals on Wheels program and then contact the individual a week later to see if he or she has successfully reached the Meals on Wheels program (individual/family level).<br>■ Work with Emergency Department (ED) nurses and home visiting nurses to develop and use a referral process for elderly individuals seen in the ED that need home healthcare services (systems level). |
| **Case Management (Wedge 2 – Green)**<br>Case management optimizes self-care capabilities of individuals and families and the capacity of systems and communities to coordinate and provide services (p. 93). | ■ Work with parents of a newborn with Down's Syndrome to identify services in their community that they can use to help them (individual/family level).<br>■ Work with a PHN and school nurse to coordinate in-home and school health services for children with severe developmental delays (systems level). |
| **Delegated Functions (Wedge 2 – Green)**<br>Delegated functions are direct care tasks a registered professional nurse carries out under the authority of a healthcare practitioner, as allowed by law. Delegated functions also include any direct care tasks a registered professional nurse entrusts to other appropriate personnel to perform (p. 113). | ■ Provide immunizations at a community flu clinic under standing orders from medical personnel (individual/family and systems levels).<br>■ Direct a peer counselor to work with a new diabetic to organize a grocery list and menu plans (individual/family level). |
| **Health Teaching (Wedge 3 – Blue)**<br>Health teaching communicates facts, ideas, and skills that change knowledge, attitudes, values, beliefs, behaviors, and practices and skills of individuals, families, systems, and/or communities (p. 121). | ■ Teach a class for teen moms about how to care for new baby (individual/family level).<br>■ Develop a program on childcare for new moms at a local high school (systems level). |

*(continues)*

**TABLE 2.1  Public Health Nursing Interventions at All Three Levels of Practice** *(continued)*

| PHN Intervention Definition | PHN Intervention Examples |
|---|---|
| **Counseling (Wedge 3 – Blue)**<br>Counseling establishes an interpersonal relationship with a community, system, family, or individual intended to increase or enhance their capacity for self-care and coping. Counseling engages the community, system, family, or individual at an emotional level (p. 151). | ■ Provide support for parents who are coping with providing care for their dying child at home (individual/family level).<br>■ Provide crisis management services to a community that has just experienced a devastating tornado (community level). |
| **Consultation (Wedge 3 – Blue)**<br>Consultation seeks information and generates optional solutions to perceived problems or issues through interactive problem-solving with a community, system, family or individual. The community, system, family or individual selects and acts on the option best meeting the circumstances (p. 165). | ■ Help a recently divorced father who has custody of his two children to problem solve balancing parenting and work responsibilities (individual/family level).<br>■ Consult with a peer-counseling group for diabetes management to help them develop strategies for working with individuals with diabetes in their community (community level). |
| **Collaboration (Wedge 4 – Orange)**<br>Collaboration commits two or more persons or organizations to achieving a common goal through enhancing the capacity of one or more of them to promote and protect health (p. 177). | ■ Partner with the nurse and social worker in an adolescent correction facility in developing a program to help inmates maintain contact with caring individuals in their family or friendship network (systems level).<br>■ Work with the county parks and playground department and local young parents group to develop a plan to provide more bike and walking paths for family use (community and systems level). |
| **Coalition Building (Wedge 4 – Orange)**<br>Coalition building promotes and develops alliances among organizations or constituencies for a common purpose. It builds linkages, solves problems, and/or enhances local leadership to address health concerns (p. 211). | ■ Develop an alliance between local environmental groups, waste management, and recycling organizations to improve community recycling (community level).<br>■ Establish a network of agencies to work together to develop a community disaster plan (systems level). |
| **Community Organizing (Wedge 4 – Orange)**<br>Community organizing helps community groups identify common problems or goals, mobilize resources, and develop and implement strategies for reaching the goals they collectively have set (p. 235). | ■ Organize a group of renters from several low-income housing developments to work together to improve the safety of their buildings (community level).<br>■ Help organize a group of low-income housing services organizations, community homeless shelters, and county human services to develop strategies to provide a more streamlined program for placing homeless people in affordable housing (systems level). |
| **Advocacy (Wedge 5 – Yellow)**<br>Advocacy pleads someone's cause or acts on someone's behalf, with a focus on developing the community, system, individual, or family's capacity to plead their own cause or act on their own behalf (p. 263). | ■ Help a client file an appeal for an insurance denial for home-care services when the client meets eligibility criteria stated in insurance policy (individual/family level).<br>■ Lobby legislators for support of community mental health programs (systems level). |
| **Social Marketing (Wedge 5 – Yellow)**<br>Social marketing utilizes commercial marketing principles and technologies for programs designed to influence the knowledge, attitudes, values, beliefs, behaviors, and practices of the population of interest (p. 285). | ■ Create a video for teen parents on how to help their infants and toddlers meet developmental milestones (individual/family level).<br>■ Participate in a televised panel discussion about the effects of drug and alcohol use during pregnancy on the fetus (community level). |

| PHN Intervention Definition | PHN Intervention Examples |
|---|---|
| **Policy Development & Enforcement (Wedge 5 – Yellow)** | |
| Policy development places health issues on decision-makers' agendas, acquires a plan of resolution, and determines needed resources. Policy development results in laws, rules and regulations, ordinances, and policies. Policy enforcement compels others to comply with the laws, rules, regulations, ordinances, and policies created in conjunction with policy development (p. 313). | ▪ Participate on a county task force to revise county human services guidelines for mandating reporting of suspected child abuse or neglect (systems level).<br><br>▪ Talk to a church group about the need to support a bill for community nutrition programs for children living in poverty (community level). |

*Source:* Definitions from MDH, Center for Public Health Nursing (2001)

## EVIDENCE EXAMPLE 2.1
### Public Health Intervention Wheel

▪ Over 600 school nurses (SNs), members of the National Association of School Nurses (NASN), completed an electronic survey on using public health interventions in their practice as defined by the Public Health Intervention Wheel. Most SNs (67%) were not familiar with the Wheel; however, participants identified interventions that were consistent with the Wheel. They used screening, referral and follow-up, case management, and health teaching more often than other interventions. In estimates of time spent at specific practices levels, SN practice was primarily at the individual level (65%). They also provided community-level interventions 22% of their time and systems-level interventions 14% of their time. SNs can use the Wheel to document and explain the interventions they provide in school nursing practice to address the health of school populations (Schaffer, Anderson, & Rising, 2016).

▪ A qualitative study explored how school nurses (n = 43) understood and used the interventions from Public Health Intervention Wheel. Data were analyzed from six focus groups conducted across the state of Minnesota. Ns represented urban, suburban, and rural schools. The SN practice stories included all interventions and levels of practice except for case management and delegation at the community level. The highest number of practice examples were for health teaching, case finding, and referral and follow-up, all at the individual level. The practice stories provide examples of how SNs can extend their practice to community and systems levels and affirm school nursing as a population-focused practice (Anderson et al., 2018).

▪ McDonald and colleagues (2015) replicated the process of identifying and defining public health interventions from the Wheel in the context of public health nursing in Ireland. Public health nursing leaders in Ireland conducted a literature review and hosted discussions on each intervention wedge at the 2011 Institute of Community Health Nursing conference. The aim was to promote visibility of the PHN role and build a common language to describe interventions. A key theme of practice stories was the importance of building trusting relationships with individuals and communities to support interventions. The Population Health Interest Group (2013) published practice stories from Irish nurses for each of the 17 interventions.

*Jaime says, "I am going to a meeting with my PHN preceptor this afternoon about how the different county agencies and the school district are working together as a team to try to reduce smoking among high school students. I guess that would be an example of collaboration, but I am not sure which level of practice that would be."*

*Abby ponders, "I think maybe when PHNs work with agencies and school districts, they are practicing at the systems level. If they use an intervention like social marketing to let teens know about the availability of a smoking cessation program at their school, then they would be practicing at the community level."*

*Jaime responds, "Teens at risk for smoking are a vulnerable population within the community, and PHNs work with populations within the community. If the team's goal is to change the smoking behaviors of individual high school students, even if they were part of a group and PHNs carried out some health teaching in the classroom, I guess those actions would be at the individual/family level. This gets kind of confusing at times."*

**TABLE 2.2  Three Levels of PHN Practice and Three Levels of Prevention With Public Health Interventions to Reduce Tobacco Use in Teens**

| Individual/Family Level of Practice | | |
|---|---|---|
| **Primary Prevention** | **Secondary Prevention** | **Tertiary Prevention** |
| *Health Teaching* | *Case Finding, Referral, and Follow-Up* | *Case Management and Collaboration* |
| ▪ Conduct classroom teaching on the dangers of tobacco use and strategies to avoid it. | ▪ Assess the health behaviors, including tobacco use, of individual students.<br>▪ Identify students at risk for tobacco use and those already using tobacco.<br>▪ Refer students who smoke to the school smoking prevention and cessation team.<br>▪ Follow up with the school nurse. | ▪ The school nurse, physical education teacher, and school psychologist team up to work with teens using tobacco and to monitor and implement a smoking cessation program. |

| Community Level of Practice | | |
|---|---|---|
| *Social Marketing and Outreach* | *Screening, Referral, and Follow-Up* | *Case Management and Social Marketing* |
| ▪ Staff a teen booth at the county fair and hand out brochures on the hazards of tobacco use and available tobacco prevention and cessation programs. | ▪ Hold health-behaviors screening, including tobacco use, for teens and young adults at the county fair. | ▪ Create a social networking site to empower teens and for teens to provide peer support for smoking cessation. |

| Systems Level of Practice | | |
|---|---|---|
| *Health Teaching/Provider Education* | *Screening, Referral, and Follow-Up* | *Case Management and Collaboration* |
| ▪ Develop and present a program to teachers and school staff about the hazards of tobacco use and available smoking prevention and cessation programs. | ▪ Develop a health-behaviors screening, referral, and follow-up program for middle school and high school students. | ▪ Develop a case management protocol for the school smoking prevention and cessation interdisciplinary team. |

PHNs take a comprehensive approach to dealing with public health problems in the community. They use multiple interventions to achieve primary, secondary, and tertiary prevention goals and, when possible, work with other members of the interdisciplinary team and members of the community. Table 2.2 outlines how primary, secondary, and tertiary interventions might be employed at all three levels of practice to reduce tobacco use in teens. (See Chapter 1 for a discussion of primary, secondary, and tertiary prevention.)

## Evidence-Based Practice

Public health organizations are expected to use evidence-based approaches in decision-making and in taking actions based on population-based evidence (Lovelace et al., 2015). This evidence-based public health approach means that PHNs use the best information available to create new interventions (Barr-Walker, 2017). This evidence-based decision process includes (Brownson, Fielding, & Maylahn, 2009, p. 177):

▪ Using the best available scientific evidence

▪ Systematically using data and information systems

▪ Applying program planning frameworks

▪ Engaging the community in assessment and decision-making

▪ Conducting sound evaluation

▪ Disseminating findings

Public health nurses' practice is expected to be evidence-based. This *evidence-based approach* means that PHNs use a problem-solving approach to find the best available scientific evidence and the best available experiential evidence and then integrate this evidence into their practice (Dang & Dearholt, 2018, p. 4).

The search for credible evidence includes knowledge gleaned from both research and nonresearch. The levels of evidence at the core of the Johns Hopkins Nursing Evidence-Based Practice Model (JHNEBP) include research and nonresearch evidence. There are five levels of evidence (see Table 2.3). You will find examples from all levels of evidence in the remaining chapters of this book. Although the levels of evidence are presented in a hierarchical manner in Table 2.3, this table does not mean that lower levels of evidence should be discounted or that randomized controlled trials (RCTs) in experimental research should be considered the only credible or most meaningful forms of evidence

**TABLE 2.3  Best Practices in Public Health Nursing by Level of Evidence**

| Evidence Level Definition | Examples |
|---|---|
| **Level I:**<br><br>Experimental study, randomized controlled trials (RCTs)<br><br>Explanatory mixed methods design | The Nurse Family Partnership involving intensive structured home visiting by PHNs reduces repeat childbirths, improves the stability of partner relationships, facilitates children's academic adjustment to elementary school, and reduces childhood mortality from preventable causes (Kitzman et al., 2010; Olds et al., 2004; Olds et al., 2007; Olds et al., 2010). |
| **Level I:**<br><br>Systematic reviews of RCTs, with or without meta-analysis | Professional organizations publish systematic reviews of medical and nursing research<br><br>▪ *The Cochrane Database of Systematic Reviews*, published online by the Cochrane Collaboration.<br><br>▪ *Worldviews on Evidence-Based Nursing*, a peer-reviewed journal published by Sigma Theta Tau International.<br><br>▪ The Joanna Briggs Institute provides an online listing of systematic reviews and meta-analysis specific to nursing practice. Systematic reviews of non-RCT research may be either Level II or Level III evidence. |
| **Level II:**<br><br>Quasi-experimental study<br><br>Explanatory mixed-method design<br><br>Systematic review of a combination of RCTs and quasi-experimental studies or quasi-experimental studies only | A prospective cohort study evaluated the impact of breastmilk expression in early postpartum period on breastfeeding duration (Jiang et al., 2015). |
| **Level III:**<br><br>Nonexperimental study<br><br>Systematic reviews of combination of RCTs, quasi-experimental, and nonexperimental studies | A descriptive study identified four significant predictors of breastfeeding attitudes: age, gender, number of breastfeeding observations in childhood, and breastfeeding beliefs (Vari et al., 2013).<br><br>A systematic review using CINAHL (Cumulative Index to Nursing and Allied Health Literature), PubMed, and Cochrane Library databases identified barriers to breastfeeding in the WIC population to make recommendations for guidelines for WIC clients (Hedberg, 2013). |
| **Level IV:**<br><br>Opinion of respected authorities and nationally recognized expert committees or consensus panels based on scientific evidence<br><br>▪ Clinical practice guidelines<br><br>▪ Consensus panels/position statements | ANA. (2013). *Public Health Nursing: Scope and Standards of Practice* (2nd ed.)<br><br>Quad Council of Public Health Nursing Organizations. (2011). *The Quad Council competencies for public health nurses*<br><br>Centers for Disease Control and Prevention. (2017). *Immunization Schedules* |
| **Level V:**<br><br>Based on experiential and nonresearch evidence<br><br>▪ Integrative reviews<br><br>▪ Literature reviews<br><br>▪ Quality improvement, program, or financial evaluation<br><br>▪ Case reports<br><br>▪ Opinion of nationally recognized expert(s) based on experiential evidence | The Best Start program supporting area-based interventions to increase breastfeeding was evaluated. Area-based interventions and community partnerships were found to have a positive influence on breastfeeding rates (Kelaher, Dunt, Feldman, Nolan, & Raban, 2009). |

*Source:* Definitions of Levels of Evidence from Dang & Dearholt, 2018, Appendix D, pp. 278–279

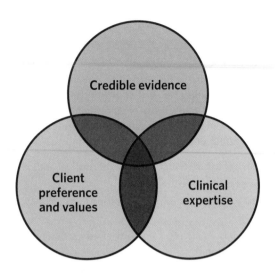

**FIGURE 2.3** Best Practice Approach to Evidence-Based Practice in Public Health Nursing
*Sources:* Based on work by Keller & Strohschein, 2009; Melnyk & Fineout-Overholt, 2014

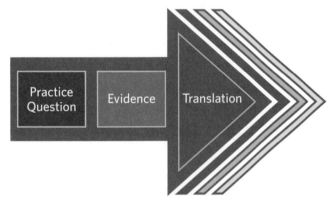

**FIGURE 2.4** JHNEBP PET Process
*Source:* Used with permission: Dang & Dearholt, 2018, p. 4

in public health. It is important to thoughtfully consider and analyze information from all levels of evidence. For example, the use of qualitative research, particularly when studying culture and ethnicity, has led to significant understanding of how diverse populations and people view themselves and the world around them.

Experiential evidence that may be found in IV and V evidence levels includes clinical expertise and client's preferences and values. PHNs know that evidence-based interventions found in the scientific literature need to fit the demographics and cultural diversity of their clients at the individual/family and community levels of practice in order to be consistent with ethical holistic nursing practice (see Figure 2.3).

These three interrelated elements occur within the context of the community—where public health nurses are expected to be lifelong learners who take the initiative to engage with their community to explore the life experiences, health status, and health determinants of diverse populations. The information PHNs gather about the individuals/families and communities they serve leads them to

question how they can positively impact the health of these individuals/families and communities.

Public health nurses use critical thinking in applying a deliberative process for identifying and implementing best practices in a timely manner. The *Johns Hopkins Nursing Evidence-Based Practice Model* (JHNEBP) includes three essential components: inquiry, practice, and learning (Dang & Dearholt, 2018):

- **Inquiry:** To question, examine, and collect information about an issue or problem (p. 36)
- **Practice:** Reflects on the translation of what nurses know to what they do (p. 36)
- **Learning:** A change in the way nurses think and behave

The movement from inquiry to learning is represented by the JHNEBP PET Process (see Figure 2.4). This process is a group effort within or across organizations. In public health, the team could be formed from members of a specific organization or be an interprofessional team at the community level with key stakeholders and community members involved. The practice team identifies the practice issue, defines and refines the practice question, searches for and evaluates the evidence, and determines which evidence can and should be translated into new or revised practices in the workplace.

*Abby wonders how PHNs know what to do when they work with their clients. She says, "The PHNs keep talking about evidence-based practice, but I am not sure exactly what that is."*

*Jaime responds, "Today, my PHN preceptor and I made a home visit to an elderly woman who lives alone. We did a fall risk assessment and a home safety check. I asked the PHN how she selected which risk assessment and home safety assessment tools to use. She told me that a committee of PHNs reviewed journal articles to find research reports on which assessment tools were effective for determining fall risks in older adults. They also looked at which home safety tools had been developed specifically for frail older adults living at home. Then they piloted the home safety assessment tools themselves and picked the tool that best fit what their PHNs needed to know about the home environment and what the elderly adults preferred. I think this is the way you do evidence-based practice, but I need to read more about it."*

*Abby comments, "One of the PHNs at my agency went to a fall prevention workshop given by an occupational therapist and a physical therapist at the local hospital. They taught the workshop participants how to screen older adults for fall risk and which types of interventions would help reduce fall risks, such as using assistive devices, installing good lighting, removing slippery rugs, and wearing nonskid slippers. Do you think this information could be considered evidence-based? The two therapists said they were reporting on what they had found worked best with their patients."*

*Jaime says, "I guess we could review the material on evidence-based practice in our textbooks and then talk more to our PHN preceptors."*

*"Good idea," says Abby. "Let's do it. We can also do a search using CINAHL to see if there are any studies that support what the PHN learned at the workshop. Do you think this information about effective interventions will be easy to find? What is an effective intervention anyway?"*

*Effective interventions* fit your client's situation and preferences and result in the desired outcomes. Using interventions that are known to be effective is important. PHNs have carried out research to demonstrate the effectiveness of many interventions provided to individuals, families, and communities. However, it is not always easy to find scientific literature on the effectiveness of PHN interventions (Swider, Levin, & Reising, 2017). Although research for evidence-based practice might be limited in public health nursing, PHNs should refer to it whenever it exists (Keller & Strohschein, 2009, from Brownson, Baker, Leet, & Gillespie, 2002). PHNs are accountable to their clients (individuals/families, communities, and systems) and to the public to determine the effectiveness of an intervention and to justify the use of resources. Your own experiences as a nursing student can also guide your choices of which interventions you can carry out effectively. You can use the evidence-based public health approach—making decisions on the best information available and creating interventions based on that evidence (Barr-Walker, 2017). Table 2.4 includes recent studies that demonstrate effective public health nursing interventions.

### TABLE 2.4 Effectiveness of Selected Public Health Nursing Interventions

| **Individual/Family Level** | |
| --- | --- |
| **Intervention** | **Results** |
| Case management | Decreased difficulty and dependence for meal preparation, telephone use, shopping, and ordinary housework (Instrumental Activities of Daily Living) were found for elders receiving home visiting in comparison with usual care (Li, Liebel, & Friedman, 2013). [Level I] |
| Case finding<br>Case management<br>Health teaching<br>Consultation counseling | Significantly higher scores on overall healthy eating and healthy eating subdimensions (i.e., food selection, preparation, and consumption) were found in elders 60 years and over in comparison to control group (Meethien, Pothiban, Ostwald, Sucamvang, & Panuthai, 2011). [Level I] |
| Counseling | Socially withdrawn students showed an increase in self-efficacy after participation in group-based counseling interventions led by school nurses (Kvarme et al., 2010). [Level II] |
| Counseling<br>Health teaching<br>Referral and follow-up | Low-income, first-time mothers who participated in the Nurse–Family Partnership (NFP) home visiting program had more beneficial breastfeeding and immunization outcomes compared to similar clients not in the program (Thorland, Currie, Wiegand, Walsh, & Mader, 2017). [Level III] |
| **Community Level** | |
| Surveillance | In response to an online survey of PHNs in 29 states, PHNs reported they conducted ongoing surveillance for tuberculosis, vaccine-preventable diseases, sexually transmitted diseases, pediculosis, foodborne diseases, and elevated blood lead levels in their communities (Schaffer, Keller, & Reckinger, 2015). [Level III] |
| Coalition building | School nurses participated in an interfaith coalition to respond to youth suicide in the community (Anderson et al., 2017). [Level III] |
| **Systems Level** | |
| Consultation<br>Screening | A maternal and child health nurse screening program for mothers experiencing domestic violence (nurse-designed model) increased safety planning among postpartum women (Taft et al., 2015). [Level I] |
| Collaboration<br>Outreach | School nurses collaborated with a hospital and a school of nursing to develop and implement an injury-prevention curriculum for helmet safety in elementary schools. Students from the intervention group reported increased helmet use after intervention in comparison with the control group (Adams, Drake, Dang, & Le-Hinds, 2014). [Level II] |

Evidence-based practice (EBP)—and nursing interventions—should be both effective and efficient. PHNs use the evidence-based public health approach and consider all evidence-based information, including the experiences of experts. Because resources are limited in both healthcare and public health, PHNs also need to consider the efficiency of interventions. Efficient interventions require the least amount of resources and achieve the desired outcomes in the shortest period of time.

Evidence-based practice supports *efficacy* (the ability to reach a desired result); *efficiency* (the achievement of a desired result with minimum expense, time, and effort); and *effectiveness* (the ability to produce a desired result). Additionally, EBP weighs risks, benefits, and costs against a backdrop of patient preferences (Dang & Dearholt, 2018, p. 4).

> *Jaime voices his concern that if he knew from the literature that an intervention was known to achieve a desired outcome, he might use it even if he did not know if it would be effective. "How do I know if it is going to work with a specific client?"*
>
> *Abby responds, "Well you can ask your preceptor what type of interventions have worked in the past with your client. You could also ask the client if he wants to try it."*

Before using an intervention, look at the literature or consult with expert PHNs to identify specific interventions that can best meet your clients' unique needs and characteristics. You also want to consider if the intervention is a good use of your time and resources and the client's time and energy. Questions you can ask to determine effectiveness and efficiency are listed in Table 2.5.

**Healthy People 2020**
healthypeople.gov

Healthy People 2020 identified 11 Leading Health Indicators (LHIs) as priority health concerns, including Nutrition, Physical Activity, and Obesity. Go to the Healthy People 2020 website, click "Leading Health Indicators," and then click "Nutrition, Physical Activity, and Obesity." Read about the most recent data and population disparities on nutrition, physical activity, and obesity. Look for the links to the science-based *Dietary Guidelines for Americans* and the *Physical Activity Guidelines*. What evidence do you find that supports a healthy eating and physical activity program for you and your family?

Just because "best practice" evidence is available does not mean that it will be adopted and used. To create a supportive evidence-based practice environment, three strategies are necessary: establishing the EBP culture, building the capacity for EBP, and ensuring sustainability (Dang & Dearholt, 2018, p. 19). A strategic plan and committed leadership are necessary to develop the organizational resources and support for a sustainable evidence-based practice culture. Staff

### TABLE 2.5 Analyzing Effectiveness and Efficiency of Interventions

| Determining Intervention Effectiveness | Determining Intervention Efficiency |
| --- | --- |
| ▪ Is the intervention culturally and developmentally congruent with the client's status and situation?<br>▪ Is the intervention acceptable to the client?<br>▪ Does the outcome of the intervention demonstrate improvement of the client's health status? | ▪ What are the costs of the intervention (money, time, people involved, and other resources) for the PHN, the other members of the health team, the agencies involved, and the client?<br>▪ Are the costs of implementing the intervention justified by the health benefits for the client and the community? |

needs include continuing education on evidence-based practice as well as initiatives to be implemented. Resources such as Internet access to useful databases and journals, evidence-based organizational mentors, and reimbursable time facilitate integration of evidence into practice.

This chapter presents an overview of evidence-based practice relevant to public health nursing practice. The term *best practices* is often used synonymously with *evidence-based practice*. A few points are helpful to keep in mind as you think about and use evidence of "best practices" in your community health clinical:

▪ Experimental research using RCTs is considered unethical when placing an individual in a control group that denies that individual treatment or interventions are already demonstrated to be effective.

▪ Public health/community health nursing agencies may be carrying out quasi- and nonexperimental research to determine the effectiveness of their programs and interventions. These activities may be a component of their ongoing quality improvement programs. Sometimes students participate in these research studies. If you are asked to participate, ask to see any informed consent or ethical guidelines that your agency is using.

▪ The policies and procedures of your public health/community agency and the professional practice standards guiding PHN practice may be considered clinical guidelines. Progress reports and annual agency reports may be considered organizational experiences.

▪ The knowledge and experiences of your preceptor and other PHN agency staff will be reflected in the practice you observe and the mentoring you receive. These represent expert opinions and clinical expertise.

▪ Clinical experiences may include both participant and nonparticipant observation. When you reflect on your observations of your preceptor or other public health/community health nurses interacting with clients by using PHN interventions, you are demonstrating *nonparticipant* observation. When you use these interventions yourself and reflect on your practice, you are demonstrating *participant* observation. Both types of experiences add to your clinical expertise.

■ Community assessments that are carried out in collaboration with community members and client satisfaction surveys provide evidence of consumer preferences. See Chapter 3, Competency #1, for information on community assessments.

## Database and Internet Searches

The sources of evidence must be as credible as the evidence itself. That is why PHNs search scientific databases. The online databases that provide the most relevant journal articles for nursing are CINAHL and PubMed. CINAHL is a proprietary database hosted by EBSCO, which means it is privately owned and available to members of subscribing institutions who pay a fee for remote access. PubMed is an open-source database that is free to the public. Other credible sources include websites maintained by professional organizations and service providers and governmental websites, such as those run by the National Institutes of Health (NIH), the U.S. Surgeon General, and the Centers for Disease Control and Prevention (CDC). The Cochrane Library is an international database of systematic reviews owned by the Cochrane Collaboration and is an open-source database that is free to use. The CDC Stacks, an excellent source for public health information, is a free digital repository of publications produced by the CDC.

The NIH provides guidelines for evaluating web-based health resources that can help you determine whether the website resource you have found is credible. One example of a credible website is a government program that reviews maternal-child health home visiting program effectiveness, called *Home Visiting Evidence of Effectiveness (HOMVEE)*. This website includes discussion of models and programs, whether they meet Department of Health and Human Services (DHHS) criteria, their target populations, and whether research shows positive effectiveness (U.S. Department of Health and Human Services, n.d.).

The goal of evidence-based practice is not to generate new knowledge, but to improve practice. Baccalaureate nursing graduates are expected to be able to find and use best practice evidence to improve their nursing practice. Hopp & Rittenmeyer (2012, p. 84) identify a five-step process known as the "5 A's." This process works well for students and PHNs alike and can be used when students partner with public health nurses during their clinical learning activities in public health. Table 2.6 outlines a process for public health nursing students to carry out the "5 A's."

## TABLE 2.6  Using the 5 A's for Evidence-Based Practice in Student Clinical Learning Activities

| The 5 A's | Students Using the 5 A's with Community Partners |
|---|---|
| **Ask:** To find the right answer, you need to ask the right question. | ■ Work with PHNs or other community partners to identify a public health practice issue about a specific health concern with a specific population and a related knowledge gap about current best practices. <br> ■ Work with PHNs or other community partners to create a specific practice question. <br> ■ Identify reasonable client outcomes that you wish to achieve with modified or new best practice evidence. |
| **Acquire:** Search for the answer by exploring all levels of evidence. | ■ Work with reference librarian, instructor, and community partners to identify credible data sources for all five levels of evidence. <br> ■ Identify appropriate databases to search and keywords for search. <br> ■ Work with instructor and community partners to identify evidence from nonscientific literature (e.g., credible websites, professional organizations, agency reports, etc.). <br> ■ Conduct key informant interviews. <br> ■ Conduct search, preferably for the past 5 years (or 10 years if there is little published information for the past 5 years). |
| **Appraise:** Critically evaluate the evidence and select the "best practice evidence." | ■ Work with fellow students, instructors, and interprofessional teams to critically review the evidence and determine what evidence answers your practice question and is applicable to the client population. <br> ■ Work with community partners to consult practice experts to determine which interventions fit what the experts know about the population and health concern. <br> ■ Work with key community stakeholders to determine population preferences and values. |

*(continues)*

**TABLE 2.6 Using the 5 A's for Evidence-Based Practice in Student Clinical Learning Activities** *(continued)*

| The 5 A's | Students Using the 5 A's with Community Partners |
|---|---|
| **Apply:** Make the evidence actionable by using the evidence to change your practice. | ■ Report credible evidence from all five levels to community partners.<br>■ Make recommendations for change in practice or new interventions.<br>■ Collaborate with community partners on modifications of current interventions or development of new interventions.<br>■ Partner with your PHN preceptor to implement the intervention if possible. |
| **Assess:** Evaluate the outcomes of the change in practice in your clinical setting. | ■ Identify how and when the client outcomes will be evaluated and determine the effectiveness and efficiency of the modified or new intervention. |

## Evidence of Best Practices

PHNs need to be critical consumers of public health and nursing research. They must use a deliberative problem-solving approach when making decisions about which evidence in the literature is strong enough to support a change in practice (Poe & White, 2010). However, public health providers often do not have adequate knowledge about evidence-based practice or the tools and resources to research current evidence-based best practices (Barr-Walker, 2017). In addition, published evidence in scientific journals is limited, and many of the sources used are from health-related statistics, government reports, and organizational or professional guidelines.

Much of the evidence for effective public health nursing comes from Evidence-Based Practice Levels III, IV, and V. It is often not ethical, possible, or practical to randomly place people in an experimental or a control group, especially if placement in either group could have a negative effect on an individual's health or well-being. An increasing body of qualitative research in public health nursing exists. Understanding the context of the family, culture, and community; the meaning of events; and the impact of these factors on the clients' health behaviors and health status is often best achieved through the use of qualitative research methods. Public health nurses also learn a great deal from their practice experiences and those of their colleagues. This evidence-based information or practice-based knowledge helps public health nurses translate evidence into practice in specific clinical care settings (Barr-Walker, 2017). Case study examples can be found in the literature, shared at professional conferences, or reported on the Internet. These anecdotal reports are also part of the practice evidence of public health nursing.

## Framing Your Evidence-Based Practice With the "5 A's"

One of the most difficult skills is knowing how to initiate the evidence-based practice process in a clinical setting. It is time to return to the "5 A's" discussed earlier in the chapter (Hopp & Rittenmeyer, 2012): ask, acquire, appraise, apply, and assess.

### Ask

When you explore the scientific literature for best practice evidence, it is helpful to first identify your clinical question so that you are focused in your search. One helpful way to frame your clinical practice question is to use the PICOT approach by identifying the patient population (P), the intervention of interest (I), the comparison intervention (C), the outcome (O), and the timeframe (T) (Stillwell, Fineout-Overholt, Melnyk, & Williamson, 2010). For example, if you wanted to research the effectiveness of teaching parents about the "Back to Sleep" program to reduce the risk of Sudden Infant Death Syndrome (SIDS), you might frame your PICOT question as outlined in Table 2.7.

The "T" in PICOT may not be necessary to include when reviewing the literature, but it may be helpful to include the time element when you plan how and when you are going to evaluate the outcome of the intervention you have selected to implement in your clinical setting. Once you find a set of articles that report on the effectiveness of the intervention you are interested in, it is time to review them to determine their usefulness.

### Acquire

After writing your PICOT question, you can identify the keywords in the sentence. A helpful way to identify keywords is to create a PCO Table (Population, Content, Outcomes). Table 2.8 demonstrates that using a PCO Table helps you to identify six keywords or phrases. If you have access to a reference librarian, you can take your keywords to the librarian who can then help you create your online literature strategy and identify the databases to search (Butler, Hall, & Copnell, 2016). Complete your search using your keywords.

### Appraise

The next step is to compare and contrast the studies and reports you have appraised. Select the best studies or reports with the most credible evidence that fits your clinical

**TABLE 2.7  The PICOT Approach to Clinical Problem Solving**

| PICOT Question Elements | Examples |
|---|---|
| P = Patient population | P = Infants at risk for SIDS |
| I = Intervention of interest | I = Teach parents to place infants on backs to sleep using "Back to Sleep" program |
| C = Comparison intervention of interest | |
| O = Outcome(s) of interest | C = No purposeful teaching about safe sleeping position of infants |
| T = Time it takes the intervention to achieve outcomes | O = Percentage of babies sleeping on back |
| | T = Evaluate at 6 weeks and 3 months |

PICOT Question: Will infants (P) whose parents are taught to place them on their backs to sleep using a "Back to Sleep" program (I) as opposed to no purposeful teaching about safe sleeping positions for infants (C) be sleeping on their backs (O) at 6 weeks and 3 months after receiving the intervention (T)?

**TABLE 2.8  Finding Keywords Using PCO**

| PCO Elements | Examples |
|---|---|
| P = Patient Population | P = Infants at risk for SIDS, parents, caretakers |
| C = Context | C = Teaching safe sleeping positions |
| O = Outcome | O = Sleeping on back |

determine efficacy of an intervention as well as a realistic expectation as to when effectiveness can be evaluated. For example, if you implemented a community-wide campaign to increase the flu vaccine in September to decrease the incidence of influenza in the fall, you would probably compare the incidence of influenza this fall to last fall in December. If you were evaluating the effectiveness of the "Back to Sleep" program, you might choose a 6-month timeframe to evaluate the outcome of the program.

It would be important to evaluate both the effectiveness and the efficiency of the intervention from a cost-benefit perspective, which would be based on the quality of life as well as the financial and human resource costs involved. This is not always easy to do. For example, if the "Back to Sleep" program reduced the incidence of crib death by one infant in a 3-month period, would any of your community partners consider the program effective and efficient?

*Jaime comments, "I think I am going to do my intervention paper on ways to reduce smoking in high school students. I have to start looking for evidence-based practice articles. I wonder how I should go about that."*

*Abby says, "I have been working with the college reference librarian to research my topic. She suggested that I use three databases: CINAHL, PubMed, and the Cochrane Database of Systematic Reviews. I have found a few good articles in each database."*

*Jaime responds, "Great! I will try those databases, too! I know that both PubMed and the Cochrane Database are in the public domain and free to users. CINAHL is privately owned, and organizations have to pay for employees to use it. I don't think my hospital has a contract to access CINAHL."*

*Abby concludes, "Don't forget to write your PICOT question first!"*

situation and addresses your specific question. Think about how you would present your findings and recommendations to the PHNs and team you are working with.

### Apply

Once you have completed the first three steps and have identified a best practice intervention, begin working with your clinical team to translate or apply the evidence into clinical practice. Before you implement a change in your practice or your clinical team's practice, you need to think about how you will evaluate the effectiveness of the change. Identify the outcome you would like to achieve.

### Assess

The timeframe for assessment of client outcomes after implementing the new intervention will depend on the urgency to

### Translating Evidence Into Practice

One of the most difficult skills is knowing how to initiate the evidence-based practice process in a clinical setting and to translate best practice evidence into practice, which means that you use the best practice evidence to evaluate and update how you practice nursing. PHNs need to make sure that their recommendations for change in practice are based on the best evidence and are appropriate and feasible for their client populations, their agencies, and their communities. Support and funding for PHN practice depends on documentation and dissemination of evidence that PHN practice makes a positive difference in the health of its communities. Evidence Example 2.2 shows step-by-step how to use an evidence-based practice approach to find best practice evidence.

## EVIDENCE EXAMPLE 2.2

**Searching for Best Practice Evidence on Optimal Breastfeeding Initiation and Translating the Evidence Into Practice**

Breastfeeding is initiated in the setting where delivery occurs. Often that is the hospital. Many new mothers are sent home from the hospital within 24 hours of delivery. So, it is important for PHNs to know the best practice evidence to share with their antepartum clients about what breastfeeding approaches work best and then to support those practices during the postpartum period. Public health nurses need to work with their nursing partners in the hospital setting to prepare their clients for breastfeeding, advocate for the preferences of the new mothers with their acute care colleagues, and provide for a seamless transition in the breastfeeding routine when the mother returns home through coordination and case management interventions. In this example, nurses in a birthing center searched for best practice evidence for initiation of breastfeeding immediately after birth. The following example shows how the "5 A's" and the PICOT process were used to identify best practice evidence and translate it into practice. The question was whether it was best practice to use a breast pump to support breastfeeding in the first 72 hours postpartum.

### Ask

A PICO(T) question was developed to frame the question to guide the literature search:

P = Efficacy of use of breast pump in early postpartum period to promote exclusive breastfeeding with mother's milk

I = Electric breast pump after breastfeeding during first 24–48 hours

C = Breastfeeding on-demand during first 24–48 hours

O = Baby fed exclusively with mother's own breastmilk

T = 6 weeks postpartum

The question: Does use of an electric breast pump after breastfeeding versus breastfeeding on-demand during the first 24–48 hours postpartum increase the likelihood a baby will be exclusively fed with a mother's own breastmilk at 6 weeks postpartum?

### Acquire

Ovid Medline, CINAHL, PubMed, and Google Scholar were searched using a variety of search terms. Although 23 articles were found, only 3 of these articles addressed the PICOT question and the actual practice question.

### Appraise

The literature reviewed suggested that while it remains unclear if pumping has any immediate impact on breastfeeding initiation and milk supply, using a breast pump in the first days and weeks postpartum is associated with a shorter breastfeeding duration (Chapman, Young, Ferris, & Perez-Escamilla, 2001; Felice, Cassano, & Rasmussen, 2016; Jiang et al., 2015).

Other important evidence was identified:

Anticipating return to work and suboptimal long-term lactation support systems increased women's dependence on expressing breastmilk with a pump (Chapman et al., 2001; Felice et al., 2016; Jiang et al., 2015).

Hand expression is more effective at expressing colostrum (first days' breastmilk supply) than an electric pump (Flaherman et al., 2013).

Developing the nurse-family relationship fosters an empowering environment where the family can experience growth and develop the skills needed to achieve successful infant feeding patterns, including direct breastfeeding and expressing breastmilk (Raile Alligood, 2010).

After reviewing the scientific evidence, the nursing team at the birthing center considered the other two evidence components: the practice and procedures of the birthing center and the preferences of the new mothers. The context of the relationship between the mother and the nursing staff was considered. The nurses' caring interaction was considered as necessary as the evidence-based knowledge to facilitate successful breastfeeding initiation.

### Apply

Supporting Breastfeeding Guidelines were developed and implemented based on the evidence. The nurse in the birthing center who initiated the quality improvement process changed jobs and became a clinical coordinator in a public health nursing agency. She was able to share the best practice evidence about the initiation of breastfeeding with the public health nursing staff.

### Assess

At the birthing center, the new guideline was instituted and evaluated at both the systems and the individual/family practice levels. Nursing staff completed a nursing practice survey before and after implementation of the new guidelines. The purpose was to measure the accuracy with which nurses were able to determine the appropriate interventions needed to support lactation (when and when not to use an electric pump) and their confidence levels of decision-making regarding when to utilize the breast pump to support lactation. The individual-level change was measured through a patient survey completed at discharge. The survey measured the breastfeeding mothers' confidence levels of continuing their breastfeeding plan of care when returning home and their perception of nursing support received for their individual infant feeding goals.

## ACTIVITY

Imagine that you are the nurse who changed jobs from the birthing center to the public health agency.

- How would you use this best practice breastfeeding initiation evidence?
- What would you want to know about the public health nurses and their antepartum and postpartum clients?
- How would you develop your PICOT question?
- How might you partner with the staff to carry out the "5 A's" process?

The evidence-based practice approach does not always entail a simple, concise process. However, through the use of various levels of evidence, clinical expertise, local context, and client preference, best practice interventions can be developed and implemented to promote and protect the health of individuals, systems, and populations.

*Jamie is continuing to work on his evidence-based practice search on how to reduce smoking in high school students.*

*Abby changed her topic. With her PHN preceptor, she has been co-visiting a first-time mom who has postpartum depression. The PHN is visiting the mom twice weekly, and the PHN has asked Abby to research best practices in working with moms with postpartum depression. Abby is going to develop her PICOT question, create her PCO Table, and then consult with her instructor and the reference librarian on how to go about searching for the best practice evidence. She is excited to be able to partner with her PHN preceptor to find the most up-to-date best practice evidence to present to the Family Health Team.*

If you follow through on the steps outlined in this chapter for researching best practices and taking steps to translate this evidence into your nursing practice, you will be practicing nursing from an evidence-based practice framework. As a professional, you are accountable for your own nursing practice, so you need to be aware of and use best practices. You will find that this book presents many levels of evidence to justify using specific interventions.

## KEY POINTS

- The public health nursing process guides the PHN's actions.
- PHNs work at all three levels of practice (individual/family, community, and systems).
- PHNs carry out 17 interventions unique to public health nursing; 16 of these interventions are practiced independently as part of professional nursing practice.
- Public health nursing practice is evidence-based.

- All five levels of evidence are used to identify best practices.
- Evidence-based practice is a deliberative process starting with a practice question, followed by an appraisal of the evidence, and then a change in practice based on credible evidence.
- Using the "5 A's" and PICOT provides a structure for practicing from an evidence-based foundation.

## REFLECTIVE PRACTICE

1. What do you think are the major differences between the nursing process and the public health nursing process?
   - What will you do differently when following the public health nursing process?
   - How will your knowledge about the determinants of health guide you in your assessments and interventions at the three levels of practice: individual/family, community, and systems?
2. Which other disciplines will you work with most often in your public health clinical?
   - What additional information do you need to know about the other health disciplines?
   - How will you find out the information that you need?
3. Which public health nursing interventions have you used in previous clinical experiences?
   - How will you carry out these interventions in your public health clinical?
   - How will this experience be the same or different from what you have done before?

4. Have you used an evidence-based practice approach in other nursing clinical experiences?
   - What have you learned in reading this chapter that you did not know before?
   - How will your past experiences and your new knowledge help you practice evidence-based public health nursing?
5. Which types of best practice evidence related to a PHN intervention would you like to explore?
   - What is your PICOT question?
   - How do you frame this as a PICOT statement?
6. Refer to the Cornerstones of Public Health Nursing in Chapter 1. Which of the Cornerstones support the use of evidence-based practice in public health nursing?

## APPLICATION OF EVIDENCE

How would you work with your PHN preceptor to identify an intervention that the staff would like to have researched to identify any new best practice recommendations?

When you search for best practice evidence, how would you implement the following steps?

- Determine which databases to use in your search.
- Carry out your literature search. Obtain help from the reference librarian if you are having difficulty with your keyword search.
- Select three to five journal articles to review. You may use articles that represent different levels of evidence.

How would you carry out the following steps to analyze the evidence?

- Compare and contrast the articles you have appraised. Are their findings and recommendations similar or different?
- Identify the articles that have the most credible evidence that best fits your clinical situation.
- What format would you use to report your evidence-based finding to the PHN staff?

## References

Adams, C., Drake, D., Dang, M., & Le-Hinds, N. (2014). Optimization of injury prevention outreach for helmet safety. *Journal of Trauma Nursing, 21,* 133–138. doi:10.1097/JTN.0000000000000047

American Nurses Association. (2013). *Public health nursing: Scope and standards of practice.* Silver Spring, MD: Author.

Anderson, L. J. W., Schaffer, M. A., Hiltz, C., O'Leary, S. A., Luehr, R. E., & Yoney, E. L. (2018). Public health interventions: School nurse practice stories. *The Journal of School Nursing, 34*(3), 192–202. doi:10.1177/1059840517721951

Barr-Walker, J. (2017). Evidence-based information needs of public health workers: A systematized review. *Journal of the Medical Library Association, 105*(1), 69–79. doi:dx.doi.org/10.5195/jmla.2017.109

Bigbee, J. L., & Issel, L. M. (2012). Conceptual models for population-focused public health nursing interventions and outcomes: The state of the art. *Public Health Nursing, 29*(4), 370–379. doi:10.1111/j.1525-1446.2011.01006.x

Brownson, R. C., Baker, E. A., Leet, T. L., & Gillespie, K. N. (Eds.). (2002). *Evidence-based public health.* New York, NY: Oxford University Press.

Brownson, R. C., Fielding, J. E., & Maylahn, C. M. (2009). Evidence-based public health: A fundamental concept for public health practice. *Annual Review of Public Health, 30*(1), 75–201.

Butler, A., Hall, H., & Copnell, B. (2016). A guide to writing a qualitative systematic review protocol to enhance evidence-based practice in nursing and health care. *Worldviews on Evidence-Based Nursing, 13*(3), 241–249. doi:10.1111/wvn.12134

Centers for Disease Control and Prevention. (2017). Immunization schedules. Retrieved from https://www.cdc.gov/vaccines/schedules/index.html

Chapman, D. J., Young, S., Ferris, A. M., & Perez-Escamilla, R. (2001). Impact of breast pumping on lactogenesis stage II after cesarean delivery: A randomized clinical trial. *Pediatrics, 107*(6), 1–7.

Dang, D., & Dearholt, S. L. (2018). *Johns Hopkins nursing evidence-based practice: Model and guidelines* (3rd ed.). Indianapolis, IN: Sigma Theta Tau International.

Felice, J. P., Cassano, P. A., & Rasmussen, K. M. (2016). Pumping human milk in the early postpartum period: Its impact on long-term practices for feeding at the breast and exclusively feeding human milk in a longitudinal survey cohort. *American Journal of Clinical Nutrition, 103*, 1267–1277.

Flaherman, V. J., Gay, B., Scott, C., Aby, J., Stewart, A. L., & Lee, K. A. (2013). Development of the breast milk expression experience measure. *Maternal & Child Nutrition, 9*(3), 425–430. Retrieved from https://doi.org/10.1111/j.1740-8709.2011.00390.x

Hedberg, I. G. (2013). Barriers to breastfeeding in the WIC population. *American Journal of Maternal Child Health Nursing, 38*(4), 244–249. doi:10.1097/NMC.0b013e3182836ca2

Hopp, L., & Rittenmeyer, L. (2012). *Introduction to evidence-based practice—A practical guide for nursing.* Philadelphia, PA: F. A. Davis.

Jiang, B., Hua, J., Wang, Y., Fu, Y., Zhuang, Z., & Zhu, L. (2015). Evaluation of the impact of breast milk expression in early postpartum period on breastfeeding duration: A prospective cohort study. *BMC Pregnancy & Childbirth, 15*, 1–13. doi:10.1186/s12884-015-0698-6

Kelaher, M., Dunt, D., Feldman, P., Nolan, A., & Raban, B. (2009). The effect of an area-based intervention on breastfeeding rates in Victoria, Australia. *Health Policy, 90*, 89–93.

Keller, L. O., & Strohschein, S. (2009). E2 evidence exchange: Your public health nursing e-source. *Public Health Nursing Faculty Conference*, Otsego, MN.

Keller, L. O., Strohschein, S., Lia-Hoagberg, B., & Schaffer, M. (1998). Population-based public health nursing interventions: A model for practice. *Public Health Nursing, 15*(3), 207–215.

Keller, L. O., Strohschein, S., Lia-Hoagberg, B., & Schaffer, M. (2004). Population-based public health interventions: Practice-based and evidence-supported. Part I. *Public Health Nursing, 21*(5), 453–468.

Kitzman, H. J., Olds, D. L., Cole, R. E., Hanks, C. A., Anson, E. A., Arcoleo, K. J., . . . Holmberg, J. R. (2010). Enduring effects of prenatal and infancy home visiting by nurses on children: Follow-up of a randomized trial among children at age 12 years. *Archives of Pediatrics & Adolescent Medicine, 164*(5), 412–418. doi:10.1001/archpediatrics.2010.76

Kvarme, L. G., Helseth, S., Sørum, R., Luth-Hansen, V., Haugland, S., & Natvig, G. K. (2010). The effect of a solution-focused approach to improve self-efficacy in socially withdrawn school children: A non-randomized controlled trial. *International Journal of Nursing Studies, 47*, 1389–1396. doi:10.1016/j.ijnurstu.2010.05.001

Li, Y., Liebel, D. V., & Friedman, B. (2013). An investigation into which individual instrumental activities of daily living are affected by home visiting nurse intervention. *Age and Ageing, 42*, 27–33. doi:10.1093/ageing/afs151

Lovelace, R. A., Aronson, R. E., Rulison, K. L., Labban, J. D., Shah, G. H., & Smith, M. (2015). Laying the groundwork for evidence-based public health: Why some local health departments use more evidence-based decision-making than others. *American Journal of Public Health, 105*(S2), S189–S197. doi:10.2105.AJPH.2014.302306

McDonald, A., Frazer, K., Duignan, C., Healy, M., Irving, A., Marteinsson, P., … McNicholas, E. (2015). Validating the "intervention wheel" in the context of Irish public health nursing. *British Journal of Community Nursing, 20*(3), 140–145.

Meethien, N., Pothiban, L., Ostwald, S. K., Sucamvang, K., & Panuthai, S. (2011). Effectiveness of nutritional education in promoting healthy eating among elders in northeastern Thailand. *Pacific Rim International Journal of Nursing Research, 15*(3) 188–202.

Melnyk, B. M., & Fineout-Overholt, E. (Eds.). (2014). *Evidence-based practice in nursing and healthcare: A guide to best practice* (3rd ed.). Philadelphia, PA: Lippincott Williams and Wilkins.

Minnesota Department of Health, Center for Public Health Nursing. (2001). *Public health interventions: Applications for public health nursing practice.* St. Paul, MN: Author. Retrieved from http://www.health.state.mn.us/divs/opi/cd/phn/docs/0301wheel_manual.pdf

Minnesota Department of Health, Center for Public Health Nursing. (2003). The nursing process applied to population-based public health nursing practice. Retrieved from http://www.health.state.mn.us/divs/opi/cd/phn/docs/0303phn_processapplication.pdf

Olds, D. L., Kitzman, H. J., Cole, R. E., Hanks, C. A., Arcoleo, K. J., Anson, E. A., … Stevenson, A. J. (2010). Enduring effects of prenatal and infancy home visiting by nurses on maternal life course and government spending: Follow-up of a randomized trial among children at age 12 years. *Archives of Pediatrics & Adolescent Medicine, 164*(5), 419–424. doi:10.1001/archpediatrics.2010.49

Olds, D. L., Kitzman, H., Cole, R., Robinson, J., Sidora, K., Luckey, D. W., … Holmberg, J. (2004). Effects of nurse home-visiting on maternal life course and child development: Age 6 follow-up results of a randomized trial. *Pediatrics, 114*(6), 1550–1559.

Olds, D., Kitzman, H., Hanks, C., Cole, R., Anson, E., Sidora-Arcoleo, K., … Bondy, J. (2007). Effects of nurse home visiting on maternal and child functioning: Age 9 follow-up of a randomized trial. *Pediatrics, 120*(4), e832–e845.

Poe, S. S., & White, K. K. (2010). *Johns Hopkins nursing evidence-based practice: Implementation and translation.* Indianapolis, IN: Sigma Theta Tau International.

Population Health Interest Group. (2013). *Public health nursing in Ireland: Demonstrating interventions from practice.* Dublin, IE: Institute of Community Health Nursing.

Quad Council of Public Health Nursing Organizations. (2011). *The Quad Council competencies for public health nurses.* Retrieved from http://www.achne.org/files/Quad%20Council/QuadCouncilCompetenciesforPublicHealthNurses.pdf

Raile Alligood, M. (2010). Family healthcare with King's theory of goal attainment. *Nursing Science Quarterly, 23*(2), 99–104.

Schaffer, M. A., Anderson, L. J. W., & Rising, S. (2016). Public health interventions for school nursing practice. *Journal of School Nursing, 32*(3), 195–208. doi:10.1177/1059840515605361

Schaffer, M. A., Keller, L. O., & Reckinger, D. (2015). Public health activities: Visible or invisible? *Public Health Nursing, 32*(6), 711–720. doi:10.1111/phn.12191

Stillwell, S. B., Fineout-Overholt, E., Melnyk, B. M., & Williamson, K. M. (2010). Evidence-based practice: Step by step. *American Journal of Nursing, 110*(5), 41–47.

Swider, S. M., Levin, P. F., & Reising, V. (2017). Evidence of public health nursing effectiveness: A realistic review. *Public Health Nursing, 34*(4), 324–334. doi:10.1111/phn.12320

Taft, A. J., Hooker, L., Humphreys, C., Hegarty, K., Walter, R., Adams, C., … Small, R. (2015). Maternal and child health nurse screening and care for mothers experiencing domestic violence (MOVE): A cluster randomised trial. *BMC Medicine, 13,* 1–10. doi:10.1186/s12916-015-0375-7

Thorland, W., Currie, D., Wiegand, E. R., Walsh, J., & Mader, N. (2017). Status of breastfeeding and child immunization outcomes in clients of the Nurse–Family Partnership. *Maternal and Child Health Journal, 21*(3), 439–445. doi:10.1007/s10995-016-2231-6

U.S. Department of Health and Human Services. (n.d.). Home visiting evidence of effectiveness. Retrieved from https://homvee.acf.hhs.gov/default.aspx

Vari, P., Vogeltanz-Holm, N., Olsen, G., Anderson, C., Holm, J., Peterson, H., & Henly, S. (2013). Community breastfeeding attitudes and beliefs. *Healthcare for Women International, 34*(7), 592–606. doi:10.1080/07399332.2012.655391

# PART II

# Entry-Level Population-Based Public Health Nursing Competencies

# COMPETENCY #1

## Applies the Public Health Nursing Process to Communities, Systems, Individuals, and Families

■ **Patricia M. Schoon**
*with Karen S. Martin, Kelly Krumwiede, and Noreen Kleinfehn-Wald*

*Kristi is listening to Beth, her public health nurse (PHN) preceptor, tell her about the client they are about to visit for the first time. The local public health agency received a maternal child health visit referral from a local OB/GYN for a 16-year-old, 20-weeks-gestation primipara. The client, Sara, has been diagnosed with anemia and is underweight with poor weight gain. Sara is single and living with her mother, mother's boyfriend, and two younger siblings. Sara and her family are uncomfortable with the idea of a public health nurse who works for the government visiting them in their home.*

*Beth says, "Well, I think the first thing we do is go and visit them. We need to get them to trust us if we are to help them."*

*Kristi responds, "I have never visited a pregnant teenager or her family in their home. I don't think I will feel comfortable. Will the family be okay with me there?"*

*Beth responds, "I asked Sara's mother if you could covisit with me and she was okay with that. We will ask Sara and her mother what their health concerns and goals are and talk with them about how to arrange our visits and what we can do to help Sara. We will open a case file on Sara and begin to do a family assessment. You can observe and listen on this visit and take a more active part in future visits."*

*Kristi says, "That sounds good to me!"*

*As they walk to Beth's car she mentions, "We can start to do a windshield survey on our way to Sara's home as part of the community assessment that you and your student work group are going to do of the local community."*

*Kristi responds, "Great. I just happen to have my camera with me."*

---

### KRISTI'S NOTEBOOK

**COMPETENCY #1** Applies the Public Health Nursing Process to Communities, Systems, Individuals, and Families

A. Identifies the population(s) for which the PHN is accountable

B. Assesses the health status of communities, systems, individuals, and families

  1) Uses a health and social determinants framework to determine risk factors and protective factors that lead to health and illness in communities, systems, individuals, and families

  2) Identifies relevant and appropriate data and information sources for the populations to which the PHN is accountable

    a. Familiar with data used in the health department

    b. Familiar with data in the programs in which the PHN works

  3) Works in partnership with communities, systems, individuals, or families to attach meaning to collected quantitative and qualitative data

  4) Works in partnership with communities, systems, individuals, and families to establish priorities

*(continues)*

## KRISTI'S NOTEBOOK
### COMPETENCY #1 *(continued)*

C. Creates public health strength, risk and asset-based diagnoses for communities, systems, individuals, and families

D. In partnership with communities, systems, individuals, and families, develops a plan based on priorities (including nursing care plans for individuals/families)

   1) Selects desired outcomes that are measurable, meaningful, and manageable

   2) Selects public health interventions that

      a. Are supported by current literature as evidence-based

      b. Reduce health determinant risk factors and strengthen health determinant protective factors

      c. Have the greatest potential for improving the health of the population

      d. Respect and are consistent with the culture and ethnic beliefs of the community

      e. Are consistent with professional standards, the Nurse Practice Act, existing laws, ordinances, and policies

   3) Selects level(s) of intervention (community, systems, individuals, and families)

   4) Selects level(s) of prevention (primary, secondary, tertiary)

E. Implements the plan with communities, systems, individuals, and families

   1) Works in partnership with communities, systems, individuals, and families to implement public health interventions

   2) Utilizes best practices when implementing the public health nursing intervention

F. Evaluates

   1) Measures outcomes of public health nursing interventions using evidence-based methods and tools

   2) Documents public health nursing process by completing forms, records, and charts for communities, systems, individuals, and families

   3) Uses information technology to collect, document, analyze, store, and retrieve the health status of communities, systems, individuals, and families

*Source:* Henry Street Consortium, 2017

### USEFUL DEFINITIONS

**Community:** Refers to (a) a group of people or population group; (b) a physical place and time in which the population lives and works; or (c) a cultural group that has shared beliefs, values, institutions, and social systems (Skemp, Dreher, & Asselin, 2006, p. 23).

**Community Assessment:** The process of systematically collecting information about a community's structure, processes, and dynamics, its physical and social environment, its populations, and its level of health and wellness to determine its strengths, its resources, its populations of interest and populations at risk, its health needs, and its health priorities.

**Electronic Health Records (EHRs):** "Longitudinal collection of clinical and demographic client-specific data that are stored in a computer-readable format" (Martin, 2005, p. 461).

**Family:** A family is defined as a social unit of two or more people who identify themselves as a family, share emotional bonds, and carry out the functions of a family including managing healthcare (Clark, 2008; Friedman, Bowden, & Jones, 2003; Martin, 2005), and family is "a group of individuals who are bound by strong emotional ties, a sense of belonging, and a passion for being involved in one another's lives" (Wright & Bell, 2009, p. 46).

**Family Assessment:** The process of systematically collecting information about clients' family structure, processes, and dynamics; their physical and social environments; and their levels of health and illness to determine their strengths, resources, health needs, and health priorities.

**Health Status Indicators:** Measures of the level of health or illness of an individual/family, community, or population, such as incidence or prevalence of disease, birth and death rates, level of independence, life satisfaction, and quality of life.

**Omaha System:** "Research-based approach to practice, documentation, and information management that incorporates the Problem Classification Scheme, Intervention Scheme, and Problem Rating Scale for Outcomes" (Martin, 2005, p. 463).

**Population:** The "total number of people living in a specific geographic area"; subpopulations (syn. groups or aggregates) "consisting of people experiencing a specific health condition, engaging in behaviors that have potential to negatively affect health, sharing a common risk factor or risk exposure, or experiencing an emerging health threat or risk" (American Nurses Association [ANA], 2013, p. 3).

**Priority Setting:** Organizing health concerns by hazard level so that health risks that place individuals/families, communities, or populations at greater risk are dealt with first.

**Public Health Informatics:** Public health informatics is the systematic application of information, computer science, and technology to public health practice, research, and learning (Centers for Disease Control and Prevention [CDC], n.d.-b).

**Public Health Nursing Process:** Integrates concepts of public health, community, and all three levels of PHN practice (i.e., individual/family, community, system) into the nursing process (i.e., assessment, diagnosis, planning, implementation, and evaluation) (Minnesota Department of Health [MDH], Center for Public Health Nursing Practice, 2003).

**System:** An organization or institution that is part of the social environmental determinant of health (i.e., healthcare, education, commerce, religion, government).

## Thinking and Doing Population Health— Nursing Process Leads the Way

PHNs work with individuals and families wherever they find them in the community and in whatever condition they find them. The priority for public health nursing is health promotion and disease prevention, but PHNs also work with individuals and families who have chronic health conditions to help them achieve their health potential and, whenever possible, manage their own lives and healthcare needs. They need to discover their clients' potential for self-care and wellness to help them reach that potential. PHNs use a strengths-based approach when using the public health nursing process. Because their clients live in the community, PHNs need to find out as much as they can about the community's support systems, resources, and resource gaps.

## Partnering With Individuals, Families, and Communities

PHNs need to understand the *story*, the context of the lives of the people in the community in which they work. PHNs must know and understand the history, culture, and lifestyle of individuals, families, populations, and the entire community. For example, in a post-clinical seminar, students were discussing the stresses and crises of the families they were visiting. They stated that they did not understand how these families could function with so much stress. One

of the students, a recent immigrant, said she thought these families were fairly well off—they had housing, food, and were safe in their homes. The country she had emigrated from was in turmoil. She had seen family members murdered, their cattle slaughtered, homes burned, and people without food or clothing. These people, she thought, had truly stressful lives. The other students reflected on her comments and came to realize that people view the world from their own experiences. Understanding and appreciating the lived experiences of people is important. Knowing about and understanding each other helps promote the opportunity for people to work together in a mutually respectful manner that can build on each other's strengths.

PHNs work in partnership with individuals, families, and communities. Partnerships are mutual relationships based on trust. PHNs establish trust with individuals, families, and communities by respecting their rights to make their own health decisions and by adapting the nursing practice to fit the lived experiences and daily lives of those individuals, families, and communities. PHNs direct their efforts to meet the priority health needs their clients identify. Public health nursing practice includes the "3 E's":

- **Egalitarian (equal)** relationships with individuals, families, and communities
- **Enhancement** of individual, family, and community strengths, resilience, and resources
- **Empowerment** of individuals, families, and communities to advocate for and manage their own healthcare needs

## Data Collection, Data Management, and the Public Health Nursing Process

Data compose the engine that drives the problem-solving process in nursing practice. Data are used to determine the health of populations and sub-populations in order to influence health priorities, health policy, and programs that promote the health and safety of communities and their populations (Allen, Soderberg, Laventure, 2017; Nelson & Staggers, 2018). A continuum of population data is used by public health agencies to improve the health of their communities (see Figure 3.1). Accurate and consistent population data can be transformed to information, which leads to population health knowledge, and then to wisdom in order to design public health interventions to create healthier communities.

Therefore, you need to have a system and process for data collection and management in place at the beginning of the nursing process. For this reason, we discuss data in this chapter before we discuss the components of the public health nursing process. Many public health and community agencies use electronic health records (EHRs) and automated health information systems (HIS). EHRs and HISs provide ways to collect, store, analyze, and share information. Community and population data can be gathered from a variety of *primary* (data collected by individuals carrying out assessment) and *secondary* (data collected and published by others) sources.

Although more than one HIS exists, a system created for public health nursing is useful as an example. The Omaha System, a standardized terminology initially developed for use in the community, provides a problem-solving approach based on the nursing process (see Figure 3.2). The Omaha System is the foundation of the HIS that interprofessional team members at many health departments and other community provider sites regularly use to collect, document, and analyze individual, family, and population clinical data. The Omaha System allows PHNs to collect and record their own evidence-based practice data, analyze the data, and generate meaningful information that can be used to improve the quality of the care they provide. By using this approach, PHNs operationalize the data-information-knowledge-wisdom continuum (Allen et al., 2017; Martin, 2005; Nelson & Staggers, 2018). They can tell their data- and evidence-driven stories about the individuals, families, and communities they serve. More than 22,000 interprofessional clinicians use the Omaha System globally (Omaha System, 2017).

The adoption of EHRs by healthcare providers, including health departments, is increasing very rapidly (American Nurses Association [ANA], 2015; Martin, Monsen, & Bowles, 2011; Office of the National Coordinator for Health Information Technology, 2017; Omaha System, 2017).

When health departments use EHRs based on the Omaha System accurately and consistently, they can aggregate individual and family data into larger data sets so that patterns can be identified within populations. Increasingly,

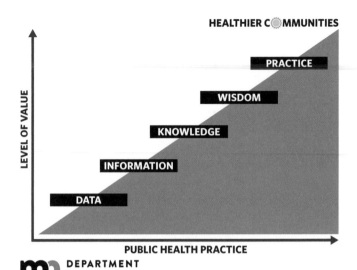

**FIGURE 3.1** Transforming Data to Practice
*Source:* Allen et al., 2017; adapted by LaVenture, 2008

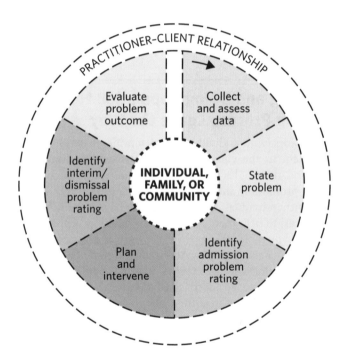

**FIGURE 3.2** Omaha System Model of the Problem-Solving Process
*Source:* Martin, 2005, p. 7, used with permission

third-party payers and accreditors require health departments to provide evidence that their programs result in improved client outcomes. Aggregate data are a powerful tool to demonstrate the value of agency programs and can be shared with the public, be used to obtain grants and other funds, and be incorporated into quality improvement and program evaluation reports. Examples of reports generated by various agencies are found at www.omahasystem.org/links.html.

## EVIDENCE EXAMPLE 3.1

### The Omaha System

The Omaha System was developed by the Visiting Nurse Association of Omaha (Nebraska) and seven test sites to enhance practice, documentation, and information management. Four federally funded research studies were conducted between 1975 and 1993 that validated appropriateness and effectiveness of the terminology. DeLanne Simmons, chief executive officer, envisioned a computerized management information system that incorporated an integrated, valid, and reliable clinical information system focused on clients who received services, not on the nurses and other interprofessional team members who provided the services (Martin, 2005; Martin et al., 2011; Omaha System, 2017). More than 400 articles, chapters, and books have been published about the Omaha System; the Listserv has more than 3,000 members located in the U.S. and 22 other countries (Omaha System, 2017).

Omaha System terms are used in documentation at the *point of care* (i.e., the time and place that care occurs). Because the terms of the Omaha System are not complex and the structure is relatively simple, nonhealthcare professionals can understand it. Clinicians see and use point-of-care terminologies in their EHRs. In 2014, Minnesota became the first state to recommend that American Nurses Association recognized point-of-care terminologies be included in all EHRs (ANA, 2015; Minnesota Department of Health [MDH], 2015). Prior to that, Minnesota Department of Health staff conducted a survey and found that 96.5% of community agencies in all counties used the Omaha System (Omaha System, 2017).

The Omaha System enables healthcare providers to analyze and exchange client-centered coded data that can be transformed to information, the first two stages of the data-to-wisdom continuum. The Omaha System was designed to be used by interprofessional clinicians to guide their practice and document and communicate information about clients from admission to discharge. It exists in the public domain (no fee or license) and is intended for use across the continuum of care nationally and globally. It is based on a conceptual model that reflects the pivotal position of the individual, family, and community as client; interprofessional partnerships; and the value of the problem-solving approach. The Omaha System encourages critical thinking, enhances communication, and operationalizes the nursing process. The problem-solving approach complements the strengths-based approach that focuses on building developmental assets and increasing the health of youth and communities (Martin, 2005; Monsen, Vanderboom, Olson, Larson, & Holland, 2017; Omaha System, 2017). The Omaha System consists of three components:

■ *Problem Classification Scheme* (client-centered assessment that engages individuals, families, and communities)—The Problem Classification Scheme is a hierarchy of terms that includes domains; individual-, family-, and community-centered problems; modifiers; and signs/symptoms.

■ *Intervention Scheme* (plans, pathways, care activities, and service delivery terms to improve safety, quality, and effectiveness)—The Intervention Scheme is a hierarchy of terms that includes categories, targets, and client-specific information.

■ *Problem Rating Scale for Outcomes* (evaluation that provides usable information for measuring and reporting client progress and change across time)—The Problem Rating Scale for Outcomes consists of Knowledge, Behavior, and Status concepts and Likert-type rating scales. Evidence Example 3.2 showcases a case study of the Omaha System used to tell the story of a nurse-client interaction.

See Appendix B for additional Omaha System resources.

"*Kristi has just finished reading about the Omaha System. Her PHN preceptor, Beth, tells her that the public health nursing agency uses the Omaha System, and Beth wants Kristi to have a basic understanding of the Omaha System before she and Beth chart on any of the clients they visit. Beth gives Kristi the case study about Anna to read to help her understand the system. Beth asks Kristi if what she read made sense.*

*Kristi reflects: "I expected to be confused about the Omaha System, but the case study helped a lot. I could see the how the nurse assessed Anna and provided nursing services to her. She could use the Problem Rating Scale for Outcomes to evaluate Anna's progress when she returns for another visit. I can see that using this system helps nurses measure the impact of their care and report how nursing care makes a difference. The one concern I have is that my instructor stresses the importance of using a strengths-based approach and the Omaha System always uses the term 'problems.'"*

*Beth comments: "I had the same concern when I started using the Omaha System, but my supervisor pointed me to the literature on how 'problem' is actually defined in the Omaha System. Here is the definition of problem that I found: 'Unique client concerns, needs, strengths, issues, foci, or conditions that affect any aspect of the client's well-being; nursing diagnosis stated from the client's perspective'\* Also, I found that the term 'problem' can be considered neutral, not negative, so a problem in the Omaha System can also be used as part of a strengths-based approach.*\*\*

*Kristi responds: "That makes me more comfortable. I am going to share with my classmates that the Omaha System term 'problem' can be used from a strengths-based perspective.*"

\* *Source*: Martin, 2005, p. 465
\*\* *Source*: Monsen, Vanderboom et al., 2017

## EVIDENCE EXAMPLE 3.2
### Omaha System Case Study

**Anna K.:** *Older woman who had a chronic cardiac condition and attended a screening clinic*

### First Visit/Encounter Data

Public health nurses at the Dakota County Public Health Department (Minnesota) developed health clinics for senior citizens. The clinics offered screening for health concerns, particularly hypertension, heart disease, and depression; accurate health information for prevention and treatment; and outreach and referral coordination for home care, equipment, medical assistance, and other community services. Because interaction time was limited, the nurses developed standardized protocols and forms based on the Omaha System to increase the efficiency and effectiveness of assessment, interventions, and documentation. When new clients visited the clinics, the nurses considered four problems, Communication with community resources, Mental health, Circulation, and Medication regimen. If those problems did not reflect clients' presenting data, the nurses selected and documented other pertinent problems, interventions, and outcome ratings.

When Anna K. came to the senior clinic for the first time, she reported that she had a history of dizziness and high blood pressure, but could not recall previous readings. When the nurse checked her vital signs, her blood pressure was 152/86 sitting and 154/82 standing; her pulse was 60 and regular. Her weight was 138 pounds, appropriate for her reported height. They talked about hypertension, blood pressure guidelines, the Circulation protocol, and Anna's data. The nurse suggested strategies to increase Anna's safety when she was dizzy. The nurse recorded Anna's vital signs on a health card, gave the card to her, and suggested that she have her blood pressure re-checked monthly and recorded on the card. She asked her to show the card to her doctor during future appointments.

Anna said she took two "heart" pills fairly regularly. She agreed to bring them with her when she returned to the Senior Clinic the following week so she and the nurse could discuss them. The nurse planned to use the Medication regimen protocol if appropriate, and record them on Anna's health card.

**Anna's Answers:** Transforming the Story into the Omaha System assessment, services, and evaluation terms

**Domain:** Physiological

**Problem: Circulation** (high priority problem)

### Problem Classification Scheme

**Modifiers:** Individual and Actual
Signs/Symptoms of Actual:

- syncopal-fainting episodes/dizziness
- abnormal blood pressure reading

### Intervention Scheme

**Category:** Teaching, Guidance, and Counseling
Targets and client specific information:

- anatomy/physiology (circulatory system)
- mobility/transfers (avoid falls)
- signs/symptoms-physical (importance of vital signs, when to notify physician, dizziness)

**Category:** Case Management
Targets and client specific information:

- continuity of care (show doctor her health card with monthly blood pressure checks)

**Category:** Surveillance
Targets and client specific information:

- medical/dental care (schedule and go to appointments)
- signs/symptoms-physical (vital signs, circulatory status, weight, blood pressure)

### Problem Rating Scale for Outcomes

**Knowledge:** 2—minimal knowledge (some information about normal/abnormal blood pressure readings but not impact on health; did not know previous readings)

**Behavior:** 4—usually appropriate behavior (usually took medications, has blood pressure checked periodically, seeks healthcare)

**Status:** 3—moderate symptoms (blood pressure exceeded expected range for non-diabetic client)

Elizabeth A. Vance, BSN, RN, PHN
RN Primary Care
Allina Health Clinics Division
Minneapolis, Minnesota

Carol A. Fish, MS, RN, PHN
Supervisor, Social Services Department
Dakota County Public Health Department
West St. Paul, Minnesota

*Source:* Vance & Fish, 2017 Omaha System case study. Personal correspondence from Karen S. Martin, Martin Associates, Omaha, NE. December 8, 2017.

# Home Visiting and the Nursing Process

PHNs carry out assessments as part of the nursing process most often in a community setting, such as a home, a school, or a clinic. Most of the information is gathered through observation and listening. When in the home setting, PHNs are guests of the family members and need to follow their lead regarding communication methods; timing, length, and place of visit; and roles of the nurse and family members. To assess the family, PHNs must first establish a trusting relationship with family members based on mutual respect and understanding (Eriksson & Nilsson, 2008; Martin, 2005; McCann & Baker, 2001). Answering questions about personal family matters and health situations requires families to disclose information they generally do not share with strangers, so the development of a trusting relationship needs to precede or occur simultaneously with the interviewing process. Andrew Gardner (2010) found that one way to engage clients and help them feel comfortable was to start by being open and friendly; this approach seems obvious but can be challenging for nurses who are learning to be professional while maintaining boundaries and creating an environment conducive to effective nursing practice. An appropriate level of openness certainly can facilitate a connection and mutual understanding, but this is sometimes a difficult balancing act, as friendship often occurs within the professional context of the nurse-client relationship. The initial visit to a family is critical in establishing the nurse-client trust relationship (see Evidence Example 3.3).

Home visiting programs may include one or more visits to a client. PHNs follow some families for months and years, depending on their health risks and needs. So you should not feel as though you have to get everything done in one visit. Table 3.1 demonstrates how a PHN would use the nursing process in making a series of home visits. The orientation phase takes one to three visits on average. The working phase might require multiple visits over a period of months or years.

---

## EVIDENCE EXAMPLE 3.3
### Public Health Nurses' Views of a Good First Meeting

Swedish researchers used focus groups to determine what public health nurses believed constituted a good first home visit with parents of newborns (Jansson, Petersson, & Uden, 2001). A good first visit is considered key to developing an effective relationship with parents. Three criteria were identified (Jansson et al., 2001):

1. **Creating trust** through good contact/reciprocal relationships; listening; being a guest; having an equal role with parents; and having time, privacy, and peace and quiet

2. **Creating a picture of the family's life situation** by getting a holistic impression of the family, seeing them in their home environment, getting a picture of what the clients are like, and taking in, consciously and unconsciously, the mood and a variety of information about the family

3. **Creating a supportive climate** by confirming and affirming parents' feelings, abilities, and responsibilities and increasing their responsibilities while providing a safety net of services until family is able to manage on its own

---

## TABLE 3.1 How the Nursing Process Occurs in Home Visits

| Home-Visiting Components | Nursing Process |
|---|---|
| **Orientation Phase**<br>▪ Introduction<br>▪ Determine purpose of visit and visit activities with client<br>▪ Engage in social conversation<br>▪ Assessment<br>▪ Identify and state client's problems | **Assessment and Diagnosis**<br>▪ Individual/family and community assessment<br>▪ Strengths-based assessment—protective factors identified<br>▪ Resources identified<br>▪ Health risks and active health problems identified<br>▪ Unmet health needs identified |
| **Working Phase: Identification**<br>▪ Client asks questions and identifies nurse as someone who can help.<br>▪ Client identifies problems.<br>▪ Nurse provides health teaching, support and counseling, follow-up assessment, referral, and advocacy. | **Planning and Implementation**<br>▪ Mutual planning, priority-setting, goal-setting<br>▪ Interventions often used include teaching, guidance, and counseling; treatments and procedures; case management; surveillance, advocacy, referral, and follow-up. |

*(continues)*

**TABLE 3.1  How the Nursing Process Occurs in Home Visits**  *(continued)*

| Home-Visiting Components | Nursing Process |
|---|---|
| **Working Phase: Mutual Relationship** <br>■ Client uses nurse as resource and accesses community resources. <br>■ Nurse engages client in mutual problem solving. | **Implementation** <br>■ Interventions often used are teaching, guidance, and counseling; treatments and procedures; case management; surveillance; collaboration; and consultation. |
| **Resolution and Termination** <br>■ Problems are solved or ongoing but stable. <br>■ Client becomes independent of nurse or continues to need support. <br>■ Relationship ends when client no longer needs nurse or no longer participates in plan (moves or refuses participation in plan or visits). | **Evaluation** <br>■ Evaluation of Knowledge, Behavior, and Status outcomes: outcomes met, partially met, or not met <br>■ Replan—change in goals, outcomes, or interventions <br>■ New priorities or emerging problems identified and nursing process continued |

*Sources:* Phases adapted from McNaughton, 2005; Omaha System terms from Martin, 2005; and interventions from Minnesota Department of Health, 2001

PHNs carry equipment they need to complete assessments on individual family members. For example, common equipment used on maternal/child health visits includes a baby scale, blood pressure cuffs, a stethoscope, paper tape measures, disposable thermometers, developmental screening tools, growth grids, and a thermometer for determining the temperature of bath water.

PHNs carry smartphones, laptops, and other electronic devices to stay in contact with others, access information, and enter family data into EHRs during their home visits. Many PHNs use automated guidelines or clinical pathways specific to individual client and family situations. For example, public health agencies have screening, assessment, and monitoring databases for newborns, infants, children, antepartum, postpartum, and family clients. PHNs collect admitting data on each client during their initial visits to their clients. They monitor and record health changes at each visit.

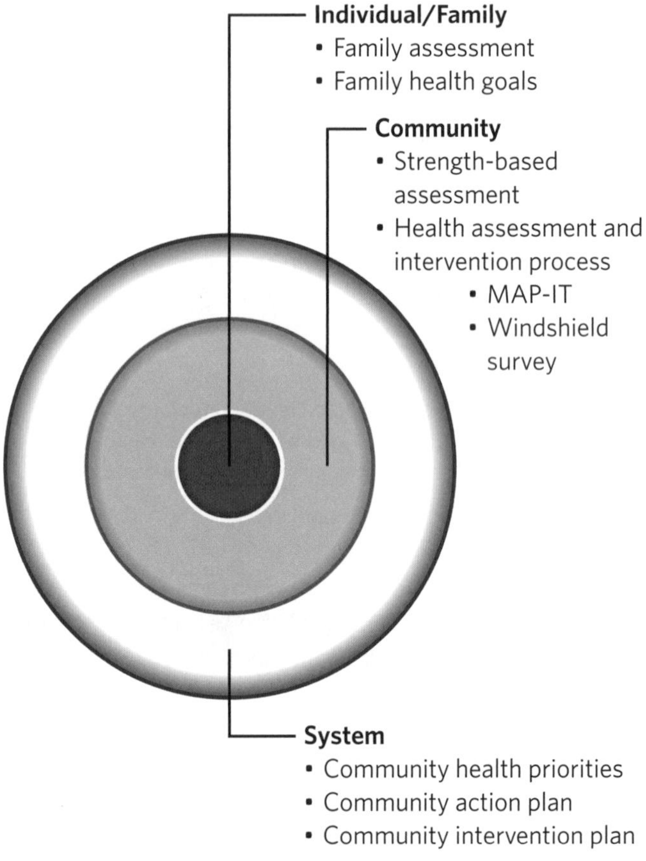

## Public Health Nursing Assessment

Public health nursing assessment is a systematic, deliberative, and holistic process of collecting data about a client (individual, family, community, or system) that leads to an understanding of the client's health determinants, health status, and priority health concerns and needs, as shown in Figure 3.3. PHNs also need to carry out strengths-based assessments so that intervention plans for health concerns and problems are based on the clients' abilities to manage their own healthcare needs. Strengths-based assessments identify clients' abilities, resources, and resilience as well as health needs (Monsen, Vanderboom et al., 2017).

**Individual/Family**
• Family assessment
• Family health goals

**Community**
• Strength-based assessment
• Health assessment and intervention process
  • MAP-IT
  • Windshield survey

**System**
• Community health priorities
• Community action plan
• Community intervention plan

**FIGURE 3.3**  How PHNs Collect Data About Individuals, Communities, and Systems

## Individual/Family Level of Practice

The family is the focus of care when PHNs work at the individual/family level of practice. The family is the primary unit of society and is responsible for carrying out the functions that allow family members to survive and thrive. In a health sense, the family is a unit of care allowing the nurse to simultaneously focus on the individual, the family, and the health issue (Hunt, 2013). Families come in many shapes and sizes and in different stages of development. Family composition is varied and changeable in contemporary society (Kaakinen, Coehlo, Steele, & Robinson, 2018). A family is "a group of individuals who are bound by strong emotional ties, a sense of belonging, and a passion for being involved in one another's lives" (Wright & Bell, 2009, p. 46).

The experience of illness or a health concern is felt by not just the individual but also by larger systems including family members and the community (Marshall, Bell, & Moules, 2010). Family-focused care has the potential to empower vulnerable and at-risk families (Rossiter, Fowler, Hopwood, Lee, & Dunston, 2011). *Family assessment* is a holistic process in which all the factors that influence a family's level of health and wellness are considered. Specifically, a family unit assessment includes collecting data on the individual, family, household, and community to identify resources, strengths, and risks (Meiers, 2016; Meiers, Krumwiede, Denham, & Bell, 2016). In addition to considering individual human development stages, PHNs consider the family's stage of development. Transitions between the stages involve rearrangement of relationships. Although it is important to note that this is a very traditional model for married families with children and would need to be adapted to a variety of diverse family structures, Carter and McGoldrick's (2005) Family Life Cycle model highlights the development of the family system over time:

- Leaving home as single young adults
- Joining of families through marriage: the new couple
- Families with young children
- Families with adolescents
- Launching children and moving on
- Families in later life

Each stage is associated with tasks that will foster each member's development. Sara's family falls in the "families with adolescents" stage. One unique aspect to this stage is that the parents face a transition with both the adolescent in terms of growing independence and the adolescent's aging grandparents. This stage requires the family to alter its parent-child relationship to accommodate the adolescent's growing independence and autonomy. This awareness of the family's stage of development can be helpful for PHNs in understanding potential family conflict as they are working through the stages. Table 3.2 outlines the components of family assessment typically included in a comprehensive family assessment using the Healthy People 2020 Health Determinants Framework.

*Beth and Kristi make their first visit to Sara. Her mother, Patricia, introduces herself at the beginning of the visit and states that she hopes the public health nurse can straighten out her daughter and help her daughter understand the poor choice she made in getting pregnant at such a young age. She is concerned because Sara is missing so much school. Sara has poor eye contact with Beth and her mother. Beth focuses on Sara and asks her what she would like help with for the rest of her pregnancy. Sara responds that she is very tired and feels uncomfortable with all of her body changes that are now becoming visible. She is afraid of how the other students at school will treat her.*

*Beth tells Sara and Patricia that she would like to get a good sense of the family before she begins any work with Sara. Beth asks if she can visit again next week to finish the family assessment she was able to start today. Before Beth and Kristi leave, Beth collects information from Sara so a case file can be opened. Beth then asks Sara if Kristi can check her height and weight to get some basic information. Sara agrees. Kristi finds that Sara weighs 100 lb. and her height is 5'3".*

*After the visit, Kristi writes in her public health nursing clinical journal. She thinks about what phases of the home visiting occurred during this first visit. She also analyzes the visit and asks herself the question, "Was this a good first visit?" Kristi also reviews the holistic family assessment framework that she and Sara will be using during the second home visit.*

**TABLE 3.2 Holistic Family Assessment Framework**

| Framework | Factors |
|---|---|
| **Family Biological and Genetic Factors** | ▪ Age<br>▪ Sex or gender identify<br>▪ Three-generation genogram<br>▪ Family-identified ethnicity<br>▪ Health status |
| **Family Behavioral Factors** | ▪ Lifestyle and daily patterns including nutrition, sleep, exercise, and recreation<br>▪ Housing and living arrangements<br>▪ Social support/ecomap<br>▪ Family and community roles<br>▪ Education, employment<br>▪ Socioeconomic status (income, poverty)<br>▪ Cultural patterns, religious affiliations<br>▪ Language and health literacy<br>▪ Health-seeking and health-limiting behaviors<br>▪ Patterns of coping and resilience<br>▪ Patterns of conformity and nonconformity |
| **Physical Environment Factors** | ▪ Home environment (use a home safety checklist appropriate to family members' age, development, and physical and cognitive abilities)<br>▪ Immediate neighborhood (observations, walkability, windshield surveys)<br>▪ Natural physical environment and weather<br>▪ Built environment, including safety<br>▪ Maintenance of sidewalks, roads, pedestrian crossing<br>▪ Transportation<br>▪ Adequate recreational resources<br>▪ Access to shopping centers<br>▪ Accessible healthcare—see the 5 A's of accessible healthcare in the community-assessment guide<br>▪ Potential or actual environmental hazards such as pollution of air, water, food, or soil |
| **Social Environment Factors (i.e., social actions, patterns, systems, healthcare access)** | ▪ Availability of health and social services resources<br>▪ Availability of quality schools and daycare<br>▪ Availability of fire and police<br>▪ Employment opportunities<br>▪ Mass media and library availability<br>▪ Cultural and social patterns of community, including potential exposure to violence<br>▪ Governmental services<br>▪ Business community and working conditions |
| **Data Analysis** | Summary of the family assessment including:<br><br>▪ Major family protective factors, major family risk factors<br>▪ Statement of family resilience and ability to manage own healthcare<br>▪ Family's priority health problems or concerns and health goals |

*During the second home visit, Kristi works with Beth to complete the family assessment. She constructs a genogram with Sara and her mother and they notice that Patricia and Sara's grandmother have a history of preterm labor. During the visit, Jimmy, Patricia's boyfriend, comes home early from work and Sara's sisters, Tara and Kara, 9-year old twins, come home from school. The home becomes loud and there are lots of interruptions during the early part of the visit. Beth asks Patricia if they can continue the visit in the kitchen and asks the twins to stay in the living room. Jimmy decides he will take a nap. The visit continues uninterrupted. By the end of the visit, information about the family health determinants of biology and behaviors have been collected. When Kristi completes her weekly clinical journal, she organizes the family data by health determinant categories.*

Table 3.3 is what Kristi recorded.

## TABLE 3.3 Sara's Family Assessment: Individual/Family Health Determinants

### Biological and Genetic Health Determinant Factors

**Sara:** is 16 years old, 20 weeks gestation, primipara, on a prenatal vitamin, diagnosed with anemia, and underweight with poor weight gain. She and her family are Caucasian.

**Patricia:** mother, is 34 years old taking hydrochlorothiazide 12.5 mg daily for hypertension.

**Jimmy:** mother's live-in boyfriend, is 37 years old and has no health conditions.

**Siblings:** Tara and Kara are 9-year-old twins; both females have attention deficit hyperactivity disorder (ADHD) and take Adderall XR 1.25 mg daily. Immunizations are up to date.

**Extended family:** Sara's grandparents, Patricia's parents, live on a farm house 30 miles away. Grandmother, 55 years old, has hypertension. Grandfather, 57 years old, has type II diabetes.

**Samuel:** Sara's boyfriend, is 17 years old, Hispanic, and has no known health conditions.

### Behavioral Factors

**Socioeconomic Status:** Sara is a full-time high school student in 10th grade, unemployed, and with no income. Patricia is a full-time factory worker and Jimmy is a full-time welder. Both have high school diplomas. Tara and Kara are full-time elementary school students. Samuel, Sara's boyfriend, is a full-time 11th-grade student and works part time at a restaurant. Although the family does not live in poverty, their income is low and they struggle to pay their monthly bills. Patricia has family health insurance and Jimmy has his own insurance.

**Cultural and Religious Affiliation:** All family members were born in the United States and are Catholic. The family attends church most Sundays.

**Family Developmental Stage:** families with adolescents' developmental stage (Carter & McGoldrick, 2005)

**Family Roles and Function:** Patricia takes on leadership and organizer role in the home and schedules Sara's prenatal check-ups. Patricia makes the decisions and Jimmy pays the bills and fixes the house. Sara babysits the twins but lacks knowledge of the difference between being an older sibling and being a parent. Patricia is tired, stressed, guilty for not being available for the family, and upset that Jimmy is not helping more at home. Samuel doesn't come over much anymore because Patricia and Jimmy are not very welcoming.

**Family Lifestyle Patterns (disrupted by health concerns):** The family is struggling to manage schedules. Sara has been missing school due to fatigue and does not want anyone to know she is pregnant. Patricia and Jimmy leave for work at 6:00 a.m., so Sara routinely takes care of the twins in the morning. Lately, Sara hasn't been helping the twins get ready for school or to the bus on time. Patricia has been contacted by both schools due to Sara's multiple absences and Tara and Kara's tardiness. Patricia has been working overtime to pay for Sara's prenatal care costs. Due to the stress of Sara's pregnancy and working overtime, the house is messy, meals are not being made or eaten together, and the twins are not taking their ADHD medication as prescribed.

**Ecomap Summary:** The family has close relationships with their neighbors and church. The twins' relationship with their school is strained due to tardiness. Sara also has a strained relationship with her school and misses Samuel and her friends. She would like to find a peer support group for pregnant and parenting teens but cannot find one.

**Health seeking behaviors:** Prior to the recent family disruptions, the family had healthy eating patterns, including eating supper together. They enjoyed weekly family bike riding. The twins and sometimes Sara got at least 8 hours of sleep most nights. No one in the family smokes; Sara does not use alcohol or other drugs.

**Health Limiting Behaviors:** The family lacks time to prepare and share meals and to go bike-riding. The twins often miss their daily ADHD medications. Sara feels like she is getting fat due to pregnancy, so she eats only one meal a day, typically a peanut butter and jelly sandwich, chips, and a soda and ice cream as a bedtime snack.

**Family Resilience and Coping Patterns:** Patricia stated she and her girls are strong and that Jimmy makes the family even stronger. Patricia went through a difficult divorce and feels her family is stronger because of the experience. Patricia and the girls talked through the experience; they "stuck together." They have a positive outlook and pray together. Sara's pregnancy has been stressful for the family. Sara is scared to give birth and depends on her mom being strong. "She has always been my rock and now I am scared because my mom is so disappointed in me. We don't talk anymore; she just yells at me all the time."

*Beth and Kristi decide that Kristi could return for a third family visit to complete the home and neighborhood portions of the family assessment if Sara and her mother are okay with this. Beth phones Patricia and gets permission for Kristi to visit. After the visit, Kristi records the data on the physical and social environmental health determinants in her clinical journal. Kristi believes that she and Beth have now completed the Orientation Phase of family visiting. She will confirm this with Beth.*

Table 3.4 shows the notes that Kristi wrote after her visit.

*Kristi goes to meet with Beth at the office before their next scheduled home visit with Sara and her family. Beth and Kristi review the data analysis of the family assessment and the summary of the family strengths and risk factors and identifies what she thinks are the family's health problems and priorities.*

*Beth comments, "It is difficult to focus on the family as a whole when we opened the case on Sara and now we are assessing and planning on intervening with the family as a whole. You did a good job focusing on the family as a unit and putting Sara in the center of that family."*

## Establishing Family Health Goals

The PHN continues the nursing process by moving into identification of the individual's or family's health priorities and mutual goal-setting. PHNs employ mutual problem-solving strategies with clients to foster self-efficacy. When working with families in the community, the PHN partners with the families in determining priorities, establishing goals, and developing an intervention plan. The plan should be congruent with and integrated into the family's culture, lifestyle, and daily routine and be within the family's potential to achieve. The plan should enhance the family's potential for self-care and autonomy. The family care plan should be realistic, understandable, measurable, behavioral, achievable, and time-limited so that the effectiveness of the plan and the nursing interventions can be determined. It is possible to develop and measure Knowledge, Behavior, and Status outcomes for a family using the Omaha System Problem Classification Scheme.

**TABLE 3.4  Sara's Family Assessment: Physical and Social Environmental Health Determinants**

| Physical Environment Health Determinant Factors (Natural and Built Environment) |
| --- |
| The family lives together in a 3-bedroom, 1-bath rambler in need of repairs in a low-income neighborhood. The twins share a room. The home safety checklist findings included: presence of smoke detectors, carbon monoxide detectors, and good lighting throughout. Cleaning products are in an unlocked cupboard under the sink. This will present a safety hazard for the new baby. Their neighborhood has sidewalks and is well lit. Traffic is light. There is a grocery store, a farmer's market, and a park nearby. The family medical clinic is 5 miles from their home. |

| Social Environment Health Determinant Factors |
| --- |
| The family feels that they live in a good neighborhood and good community. The neighborhood has a neighborhood watch committee and a few retired neighbors have a Safe Home sign in their window, which means that any child who needs help can go to those homes. The local schools have good teachers and are safe. Patricia and Sara are relieved that a PHN can come to see Sara at home. The PHN is working with the school nurse and social worker to plan for Sara's return to school once she has the baby. There is no peer support program for pregnant and parenting teens at the school. The City Council has recently started a marketing program to attract new businesses, which will give Patricia and Jimmy opportunities for better jobs. |

| Data Analysis—Summary of Family Assessment |
| --- |
| **Family Strengths (Protective Factors):** The family has a good history of resilience and healthy family roles and functions. The family has good community support systems. Patricia and Jimmy expressed the desire to support Sara in her pregnancy. Sara plans to complete high school and go to college; she does not use substances such as tobacco, drugs, or alcohol. The family is working with the PHN, school nurse, and social worker to help Sara achieve her goals. |
| **Family Risk Factors:** Sara's unexpected pregnancy has placed a stress on the family functions that has resulted in interruptions in some family processes. Key areas for improvement are meal preparation, Sara's difficulty with caretaking the twins in the morning, and Sara's poor eating habits. The family history of preterm labor is an added risk factor for Sara's pregnancy. Sara has experience caring for her younger siblings and has a desire to learn about prenatal care; however, she has a lack of knowledge about pregnancy and caring for an infant. The relationship between Patricia and Sara is strained, and Sara does not feel she is receiving the support she needs from her mother. The relationship between Samuel and the family is strained. The twins are not receiving their daily ADHD medications and are often tardy at school, while Sara has frequent absences from her school. |

"*Kristi and Beth carry out a home visit with Sara and her family to identify the family's priority health goals. During the visit, they work collaboratively with the family to identify two family health goals and then translate them into the Omaha System Problems.*

- *Goal One: Have a healthy baby to add to the family → Problem: Pregnancy.*

- *Goal Two: Work on supporting each other by improving their relationships and communications and get back into a scheduled routine → Problem: Interpersonal Relationship.*

*Kristi and Beth return to the office to input the family data for their family health goals using the Omaha System Problem Classification Scheme. In order to measure health outcome improvements over the time of the home visiting, Beth assigns a Knowledge, Behavior, and Status (KBS) rating starting for the primary family health problems.*"

Kristi's KBS rating for Sara and her family is shown in Table 3.5.

"*Beth says, "The next step will be to develop care plans." Kristi states, "I just reviewed Anna's case study and the Intervention Scheme. Was that a care plan?"*

*Beth suggests, "The Omaha System Intervention Scheme is used to describe care plans and services. For simplicity, Anna's case study documents services so readers can 'match' the services to the text in Anna's story. Why don't you take the next half hour and go online to the Omaha System Community of Practice (http://omahasystemmn.org/data.php)? Watch 'An Introduction to the Omaha System'* and 'How to Read an Omaha System Pathway.' You will see that the term 'pathway' is used to suggest various Intervention Scheme categories, targets, and client-specific information for specific problems. Then we can work together to develop pathways for the Pregnancy and Interpersonal relationship problems.""

*Kristi responds, "That sounds like a great idea. I am concerned though that Sara has a lot of other health problems related to her pregnancy: her eating habits and not gaining any weight, anxiety, isolation from her friends and her boyfriend, Samuel. The list goes on and on! When will we deal with those issues?"*

*Beth responds, "With home visiting, we take things one small step at a time. We are still in the Identification Phase of the Home Visiting Process. As we work with Sara and her family, we will deal with all of these issues using many interventions. Once we have developed a working relationship with the family we will move into the Mutual Relationship Phase. Then we will be able to have more of a consultative relationship and help them connect with community resources and decide how they want to manage the challenges of the birth of Sara's baby.*"

Health teaching, counseling, consultation, and case management are interventions commonly used to build on and enhance the families' strengths and encourage them to manage their healthcare. PHNs use advocacy to facilitate the individual's and family's ability to access health and social resources. They also use advocacy when populations are found to be at risk for a specific health hazard.

Whether individuals live alone or with others, the same family functions are relevant. If you are working with an individual who lives alone or whose extended family lives

## TABLE 3.5  Sara's Pregnancy and Family Stress in the Omaha System

| DOMAIN: Physiological | DOMAIN: Psychosocial |
|---|---|
| **PROBLEM:** Pregnancy (high-priority problem) | **PROBLEM:** Interpersonal Relationship |
| **Modifiers:** Individual and Actual | **Modifiers:** Family and Actual |
| Signs/Symptoms of Actual | Signs/Symptoms of Actual: |
| ■ Difficulty with prenatal exercise/rest/diet/behaviors | ■ Difficulty establishing/maintaining relationships |
| ■ Difficulty coping with body changes | ■ Incongruent values/goals/expectations/schedules |
| ■ Inadequate social support | ■ Prolonged, unrelieved tension |
| ***Problem Rating Scale for Outcomes*** | **Knowledge: 3**—Basic knowledge (describes importance of positive communication but not methods) |
| **Knowledge: 2**—Minimal knowledge (interested in information about appropriate rest, exercise, and diet patterns) | **Behavior: 3**—Inconsistently appropriate behavior (great decrease in number and increase in length of relationships, increase in repairing relationship) |
| **Behavior: 1**—Not appropriate behavior (no prenatal care; high-risk behaviors) | **Status: 2**—Severe symptoms (limited, brief communication and interaction, often tense) |
| **Status: 1**—Extreme signs/symptoms (anemia and is underweight with poor weight gain) | |

elsewhere, you still need to use the same family assessment approach. Sometimes a complete family assessment is not needed or impossible to collect. In that case, the PHN would select the assessment components that relate to the specific family health problem or priority concern. It would be important to include the following components in this focused family assessment: the health problem or issue and the related risk factors and protective factors, the family goal related to the health problem or concern, necessary access to health and social services, and the family's ability to manage healthcare needs and resources.

## Community Level of Practice

PHNs assess communities to determine their levels of health and wellness. These assessments are carried out in partnership with the community. Many geographic communities, such as cities, counties, and states, conduct a community assessment on a periodic basis. They do this to monitor changing health conditions of the populations in their communities and to establish community priorities for health goals, funding, and actions. The governmental agencies conducting the assessment partner with other community organizations and members to ensure that the diversity of the community and all points of view are reflected in the assessment. PHNs are part of the team that collects and analyzes the community data.

It is important to conduct a strengths-based assessment as part of the community-assessment process. PHNs work to enhance community strengths so that communities can be as independent as possible in solving their own healthcare problems and managing their own healthcare needs. See Chapter 8 for a discussion of the formation of community partnerships and building on community assets to strengthen the community's ability to manage its own healthcare needs.

The population data collected in public health includes population health status, health differences or health status gaps between populations (health disparities), and health determinants (causes of health and illness within the population). Population health status data, also known as global health status measures, are the "vital signs" of the population. These global health measures include:

- Mortality (death rates) data
- Life Expectancy (average years lived for someone born in a specific year)
- Years of Potential Life Lost (life expectancy–age of death = YPLL)

- Morbidity (illness rates) data
- Health behaviors data (e.g., smoking, exercise, obesity, use of seatbelts)
- Health and life satisfaction data (how satisfied one is with current health and lifestyle)
- Functional health data (ability to live independently and manage own healthcare needs)

*Kristi is just starting her community-assessment project with three of her classmates. They are conducting an aggregate assessment (focusing on a specific portion of the population). Because of the home visits to Sara and her family, Kristi is interested in looking at the needs of pregnant and parenting teens and identifying existing resources and resource gaps. She finds out that Sara's mother's church is considering starting an outreach program for pregnant and parenting teens. She asks Beth what information the health department might have to help her and the church members decide what to do. Did the PHNs have any data that would help?*

*Beth responds, "The public health department carries out a community assessment every five years to determine the priority health problems of the people living in the community. We want to know what the major health needs are and which needs are met and which are unmet. We also look at the assets or resources of the community to determine the community's capacity to manage its own healthcare needs and solve its own problems. Then we prioritize and decide which services to offer, what the funding should be, and how to allocate resources to our different programs. During the last community-assessment process, we found out that while our teen pregnancy rate had decreased, we still did not have the outreach and health promotion services to meet their needs. One area we identified as a priority was peer support groups for pregnant and parenting teens. Many of our public health nurses provide health teaching and case management interventions for pregnant and parenting teens in the home, and they found that until the teens return to school, they are quite isolated. We aren't sure if this is affecting their ability to parent their newborns. So, we are in the process of using Omaha System data to see if there are services we need to provide. When you organize your aggregate assessment, you should consider looking at what other churches and community organizations are doing or if they have the resources to develop new programs."*

## Community Health Assessment and Intervention Process

Community assessment and intervention is an inclusive process that involves all relevant stakeholders such as health and social services providers, spokespeople for the community and its sub-populations, and key decision-makers in the community. The MAP-IT 5-step process (see Figure 3.4) is a Healthy People 2020 tool that helps people unite to improve the health of their communities (CDC, n.d.-a). It may be used as a community-assessment tool and as a community planning process tool. MAP-IT resources are found at http://www.healthypeople.gov/2020/implement/MapIt.aspx.

Before starting the data-collection process, an assessment tool must be selected or developed. The community-assessment tool presented in Table 3.6 is based on the determinants of health (see Chapter 1). The community-assessment project you participate in as a student may include many of these components. Remember that all data sources, both primary and secondary, must be documented.

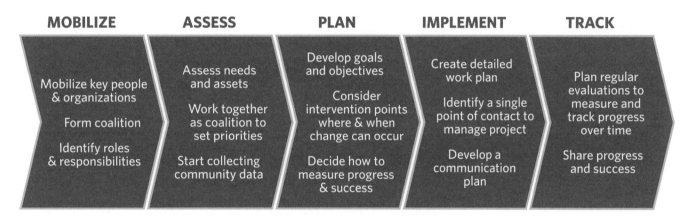

**FIGURE 3.4** Community Planning Process: MAP-IT
*Source:* Adapted from MAP-IT (CDC, n.d.-a)

## TABLE 3.6 Community-Assessment Guide

### Part I: Defining Target Population

- *Entire Population of a Geographic Area:* Population by census track, community, county, state, country
- *Sub-Population or Aggregate:* Population who share common character (i.e., ethnic, cultural or religious group, age or developmental stage, common health risk [potential or actual])
- *Population of Interest:* Population who is essentially healthy but could improve factors that promote or protect health (MDH, 2001)
- *Population at Risk:* Population with a common identified risk factor or risk exposure that poses a threat to health (MDH, 2001)

### Part II: Identifying Population Health Status

**Levels of Health and Illness**
- Birth and Death (Mortality) Rates
- Accidents and Injuries: accidental, intentional, homicide, and suicide
- Communicable and Infectious Disease Incidence and Prevalence Rates
- Acute and Chronic Disease Rates (physical, mental)

**Health Risk Behaviors (may also be listed under Behavioral Health Determinants)**
- Rates of smoking or chewing, drinking, drug use, obesity, drinking and driving, sexual behaviors and unprotected sex, use of seatbelts and helmets, interpersonal abuse, participation in antisocial or illegal behaviors

Levels of Independence by age, gender, health status, socioeconomic status

Levels of Life Satisfaction by age, gender, health status, socioeconomic status

*(continues)*

**TABLE 3.6  Community-Assessment Guide**  *(continued)*

### Part III: Assessing Population Determinants of Health

*Population Biological and Genetic Factors*

■ Population at last census and population changes in last decade

■ Demographics: Age, gender, race, and ethnicity (may use population pyramids)

■ Physical characteristics

■ Genetic factors

■ Health conditions: Acute and chronic

*Physical Environment Factors*

■ Natural Environment: Geography, climate, weather, air and water and other natural resources, agriculture, animal life, urban, rural, suburban

■ Built Environment: Infrastructure of community (roads, bridges, transportation, public spaces, and recreational areas), public, and governmental buildings; housing stock and density; industries and workplaces; educational and religious facilities; healthcare facilities; shopping and entertainment; accessibility; and environmental adaptation

**Social Environmental Factors: Social Actions and Social Patterns**

*Population Behavioral Patterns*

■ History of the community

■ Social, economic, and political patterns

■ Socioeconomic status (income, poverty), education, employment, and work patterns

■ Housing and living arrangements

■ Lifestyle patterns

■ Cultural patterns, diversity, and religious affiliations

■ Community roles and engagement

■ Language

■ Health insurance

■ Health literacy

■ Health-seeking behaviors

■ Health-limiting behaviors

■ Patterns of coping and resilience

■ Patterns of conformity and nonconformity

*Community Systems (Institutions)*

■ Cultural and ethnic organizations

■ Education (public, private, religious)

■ Commerce and job opportunities

■ Media and forms of communication including mail delivery, phone, radio, television, and Internet

■ Libraries and public information

■ Governmental systems and services: public health and social services; police and protective services; environmental services (water, air quality, sanitation, waste management, recycling services, vector control); emergency preparedness and response

■ Laws, regulations, ordinances

■ Community safety net programs (public and private)

■ Community support systems (formal and informal)

■ Community networks, coalitions

■ Health services and health services access (physical, mental, chemical, dental, pharmaceutical)

*Access to Healthcare*

Assessing the "7 A's of Access"

(Truglio-Londrigan & Lewenson, 2013, p. 93)

1. Is the individual, family, or population *aware* of its needs and the services available in the community?

2. Can the individual, family, or population gain *access* to the services it needs?

3. Are services *available* and convenient for the individual, family, or population in terms of time, location, and place for use?

4. How *affordable* are the services for the individual, family, or population?

5. Are the services *acceptable* to the individual, family, or population in terms of choice, satisfaction, and congruency with cultural values and beliefs?

6. How *appropriate* are the services for the individual, family, or population?

7. Are the services *adequate* in terms of quantity or degree for the individual, family, or population?

### Part IV: Analysis of Population Health Data

■ Summarize the population demographics and health status

■ Summarize the physical and social environmental factors

■ Identify the major protective factors for population health

■ Identify the major risk factors for population health

■ Identify the key health disparities within the population as a whole and between sub-groups

## Windshield Survey

The *windshield survey* is a first look at a community through a car's windshield. Observers are asked to use their senses (sight, hearing, and smell) to learn about a community as they drive, walk, or use public transportation to get around the community. They then make observations about the physical and social environments and the natural and built environments. The windshield survey is sometimes referred to as a familiarization survey because it helps establish the community context of care for PHNs. It can also be an initial step to a more comprehensive community assessment by raising awareness of issues for further exploration. Table 3.7 includes a list of questions you might ask yourself to help guide your windshield survey and analyze your findings.

Other types of windshield surveys may also be carried out, such as environmental hazard surveys (see Chapter 5) and walkability surveys to assess areas not accessible by car such as sidewalks, paths, parks, playgrounds, campuses, and malls.

### TABLE 3.7  Windshield Survey—Snapshot of Community Assessment

**Windshield Survey**

The first steps of a windshield survey require identifying the community boundaries and determining whether you will conduct the survey by car, by public transportation, or partially on foot to determine feasibility of your possible travel routes. It is best to conduct the survey in pairs or as a group. As you drive or ride through the community, pay careful attention to as many characteristics of the community as possible. You may wish to take photos or videotape your windshield survey. Make sure that you are only taking photos of people in public places. Be sensitive to the privacy of others; avoid taking pictures of people where they could be identified.

- Which resources/assets do you see available in the community? Resources may include libraries, clinics, thriving local businesses, and other features that may provide support to community members.
- Which types of services for families do you see in the community?
- Are there other organizations, such as youth centers, churches, or Head Start programs that might provide activities for children/families?
- Where do people live in the community? Is the housing primarily single-family housing or apartments? What is the condition of the housing?
- What types of jobs are available in the community? Would these jobs likely be held by people in the area?
- Where do people shop? Which types of stores are available: locally owned or chain stores?
- How do people get around in the community? Is public transportation available?
- What do you notice about ethnic diversity in the community? Which age range seems predominant?
- What is the geographic environment? Which types of opportunities are available for exercise? Are parks available? Is there green space?
- Which options are available for eating out?
- What did you learn about the health status of population groups in the community that augments published population health data?
- Where can people go for healthcare services?
- Based on your observations, what would you identify as assets in this community?
- Overall, how did you feel about being in the community (e.g., safe, comfortable, uneasy)?

**Reflection and Analysis Questions**

- What is the story of each photo you have taken? What do the photos tell you about the life and health of the community?
- What are the community's outstanding assets? Is there a relationship between these assets and the health of the community?
- What appear to be the community's major challenges? Is there a relationship between these challenges and the health of the community?
- What do you see as the most striking characteristic about the community? Would this characteristic influence your approach to providing care to the community?
- What did you find to be the most unexpected? Would the unexpected be an asset or a challenge to providing care to the community?

*Source:* Modified from Hargate, 2013

### EVIDENCE EXAMPLE 3.4
**Windshield Survey**

A total of 284 windshield surveys were carried out by nursing students in Mexico, New Zealand, Norway, Turkey, and the United States. The Omaha System Problem Classification Scheme was used to evaluate the windshield survey data. The students were able to input the community-assessment data into electronic records using an online checklist of 11 Omaha System problems. This framework for collecting and analyzing community data was found to be an effective teaching-learning tool for students.

*Source: Kerr et al., 2016*

## PHN Assessment at the Systems Level of Practice

Systems are part of the social environmental category of health determinants. Systems can be assessed to determine their ability to respond to public health priorities in the community. Systems that PHNs interact with on an ongoing basis include healthcare systems; public and governmental agencies; schools and school systems; community health and social service agencies; local and state governments, including elected and appointed officials; insurance companies; and faith-based organizations. PHNs assess systems to identify the extent to which they can meet community health needs and, if gaps exist, to identify the additional resources that are needed. Kristi's discussion about the local Catholic church, the Salvation Army, and county public health nurses working together demonstrates how public-private partnerships can often fill the gap when one organization cannot meet the need alone.

*Kristi and her fellow students find that two organizations in the community are interested in developing some outreach services to pregnant and parenting teens: a local Catholic church and the Salvation Army. She asks her PHN preceptor if two such different organizations might be able to work together.*

*Beth advises, "You might want to divide your group of four students into two and ask each pair to assess one of the organizations. You would want to look at their values, goals, resources, and willingness to work with each other.*

*If you find common ground based on an interest in helping pregnant and parenting teens, then you can arrange a meeting of the two organizations. You could let them know that the PHNs in our agency would be willing to help them."*

*Kristi responds, "Wow! We might be able to do something valuable for the community while we are carrying out our clinical assignment. I am going to call my classmates and set up a meeting to get started. Thanks."*

## Identifying Community Health Priorities

PHNs employed in governmental public health agencies are accountable to the public for the health priorities they select, the populations they serve, and the services they provide (see Chapter 7). PHNs consciously make the connection between the health needs of the community as a whole and the health needs of individuals and families within the community. The priority health needs identified through the community-assessment process help PHNs determine the most vulnerable and underserved populations in their communities and target those with greatest need for services.

PHNs also identify health priorities in the community by determining health and illness patterns among their individual clients and families by aggregating data on all the families whom their agency serves. PHNs look at multiple interacting health determinants, including the social determinants of health, to identify population health patterns and causes when working with individual clients and community partners (Monsen, Swenson, & Kerr, 2016; Monsen, Brandt et al., 2017; Monsen, Swenson, Klotzbach, Mathiason, & Johnson, 2017). PHNs also conduct research to identify health concerns in known vulnerable populations. For example, a study of early care and education programs identified the following health needs of the centers and enrolled children: hygiene and hand-washing; sanitation and disinfection; supervision; and safety of indoor and outdoor equipment (Alkon, Rose, Wolff, Kotch, & Aronson, 2016). PHNs can determine community health priorities by reviewing the community-assessment data to determine which health problems have the greatest potential for harm and have effective interventions. Questions to consider when establishing health priorities are listed in Table 3.8.

PHNs are ever-vigilant community watchers who are often the first to notice when a new health concern emerges or when a service gaps exists in the community. An example of a health concern identified by a PHN intake nurse, explored by agency staff, and taken to a group of community partners for a systems-level intervention is found in Evidence Example 3.5.

## TABLE 3.8  Determining Community Health Priorities

1. What is the incidence and prevalence of major diseases, health risk behaviors, and health concerns in the community (e.g., heart disease, teen pregnancy, drinking and driving, smoking, depression, influenza)?

2. What are the major causes of death and disability in the community (e.g., heart attacks, stroke, cancer, dementia, car accidents, and homicide)?

3. Which populations in the community are most affected by these health problems (health disparities)?

4. What are the major health risks in the community (e.g., obesity, air pollution, homes with lead-based paint, seasonal flooding, homelessness, lack of health insurance)? Consider level of risk and proportion of population affected. What are the key social determinants of health affecting vulnerable populations in the community?

5. Which health needs are met by community resources?

6. Which health needs are not met?

7. Are affordable and effective interventions available for these health needs?

8. Who is responsible for meeting these health needs?

9. Rank order priorities by level of risk or hazard to community population or sub-populations.

## EVIDENCE EXAMPLE  3.5
### Determining Population Needs in a Rural/Suburban County

The intake nurse at the public health agency was responsible for logging referrals and conversations of significant public health concern. The agency she worked at was small and lacked an on-site physician or walk-in clinic services. It was a 50-mile drive to the larger metropolitan community where low-cost clinics were available. An analysis of the monthly logs included calls from uninsured adults with a variety of acute and chronic healthcare conditions. The intake nurse found a trend of increasing numbers of working adults lacking access to care. She compiled a brief report summarizing two months of log entries and presented it to her public health director. At the next community partner committee meeting with local medical clinics and hospitals, the director shared the intake nurse's report. After consulting with other community partners, the committee proposed establishing a nursing center. The hospital agreed to fund the part-time center staffed by a PHN for one afternoon a week for two years. Services focused on screening, referrals, and health promotion. A review of client data after several months identified a need for limited physician services. A local medical clinic offered to see patients referred by the nursing center free of charge. Another healthcare provider purchased a mobile health unit to do mammography outreach. The committee worked with this provider to use the mobile unit to visit several community sites on a monthly basis. These services were the direct result of systems-level collaboration and advocacy for those lacking access to healthcare.

*Source:* Kleinfehn-Wald, 2010

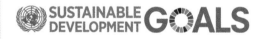 SUSTAINABLE DEVELOPMENT GOALS

**Decline in Child Mortality**

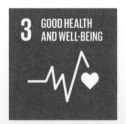
**3** GOOD HEALTH AND WELL-BEING

**GOAL 3**  Significant progress has been made in reducing child mortality. In 2015, the mortality rate for children under age 5 worldwide was 43 deaths per 1,000 live births—a 44% reduction since 2000. This translates to 5.9 million under-5 deaths in 2015, down from 9.8 million in 2000. But despite progress in every region, wide disparities persist. Sub-Saharan Africa continues to have the highest under-5 mortality rate, with 84 deaths per 1,000 live births in 2015—about twice the global average.

Children are most vulnerable in the first 28 days of life (the neonatal period). To reduce child deaths even further, greater attention must be focused on this crucial period, where progress has not been as rapid. In 2015, the global neonatal mortality rate was 19 deaths per 1,000 live births, a 37% reduction since 2000. This means that, in 2015, about 2.7 million children died in the first month of life. Neonatal mortality remains highest in Central and Southern Asia and in sub-Saharan Africa: 29 deaths per 1,000 live births in 2015 in both regions.

The share of newborn deaths in all under-5 deaths grew from 40% in 2000 to 45% in 2015, due to the slower pace of progress among newborns. It is estimated that 40% of neonatal deaths could be prevented by providing high-quality care for both mother and baby around the time of birth (United Nations, n.d.).

Public health diagnoses for populations are often written as population risk diagnoses. The traditional risk diagnoses have four components: health risk, population at-risk, modifiable risk factors, and bio-statistical data. This traditional population risk diagnosis has been modified to create an asset-based risk diagnosis by adding the component of modifiable protective factors (see Table 3.9). This approach helps to build on existing community resources and involve community members when creating an intervention plan.

If you wish to write an asset-based public health risk diagnosis using the Omaha System taxonomy, you would include Domain, Problem, and Signs/Symptoms in the health risk area and could use the KBS ratings as a way to measure outcomes. The category of Problem as discussed in Chapter 2 may also be used to identify strengths.

## Public Health Nursing Community Action Plan

When the PHN is working with the community, the planning process and intervention process involves an interprofessional team and key community members. After the team has established priorities and formulated clear statements of the health priorities to be addressed, it is time to determine goals. Community goals are based on community values, beliefs, and the willingness of community members and elected and appointed officials to make changes; the resources available; and a consensus of what is achievable in the given time frame. Specific outcomes are then established. An example of a goal and an outcome for a community follow (sometimes the words *goal* and *outcome* are used interchangeably):

- Goal: Reduce obesity in our community
- Outcome: Reduce obesity in adults in our community by 10% by 2020

## Population Health Goals

The United States has established population health goals each decade since 1990. The purpose of the goals is to encourage communities to work together to improve the health of their citizens and to empower individuals to make better health decisions (U.S. Department of Health and Human Services [U.S. DHHS], 2010). These measurable outcomes, called *health status indicators,* are determined by reviewing existing population health outcomes, comparing specific population outcomes with outcomes from other populations, and analyzing evidence from the literature on acceptable outcomes. They are time-specific and stated as a percent. For example, scientific evidence suggests that obesity is a risk factor for many diseases, so reduction of obesity in adults within the U.S. population by 2020 would be a positive health outcome. Healthy People 2020 was based in part on the level of achievement of Healthy People 2010 goals (Reinberg, 2010; U.S. Department of Health and Human Services [U.S. DHHS], 2010). Healthy People 2030 will be based on the population progress toward achievement of Healthy People 2020 goals. Evidence Example 3.6 illustrates the ongoing monitoring of level of achievement of Healthy People 2020 goals.

**TABLE 3.9  Asset-Based Public Health Population Risk Diagnosis**

| Components | Example |
| --- | --- |
| Health risk | **Increased risk of** infection (pertussis) |
| Population at risk | **Among** nonimmunized or partially immunized infants and children in (specify geographic area, community, or county) |
| Modifiable risk factors | **Related to** contact with nonimmunized children and adults who may have pertussis, health beliefs opposing childhood immunizations, knowledge deficit about benefits of immunization, lack of access to health resources |
| Modifiable Protective Factors | **Related to** increased funding for outreach and immunizations to at-risk populations through the public health department, coalition with local religious organizations and safety net organizations to immunize children. |
| Bio-statistical data (for geographic area, community, city, county, state, national) | **As evidenced by** lack of herd immunity (80–90% immunization) in preschool population (state immunization rate) in (geographic area or city, county, state, country) with (insert number of cases) reported cases of pertussis in the last month in infants and children ages (insert age range). |

### EVIDENCE EXAMPLE 3.6
**Healthy People 2020 Goals**

A mid-decade review of progress toward Healthy People 2020 goals identified that Healthy People 2020 goals would be more modest than the 2010 goals. Only 19% of Healthy People 2010 goals were met, and progress was made on only 52% of them. Some, like obesity, had become worse since 2000. U.S. obesity rates increased from 25% to 34% between 2000 and 2010 (Reinberg, 2010), and the prevalence of obesity in the U.S. was 35.6% between 2011 and 2014 (CDC, 2015).

🌐 **Online Activity**

Go to Healthy People 2020 and study a goal of interest to you.

- Identify an objective and then click "National Snapshots" to see how progress has been made on that goal.

- Go to the "Interventions & Resources" tab to find evidence of interventions that have been effective in working to achieve this goal.

Public health nurses and other public health professionals use Healthy People goals as well as their community-assessment data to establish organizational and program goals for their communities and the clients they serve. The focus in Public Health is primary prevention; however, PHNs will include secondary and tertiary prevention goals when appropriate to meet unmet community needs. PHNs often work at more than one level of practice simultaneously. For example, if there is a primary prevention goal to reduce childhood obesity, the PHNs might do the following.

- **Community Level:** Collaborate with local television stations to have a media campaign to increase community level of awareness for the need to increase children's activity levels and to develop more afterschool sports and activity programs for children.

- **Systems Level:** Consult with schools to increase the physical activities of students within the curriculum.

- **Individual/family Level:** Provide health education and counseling to children and families to empower them to develop healthier lifestyles.

## The Public Health Nursing Community Intervention Plan

PHNs work collaboratively with multiple community partners to establish population health goals and to develop intervention plans. These plans need to be consistent with the demography, culture, and health status of the target population and be in language that is clear to interprofessional partners and the community. It may be more appropriate to label the plan a population health plan rather than a nursing care plan. However, the framework of the public health nursing process can be used effectively with interprofessional as well as lay groups. Public health interventions for population health:

- Modify the health determinant risk factors that are causing the population health problems or disparities by weakening or eliminating the risk factors

- Modify health determinant protective factors that will improve the ability of at-risk and vulnerable populations to better manage their own healthcare

## THEORY APPLICATION
### Population-Based Models for PHN Interventions and Outcomes

Twelve conceptual models of population-based PHN interventions and outcomes published between 1981 and 2003 were identified and compared (Bigbee & Issel, 2012). Four of the twelve models are very consistent with the PHN community assessment and intervention model presented in this chapter. The following table demonstrates how these models reflect essential components of this book's population-based PHN intervention plan.

| Model | Major Components | PHN Concepts |
|---|---|---|
| PHN Conceptual Model (White, 1982) | Determinants of health impacted by nursing process at individual/family, and population levels | PHN process, levels of practice, determinants of health, PHN interventions, outcomes |
| Community as Partner Model (Anderson & McFarlane, 1988, 2011) | Based on Neuman's systems model and includes assessment wheel and interventions based on Intervention Wheel | PHN process, levels of prevention, PH interventions from the Intervention Wheel, outcomes |
| Public Health Intervention Model (Keller-Olson et al., 1998) | Population-based model including 17 interventions at individual, community, and systems levels | Population focus, levels of practice, interventions, interprofessional aspects |
| LA Public Health Nursing Practice Model–LA Model (Smith & Bazini-Barakat, 2003) | Population-based model using nursing process to address health indicators using Intervention Wheel | PHN process, population focus, levels of practice, interventions from Intervention Wheel, outcomes, interprofessional aspects, client participation |

*Source:* Abstracted from Bigbee & Issel, 2012

The Public Health Nursing Community Intervention Plan includes the following components:

- Public health asset-based population risk diagnosis
- Population health goal and level of prevention focus
- Client focus: individual/family, community, system
- SMART behavioral outcomes that are measurable and attainable and understandable to the family. SMART outcomes are:
  - **S**pecific: What needs to be accomplished?
  - **M**easurable: How will the nurse, client, and family know the goal has been met?
  - **A**ttainable: Can the goal be met with the resources available?
  - **R**ealistic: Does the client (and family) have the physical, emotional, and mental capacity to meet the goal?
  - **T**ime-Bound: When will the goal be achieved?
- **Evidence-Based Public Health Interventions:** Public Health Intervention Wheel (Keller, Strohschein, Lia-Hoagberg, & Schaffer, 2004; refer to Chapter 2) or Omaha System (Omaha System, 2017) interventions may be used. Include the intervention, the strategy or process to be used, and the provider(s) of the intervention
- **Evidence-Based Rationale** for each intervention: Include the scientific rationale with citations as well as population preferences
- **Evaluation of Outcomes:** Use quantitative measures to determine the progress made toward achievement of the outcome. These measures to be used should be selected during the planning process.

Implementing population-based interventions in a community often includes collaborative efforts of many providers, organizations, and community members. Usually, a core team develops the implementation plan timeline and selects or designs public health intervention strategies. For example, if social marketing is selected for a program to encourage parents to have their children immunized, potential strategies could be billboards, development of online and printed media, and radio and television adds or other forms of media. It would be important to know when the best time (i.e., window of opportunity) would be to start a social marketing campaign and where (before school starts in the fall, during spring preschool enrollment, etc.).

> *Kristi and her classmates complete an assessment of the sub-population of pregnant and parenting teens in their community and identify an unmet need for a pregnant and parenting peer support group. They work with a group of local churches and the Salvation Army to plan a community-wide outreach effort with the Salvation Army for the meeting site. The church groups and local high school are ready to start recruiting teen participants. They work with Kristi's preceptor, Beth, to identify the best time to recruit teens and start the program. They decide to recruit teens at the time the pregnancy is confirmed, and decide that the beginning of the next school year is a good time to launch the program.*

---

## EVIDENCE EXAMPLE 3.7

### Evaluation of a Home Visiting Program for Pregnant and Parenting Teens

After interventions are implemented, it is necessary to assess the effectiveness of the program and the progress of the target population toward goal and outcome achievement.

Four commonly used public health evaluation methods identified by Spiegelman (2016) are:

- **Feasibility evaluation:** Assess whether something will work and be effective in the "real world"
- **Impact evaluation:** Assess the efficacy and effectiveness of an intervention on health outcomes

- **Program evaluation:** Assess a program's processes to improve them (quality improvement approach)
- **Comparative effectiveness:** Assess and compare interventions to see which work best for whom, in what situations, and from a cost-effectiveness perspective

The Pregnant and Parenting Teen program, discussed in Evidence Example 3.8, demonstrates the effectiveness of using all four of these evaluation methods.

### EVIDENCE EXAMPLE 3.8

**PHN Home Visiting Program for Pregnant and Parenting Teens**

A visiting nurse association created and implemented a Pregnant and Parenting Teen Program to promote family and child health and family self-sufficiency for teen moms 19 years of age or younger. The pillars of the program are: a trusting relationship between the PHN and the teen; outreach and coordination with schools, clinics, and human service agencies; a comprehensive and intensive maternal mental health curriculum; and community support and caring by provision of needed resources. A comprehensive evaluation of the program's effectiveness and client outcomes's success was completed after two years (Schaffer, Goodhue, Stennes, & Lanigan, 2012). Key outcomes presented by four public health evaluation methods follow.

- **Feasibility evaluation:** 78% of the teens referred to the program accepted the services.

- **Impact evaluation:** 76% of teens with 10 or more visits continued or graduated high school compared to 56% of teens who received 9 visits or less; 97% were up-to-date on well-child check-ups; 95% were up-to-date on immunizations; and 96% had healthy birth weight babies.

- **Program evaluation:** 69% referred to community resources; 47% received needed resources.

- **Comparative effectiveness:** Teens with 10 or more visits were more successful in achieving expected outcomes than teens who had 9 or fewer visits.

*Kristi asks her neighbor, a county commissioner, if she would help to find funds for the pregnant and parenting teen peer support group that will be held at the Salvation Army. The group needs funding for transportation for the teens and their babies to attend a support group meeting once a week for 6 months. The commissioner asked Kristi if she has data to support the need for transportation services. Kristi assures her that she does. There are 20 teens interested in joining such a group, and only two of them have transportation. Although the local bus service has a stop only a block away from the Salvation Army, only five of the girls are on a bus line. That leaves 13 teens without transportation. In addition, the PHNs have assessed all the teens and have data that support the need for socialization and peer group support for these pregnant and parenting teens. The commissioner is not sure if these teens can make a commitment to attend the group or if attending the group would really make a difference. Kristi tells the commissioner that PHNs from the county are going to be group facilitators and would be using the Problem Rating Scale for Outcomes to determine if the outreach and counseling efforts are effective. Of course, she has to explain to the commissioner what the Problem Rating Scale for Outcomes is! The commissioner asks Kristi and her classmates to come to a council meeting to present their proposal. Kristi says they can do that and she will also ask her PHN preceptor to come to the meeting.*

## Ethical Application

Community assessment and program evaluation involves collecting data on individuals. These data are then aggregated to provide for confidentiality and anonymity. However, when the group size is small or the members of the group are easily identified, ethical issues related to privacy rights can arise.

*Kristi is concerned because there are only 20 teens who will be participating in the initial pregnant and parenting teen peer support program. Most of these teens are well known in the community. She is worried that when the program evaluation occurs, the teens will be evaluated as individuals. Even though their outcome data will be aggregated, it will be difficult to provide for anonymity if there is a need to present program outcomes to the county commissioners.*

Use the ethical framework in Table 3.10 to determine how you would use ethical principles to make decisions about this ethical problem.

**TABLE 3.10 Ethical Application of the Nursing Process in Public Health Nursing**

| Ethical Perspective | Application |
|---|---|
| Rule Ethics (principles) | ■ Respect the rights of individuals related to privacy, autonomy, and self-determination. <br> ■ Critique selected actions and interventions for possible unintended harmful consequences that might occur for diverse populations in a community. <br> ■ Select interventions that promote justice through reducing health disparities. |
| Virtue Ethics (character) | ■ Maintain the dignity and confidentiality of individuals, families, populations, and communities when assessing their health needs. <br> ■ Be honest in communicating the purpose of selected interventions to individuals, families, populations, and communities. <br> ■ Be an advocate for assessing the public health needs of vulnerable populations. |
| Feminist Ethics (reducing oppression) | ■ Include voices of vulnerable populations in community assessments and in setting priorities for action. <br> ■ Emphasize the contribution of the assets that communities and diverse populations bring to resolving public health concerns. |

Table based on work by Volbrecht (2002) and Racher (2007)

## KEY POINTS

- PHNs are accountable to the individuals and families they serve, and the communities in which they live and work, to take action to maintain or improve their health status.

- PHNs work in partnership with individuals, families, communities, and systems.

- The public health nursing process is used to assess and intervene with individuals, families, communities, and systems.

- PHNs collect demographic and health determinant data when carrying out family and community assessments.

- PHNs use public health nursing interventions to provide nursing services to individuals, families, communities, and systems.

- PHNs use EHRs and HIS to assist them in assessing and monitoring their clients' health status, evaluating their clients' progress, and determining the effectiveness of interventions and programs. The Omaha System is the only ANA-recognized standardized terminology that has integrated those components.

## REFLECTIVE PRACTICE

It is difficult for public health nursing students to adapt to providing nursing care in the unstructured environment of the home and community. When students are in family homes, they are visitors in someone else's personal space. Visits often do not go as planned. It takes time to develop trust with family members who may initially be uncomfortable with a nurse in their home. Think about Kristi's co-visits with her PHN preceptor Beth to Sara, the pregnant teen, and her mother and then the individual visit Kristi made to complete the home environmental assessment. If you were making that visit alone as Kristi was, consider how you would carry out the home environmental assessment with Sara and her mother.

- How would you prepare for the visit? What would you wear? Do you think you should phone Patricia or Sara to confirm the visit?

- How would you introduce yourself to Sara and her mother and review the purpose of the visit?

- This is your first visit alone with Sara and her mother. Think about what makes a good first visit. What would you want to do to make your visit a good one?

- When you carry out the home environmental assessment, you will probably be going into some private areas of the home. What can you do to make Sara, her mother, and yourself comfortable in these private spaces?

- What will you do if you are told you cannot go into certain rooms?

- Will you share your assessment of the family home environment as you conduct the assessment, or will you wait until the end of the visit?

- How will you end the visit with Sara and her mother?

## APPLICATION OF EVIDENCE

Think about the community assessment you and your classmates are going to complete. You are interested in determining the need for and the resources for a teen pregnant and parenting peer support group. Your assessment is going to be assessing a sub-group of the community (i.e., aggregate), so you need to think about whom you will want to work with and what data you need to collect.

Review Figure 3.4 (Community Planning Process: MAP-IT):

1. How would you use this tool to plan a community assessment?

2. How would you carry out the community assessment?

3. When you develop your intervention plan, you need to consider your "window of opportunity" for implementation. How would you find your "window of opportunity"?

4. The implementation phase requires a detailed work plan. What would you include in your work plan?

5. The tracking phase includes measuring the effectiveness of your intervention plan. How would you measure the effectiveness of your plan?

6. Review Evidence Example 3.7. What type of evaluation would you want to include? What measures might you use?

Review the Community-Assessment Guide. This is an aggregate assessment. You do not have to collect all of the community data. Think about what you need:

1. What community demographic data would you want to collect?

2. What biological and genetic health determinant data would you want to collect?

3. What physical environmental health determinant data would you need?

4. What social environmental health determinant data would be most important?

5. How would you collect information about healthcare access?

6. Once you have all of your data collected, how would you analyze it?

7. What would be effective methods to communicate your community-assessment data to others?

## References

Alkon, A., Rose, R., Wolf, M., Kotch, J., & Aronson, S. (2016). Health and safety checklist for early care and education programs to assess key national health and safety standards. *Maternal and Child Health Journal, 20*, 114–127. doi:10.1007/s10995-015-1809-8

Allen, B., Soderberg, K., & Laventure, M. (2017). Connecting community data for population health: Supporting use of EHR data for community health assessments. *NACCHO Voice*. Retrieved from https://nacchovoice.naccho.org/2017/06/22/connecting-community-data-for-population-health-supporting-use-of-ehr-data-for-community-health-assessments/

American Nurses Association. (2013). *Public health nursing: Scope and standards of practice*. Silver Spring, MD: Author.

American Nurses Association. (2015). *Inclusion of recognized terminologies supporting nursing practice within EHRs and other health information technology solutions*. Retrieved from https://www.aorn.org/-/media/aorn/guidelines/position-statements/posstat-endorsed-ehr-hit-terminologies.pdf

Bigbee, J. L., & Issel, M. (2012). Conceptual models for population-focused public health nursing interventions and outcomes: The state of the art. *Public Health Nursing, 29*(4), 370–379. doi:10.1111/j.1525-1446.2011.0100.x

Carter, B., & McGoldrick, M. (2005). *The expanded family life cycle: Individual, family, and social perspectives* (3rd ed.). Boston, MA: Allyn & Bacon.

Centers for Disease Control and Prevention. (n.d.-a). *MAP-IT: A guide to using Healthy People 2020 in your community*. Retrieved from http://www.healthypeople.gov/2020/implement/MapIt.aspx

Centers for Disease Control and Prevention. (n.d.-b). *Public health 101 series: Introduction to public health informatics*. Retrieved from https://www.cdc.gov/publichealth101/documents/introduction-to-public-health-informatics.pdf

Centers for Disease Control and Prevention. (2015). *Prevalence of obesity among adults and youth: US 2011–2014*. Retrieved from https://www.cdc.gov/nchs/data/databriefs/db219.pdf

Clark, M. J. (2008). *Community health nursing*. Upper Saddle River, NJ: Pearson/Prentice Hall.

Eriksson, I., & Nilsson, K. (2008). Preconditions needed for establishing a trusting relationship during health counseling—An interview study. *Journal of Clinical Nursing, 17*(17), 2352–2359.

Friedman, M. M., Bowden, V. R., & Jones, E. (2003). *Family nursing: Research, theory, and practice* (5th ed.). Hoboken, NJ: Pearson Education, Inc.

Gardner, A. (2010). Therapeutic friendliness and the development of therapeutic leverage by mental health nurses in community rehabilitation settings. *Contemporary Nurse, 34*(2), 140–148.

Hargate, C. (2013). *Survey*. Unpublished manuscript, Bethel University, St. Paul, MN.

Henry Street Consortium. (2017). *Entry-level population-based public health nursing competencies.* St. Paul, MN: Author. Retrieved from www.henrystreetconsortium.org

Hunt, R. (2013). *Introduction to community-based nursing.* Philadelphia, PA: Wolters Kluwer Health/Lippincott Williams and Williams.

Jansson, A., Petersson, K., & Uden, G. (2001). Nurses' first encounters with parents of new-born children—Public health nurses' views of a good meeting. *Journal of Clinical Nursing, 10,* 140–151.

Kaakinen, J. R., Coehlo, D. P., Steele, R., & Robinson, M. (2018). *Family health care nursing: Theory, practice, and research* (6th ed.). Philadelphia, PA: F. A. Davis.

Keller, L. O., Strohschein, S., Lia-Hoagberg, B., & Schaffer, M. A. (2004). Population-based public health interventions: Practice-based and evidence-supported. Part I. *Public Health Nursing, 21*(5), 453–468.

Kerr, M. J., Flaten, C., Honey, M. L., Gargantua-Aguila, S. D. R., Nahcivan, N. O., Martin, K. S., & Monsen, K. A. (2016). Feasibility of using the Omaha System for community-level observations. *Public Health Nursing, 33*(3), 256–263. doi:10.1111/phn.12231

Kleinfehn-Wald, N. (2010). *Determining population needs in a rural/suburban county.* Unpublished manuscript, Scott County Public Health, Shakopee, MN.

LaVenture, M. (2008). *Building public health/clinical health information exchanges: The Minnesota experience. PHDHC, HRSA Panel* [PowerPoint]. Minnesota Department of Health, St. Paul, MN. Retrieved from http://www.google.com/url?sa=t&rct=j&q=&esrc=s&source=web&cd=8&ved=0ahUKEwiPq_TSwvvXAhXszIMKHRv_CVwQFghWMAc&url=http%3A%2F%2Fwww.phdsc.org%2Fabout%2Fcommittees%2Fpresentations%2FPHDSC_HRSA_Panel_%2520Marty_LaVenture.ppt&usg=AOvVaw23pM-1bJ1ZQ96G_krsLMNx

Marshall, A., Bell, J., & Moules, N. (2010). Beliefs, suffering, and healing: A clinical practice model for families experiencing mental illness. *Perspectives in Psychiatric Care, 46*(3), 197–208. doi:10.1111/j.1744-6163.2010.00259x

Martin, K. S. (2005). *The Omaha System: A key to practice, documentation, and information management* (2nd ed.). Omaha, NE: Health Connections Press.

Martin, K. S., Monsen, K. A., & Bowles, K. H. (2011). The Omaha System and meaningful use: Applications for practice, education, and research. *CIN: Computers, Informatics, Nursing, 29*(1), 52–58. doi:10.1097/NCN.0b013e3181f9ddc6

McCann, T. V., & Baker, H. (2001). Mutual relating: Developing interpersonal relationships in the community. *Journal of Advanced Nursing, 34*(4), 530–537.

McNaughton, D. B. (2005). A naturalistic test of Peplau's theory in home visiting. *Public Health Nursing, 22*(5), 429–438.

Meiers, S. J. (2016). Using family theory to guide nursing practice. In S. Denham, S. Eggenberger, P. Young, & N. Krumwiede (Eds.), *Family-focused nursing care.* Philadelphia, PA: F. A. Davis.

Meiers, S. J., Krumwiede, N. K., Denham, S. A., & Bell, S. E. (2016). Family assessment. In S. Denham, S. Eggenberger, P. Young, & N. Krumwiede (Eds.), *Family-focused nursing care.* Philadelphia, PA: F. A. Davis.

Minnesota Department of Health. (2001). *Public health interventions: Application for public health nursing practice.* St. Paul, MN: Author. Retrieved from http://www.health.state.mn.us/divs/opi/cd/phn/docs/0301wheel_manual.pdf

Minnesota Department of Health, Center for Public Health Nursing Practice. (2003). The nursing process applied to population-based public health nursing practice. Retrieved from http://www.health.state.mn.us/divs/opi/cd/phn/docs/0303phn_processapplication.pdf

Minnesota Department of Health. (2015). Recommendations regarding the use of standard nursing terminologies in Minnesota, 2014. Retrieved from http://www.health.state.mn.us/e-health/standards/docs/nursingterminology082114.pdf

Monsen, K. A., Brandt, J. K., Brueshoff, B., Chi, C. L., Mathiason, M. A., Swenson, S. M., & Thorson, D. R. (2017). Social determinants and health disparities associated with outcomes of women of childbearing age receiving public health nurse home visiting services. *Journal of Obstetric and Gynecological Neonatal Nursing, 46*(2), 292–303. doi:10.1016/j.jogn.2016.11.014.

Monsen, K. A., Swenson, S. M., & Kerr, M. J. (2016). The perceptions of public health nurses on using standardized care plans to translate evidence-based guidelines into family home visiting practice. *Kontakt, 18*(2), e75–e83. doi:10.1016/j.kontakt.2016.04.001

Monsen, K. A., Swenson, S. M., Klotzbach, L., Mathiason, M. A., & Johnson, K. E. (2017). Empirical evaluation of change in public health nursing practice after implementation of an evidence-based family home visiting guideline. *Kontakt, 19*(2), e75–e85.

Monsen, K. A., Vanderboom, C. E., Olson, K. S., Larson, M. E., & Holland, D. E. (2017). Care coordination from a strengths perspective: A practice-based evidence evaluation of evidence-based practice. *Research and Theory for Nursing Practice, 31*(1), 39–55. doi:10.1891/1541-6577.31.1.39.

Nelson, R., & Staggers, N. (2018). *Health informatics: An interprofessional approach* (2nd ed.). St. Louis, MO: Elsevier.

Office of the National Coordinator for Health Information Technology. (2017). *Standard nursing terminologies: A landscape analysis.* Washington, DC: Author. Retrieved from https://www.healthit.gov/sites/default/files/snt_final_05302017.pdf

Omaha System. (2017). Omaha System website. Retrieved from http://www.omahasystem.org

Racher, F. (2007). The evolution of ethics for community practice. *Journal of Community Health Nursing, 24*(1), 65–76.

Reinberg, S. (2010). U.S. government sets new health goals for 2020. Retrieved from http://consumer.healthday.com/Article.asp?AID=646932

Rossiter, C., Fowler, C., Hopwood, N., Lee, A., & Dunston, R. (2011). Working in partnership with vulnerable families: The experience of child and family health practitioners. *Australian Journal of Primary Health, 17*(4), 378–383. doi:10.1071/PY11056

Schaffer, M. A., Goodhue, A., Stennes, K., & Lanigan, C. (2012). Evaluation of a public health nurse visiting program for pregnant and parenting teens. *Public Health Nursing, 29*(4), 218–231. doi:10.1111/j.1525-1446.2011.01005.x

Skemp, L. E., Dreher, M. C., & Asselin, M. (2006). *Healthy places, healthy people.* Indianapolis, IN: Sigma Theta Tau International.

Spiegelman, D. (2016). Evaluating public health interventions: 1. Examples, definitions, and a personal note. *American Journal of Public Health, 106*(1), 70–73. doi:10.2105/AJPH.2015.302923

Truglio-Londrigan, M., & Lewenson, S. B. (2013). *Public health nursing: Practicing population-based care.* Sudbury, MA: Jones and Bartlett.

United Nations. (n.d.). Goal 3: Ensure healthy lives and promote well-being for all at all ages. *Sustainable Development Goals.* Retrieved from https://unstats.un.org/sdgs/report/2017/goal-03/

U.S. Department of Health and Human Services. (2010). Introducing Healthy People 2020. Retrieved from http://www.healthypeople.gov/2020/about/default.aspx

Vance, E. A., & Fish, C. A. (2017). Omaha System case study. Personal correspondence from Karen S. Martin, Martin Associates, Omaha, NE. December 8, 2017.

Volbrecht, R. M. (2002). *Nursing ethics: Communities in dialogue.* Upper Saddle River, NJ: Pearson/Prentice Hall.

Wright, L. M., & Bell, J. M. (2009). *Beliefs and illness: A model for healing.* Calgary, Alberta, Canada: 4th Floor Press.

# Utilizes Basic Epidemiological (The Incidence, Distribution, and Control of Disease in a Population) Principles in Public Health Nursing Practice

■ **Carolyn M. Porta**

*with Noreen Kleinfehn-Wald, Linda J. W. Anderson, and Madeleine Kerr*

> *Elizabeth has worked as a public health nurse (PHN) doing home visits on the maternal child health team for approximately a year. One day as she is having lunch with her co-workers, someone mentions that an outbreak of pertussis had occurred in an adjacent county. In fact, there are 42 cases! Two days later, Elizabeth's supervisor asks whether she can help the Disease Prevention & Control (DP & C) team investigate 10 probable cases of pertussis.*
>
> *DP & C nurses operate the immunization clinic and work with infectious disease issues, such as tuberculosis. Other than these activities, Elizabeth knows very little of what their day-to-day work is like. Her supervisor explains that disease investigation is case management work. She will most likely not be required to do any additional home visits. (Sometimes follow-up visits are necessary when it is difficult to locate people.) She will need to plan on a limited amount of time to place phone calls, review records, and work with community partners, such as school nurses. Elizabeth agrees to take the additional assignment and arranges to receive orientation from the lead nurse. During this briefing, the lead nurse explains the state's data-privacy laws, the state health department's infectious disease reporting requirements for pertussis, and the report form that needs to be completed by the healthcare provider or the lab associated with the clinic for each suspect or confirmed case. This is a lot of new information!*

---

**ELIZABETH'S NOTEBOOK**

**COMPETENCY #2** Utilizes Basic Epidemiological (The Incidence, Distribution, and Control of Disease in a Population) Principles in Public Health Nursing Practice

A. Understands the relationship between community assessment and health promotion/disease prevention programs, especially the populations and programs with which the PHN works

B. Understands the relationships between risk/protective factors and health issues

C. Obtains and interprets information regarding risks and benefits to the community

D. Applies an epidemiological framework when assessing and intervening with communities, systems, individuals, and families

*Source:* Henry Street Consortium, 2017

(continues)

**ELIZABETH'S NOTEBOOK** *(continued)*

### USEFUL DEFINITIONS

**Agent:** The primary cause of the health-related condition. Agents are most often classified into six main types: physical agents, chemical agents, nutritive agents, infectious agents, genetic agents, and psychological agents (Valanis, 1999). [Note that the term *infectious agent* has been replaced with *causative factors* (Merrill, 2017, p. 11).]

**Communicability:** The ability of a disease to be transmitted from one person to the next; communicability is determined by how likely a pathogen or agent is to be transmitted from a diseased or infected person who is not immune and is susceptible (Merrill, 2017, p. 43).

**Environment:** Reflects the aggregate of those external conditions and influences affecting the life and development of an organism . . . physical, chemical, biological, and social factors that affect the health status of people (Merrill, 2017, p. 214); factors external to the human or animal that cause or allow transmission (p. 8).

**Epidemic:** Occurrence of cases of an illness, specific health-related behavior, or other health-related events clearly in excess of normal expectancy in a community or region (Merrill, 2017, p. 5).

**Epidemiological Triangle:** Shows the interaction and interdependence of the agent, host, environment, and time (Merrill, 2017, p. 8).

**Epidemiology:** The study of the distribution and determinants of health-related states or events in human populations and the application of this study to the prevention and control of health problems (*Stedman's Medical Dictionary for the Health Professions and Nursing* (5th ed.) in Merrill, 2017, p. 2).

**Herd Immunity:** Resistance a population has to the invasion and spread of an infectious disease. Herd immunity is accomplished when the number of susceptible people is reduced and the number of protected or non-susceptible people dominates the herd (population); provides barriers to direct transmission of the disease; occurs when 85% level of immunity exists (Merrill, 2017, p. 53).

**Host:** The human being affected by the particular condition under investigation. Factors that the host brings to the triangle include intrinsic factors (age, gender, race, etc.), physical and psychological factors, and the presence or absence of immunity (Clark, 2008). Host can be a human or animal that is susceptible to disease (Merrill, 2017, p. 8).

**Immunity:** The state of nonsusceptibility to a disease or condition. Types include (a) *active immunity*, where the host is exposed to the antigen through having the disease or via immunization; and (b) *passive immunity*, where antibodies are provided to the host via immune globulin or mother-to-fetus transfer across the placenta—passive immunity is short-lived (Merrill, 2017, p. 52).

**Incidence:** The number of individuals who develop the disease over a defined period of time (Le, 2001) or the number of new cases of a particular health-related state or event reported over a specific period of time (Merrill, 2017, p. 74).

**Life Course Epidemiology:** The study of long-term effects on later health or the risk of disease due to physical or social exposures during gestation, childhood, adolescence, young adulthood, and later adult life (Kuh, Ben-Shlomo, Lynch, Hallqvist, & Power, 2003, p. 778).

**Prevalence:** The presence of a disease or health condition in a given population at a given point in time divided by the number of persons in that population (Friis, 2018, p. 64).

**Protective Factor:** Health determinants that protect one from illness or assist in improving health (see Chapter 1).

**Risk Factor:** A condition that is associated with the increased probability of a health-related state or event (Merrill, 2017, p. 3). Risk factors are also health determinants (see Chapter 1).

**Surveillance:** The ongoing systematic collection, analysis, interpretation, and dissemination of health-related data to improve the health of populations (Centers for Disease Control and Prevention [CDC], 2001). Public health surveillance is the systematic ongoing collection, analysis, interpretation, and dissemination of health data (Merrill, 2017, p. 112).

## Using Data to Solve Health and Disease Mysteries

Nurses often want to know why something happens or does not happen. This inquisitive nature is useful when nurses are working to prevent something from happening or to intervene before something gets worse. In some situations, if questions are not asked, credible solutions might be overlooked, and health outcomes might not be optimal. In a worst-case scenario, lives might be lost or seriously harmed if the status quo is maintained and curious questions are not asked and acted upon. At the foundation of effective population-based public health nursing is the science of epidemiology. *Epidemiology* guides the questions that PHNs ask and the steps that they take to find answers and solutions. Following is a list of questions nurses ask or should ask regularly:

- When did the problem start (end, worsen, improve)?
- What has contributed to the change? Triggered a response?
- Why have x, y, z not improved?
- How did this occur?
- Who should be involved to contribute to the solution?
- Where are available resources to aid in addressing this situation?

- Which interventions can reduce the spread of this occurrence/disease?
- Will I be working at the individual/family, community, or systems level?
- Do I need to consider any ethical issues?
- How will I know whether the interventions are effective?
- What could have prevented this outcome?

At its core, epidemiology is the study of solving mysteries—of understanding where and to what extent diseases, events, and behaviors are influencing the health of populations. Epidemiology is more than simply understanding what is going on. It also involves acting on what you learn to prevent or control problems. Similarly, a PHN should be committed not only to understanding what is contributing to a problem and the extent of the problem but also to identifying and implementing disease prevention and health promotion strategies. In fact, this use of core epidemiological tools—namely, mathematics and data analysis—contributed to advancing the role and view of nursing in the 19th century (Earl, 2009). See Evidence Example 4.1 to examine how Lillian Wald and Florence Nightingale used data gathering and analysis to understand and address key health problems. By doing so, they advanced the profession of nursing beyond what had, up until that time, been a fairly ill-considered occupation.

### EVIDENCE EXAMPLE 4.1
#### Origins of Epidemiology and Nursing

Catherine Earl (2009) has written a fascinating and thorough historical article that describes the influence of epidemiology in the developing role of public health nursing. Beginning in the early 19th century, Earl presents a summary of history that reminds the reader of how far nursing and science have come in the past 200 years. Not that long ago, diseases were addressed solely within the individual, with little appreciation given for trends among the group or population. Advances in mathematical theories caused a shift, notably when Pierre Charles Alexandre Louis, a leading 19th-century physician, declared that the practice of bloodletting (often with the help of leeches) was ineffective and used statistics to support his claims. It is intriguing that, according to Earl, the use of quantitative methods was not well supported at that time and was poorly understood. In the 21st century, quantitative analyses are core to randomized controlled trials (RCTs), which are considered the gold standard for establishing evidence.

Lillian Wald used this advance in health and science to support her work with families in New York. She advocated for nurses to live and work near and among those they were also serving. She used numbers to support her need for resources, including the number of nurses. Her successes are many, and they are in part based on her foresight and wisdom in recognizing the need for data to accomplish goals and meet the health and social needs of society. Earl summarizes well the contribution PHNs—led by Lillian Wald—made in addressing tuberculosis, because they collected and reported critical data: "Nurses' involvement in the care of TB [tuberculosis] patients in 1914 was considered a major advancement in the use of statistical methods, because nurses became involved in improving health through their role as data collectors" (p. 262).

Florence Nightingale, considered by many to be the first biostatistician and the first epidemiologist, also used data to support her efforts to address health and sanitation. In her era, it was not common for women to be educated, yet her father encouraged her to learn varied subjects, including mathematics. As a result, Nightingale had skills that enabled her to identify causes of problems and to intervene not only to heal or cure but also to prevent. As Earl states, "With an epidemiological perspective and further discussions of mortality and morbidity rates and the importance of sanitary conditions as described by Florence Nightingale, the first preventorium, a program established to save children, was designed for the prevention, not the treatment, of TB" (p. 263). Both Lillian Wald and Florence Nightingale contributed to a significant shift from solely focusing on treatment to also concentrating on prevention, which today is also a primary focus of PHNs all over the world.

Although most PHNs are not epidemiologists, many activities that PHNs engage in parallel the work of epidemiologists. Often, epidemiologists work at the systems level of a healthcare facility or state health department and are responsible for the data collection, analysis, and program development related to a particular health/medical issue. Conversely, PHNs are frequently found in the grassroots level of healthcare, working with local vulnerable populations and community partners, interpreting and promoting the recommendations, protocols, and policies that have been developed by an authoritative body. See Table 4.1 for a sample list of activities that an epidemiologist often engages in, and note the similarities to many public health nursing activities and interventions.

*Elizabeth realizes she needs to have a better understanding of terms that she is reading as she investigates state and county reports about infectious disease threats in her community. She is getting confused by the different labels for cases and isn't exactly clear on the difference between quarantine and isolation. She finds the following definitions that provide clarity and adds them to her notebook:*

✔ **Case:** Person or population identified as having a particular disease, disorder, injury, or condition (Merrill, 2017, p. 7)

  • **Primary case:** The first disease case in the population (p. 7)

  • **Index case:** The first disease case brought to the attention of the epidemiologist (p. 7)

  • **Secondary case:** Persons who have become infected and ill after contact with a primary case (p. 7)

✔ **Incubation period:** Time interval between the invasion by an infectious agent and the appearance of the first signs or symptoms (Friis, 2018, p. 284)

✔ **Isolation:** Persons who have a communicable disease are kept away from other persons for a period of time that corresponds generally to the interval when the disease is communicable (Friis, 2018, p. 284)

✔ **Quarantine:** Persons, animals, or objects that have been exposed to a contagious disease are kept away from other persons for a specified period of time (adapted from Merrill, 2017, p. 57)

Historically, nurses participated in epidemiological investigations to determine the cause of a recurring problem, such as cholera outbreaks. As part of that process, nurses realized very early on that numerous risk factors often contributed to the spread of disease. This realization led to creative interventions that had multiple components to aid those already sick or affected and to prevent others from becoming sick. Quarantine (i.e., separation of an exposed individual from the rest of the community) laws are a good example of a specific effort to contain the spread of disease in the absence of other strategies. Interestingly, quarantine strategies are still used today, because some infectious viruses can spread

during an incubation period before symptoms are present. Examples of such illnesses in the 21st century include pertussis, chicken pox, measles, Ebola, avian influenza, and seasonal flu. When an individual is diagnosed with pertussis and other family members have been exposed, the pertussis case is strongly encouraged to stay isolated from the

**TABLE 4.1 Alignment of Epidemiologist Activities With PHN Intervention Wheel**

| Epidemiologist Activities | Public Health Nursing Activities and Interventions |
|---|---|
| Identifying risk factors for disease, injury, and death | Disease and Health Event Investigation |
| Describing the natural history of disease | Health Teaching |
| Identifying individuals and populations at greatest risk for disease | Outreach<br><br>Screening<br><br>Referral and Follow-Up<br><br>Advocacy<br><br>Case Management |
| Identifying where the public health problem is greatest | Surveillance<br><br>Disease and Health Event Investigation |
| Monitoring diseases and other health-related events over time | Surveillance |
| Evaluating the efficacy and effectiveness of prevention and treatment programs | A key part of the nursing process, but not a specific component of the intervention wheel |
| Providing information useful in health planning and decision-making for establishing health programs with appropriate boundaries | Consultation<br><br>Collaboration<br><br>Community Organizing<br><br>Policy Development and Enforcement |
| Assisting in carrying out public health programs | Most interventions on the Public Health Intervention Wheel |
| Serving as a resource | Consultation |
| Communicating health information | Outreach<br><br>Health Teaching<br><br>Social Marketing<br><br>Consultation |

*Source:* Adapted from Merrill, 2017

broader community until five days of antibiotic treatment have been completed. During the Sudden Acute Respiratory Syndrome (SARS) event in 2002 and 2003, quarantine of exposed individuals was key to containing the epidemic. Individuals placed under quarantine were monitored twice daily by public health workers until the SARS incubation period was completed. Although quarantines are not always enforced as they were years ago and in the SARS event, they can be effective when they are followed and when individuals and families adhere to the restrictions.

More broadly, Lillian Wald offers a great example of a PHN using a variety of intervention tools to address uncontrolled disease and unnecessary deaths in New York City tenements, as shown in Figure 4.1. At the individual level, she provided direct care for sick individuals in crowded apartments. At the community level, she organized community care for neighborhood children in need of a place to engage in physical activity. At the systems level, she advocated for programs that would meet the needs of many (e.g., welfare, food accessibility, child labor laws).

Today's PHN needs a repertoire of intervention strategies so that when health improves, it can be maintained over time—which is sometimes hard to do, especially in the presence of poor health determinants. For example, if a child recovers from an illness that worsened as a result of malnourishment and lack of warmth, but the family home environment remains unchanged, the child's recovery might not be maintained. In this case, the nurse might link the family to resources such as financial heat assistance, food banks, food stamps, etc. The nurse might begin to create long-term solutions by helping adult family members to explore financial management strategies as well as possibilities for higher-paying employment or more affordable, reliable housing. Finally, the nurse might advocate for legislation that prohibits companies or landlords from turning off heat sources during cold winter months. Nurses encounter numerous possible mechanisms for influence when they face a problem that might appear to have a simple solution but often requires complex intervention approaches to keep that problem from recurring.

## Understands the Relationship Between Community Assessment and Health Promotion and Disease Prevention Programs, Especially the Populations and Programs With Which the PHN Works

Many public health agencies and community organizations use community assessments to prioritize their resources and subsequent programs and services. Fundamental to the community assessment is the understanding of the incidence and distribution of disease in the community. The PHN might begin by reviewing the birth and death (mortality) data available through the state department of health. Morbidity (illness/disease/injury not resulting in death) data can also be reviewed to determine trends in reportable diseases (such as tuberculosis or sexually transmitted infections) or conditions such as cancers or motor vehicle fatalities. A comprehensive review of data sources generally leads and directs the community assessment process.

A variety of other strategies (e.g., needs assessment via focus groups or key-informant interviews, windshield survey) can be used to expand the community assessment. (See Chapter 3 for more information on community assessment.) PHNs work collaboratively in conducting assessments and using the resulting data for informing priorities and actions. Although it might be natural to focus on needs because the nurse is trying to address a problem, it is extremely valuable to take an asset-based approach toward the issue (Lind & Smith, 2008). An asset-based approach ensures that the assessment includes documentation of existing or potential strengths. In this way, the possible problem-solving strategies will ideally build on identified strengths and assets. If nurses focus only on problems, they might reach a solution that consists of outside resources rather than builds on what is available. Asset-based perspectives inherently encourage capacity building as well as self-care among individuals and families, communities, and populations. (See Chapter 8 for discussion of incorporating community assets.)

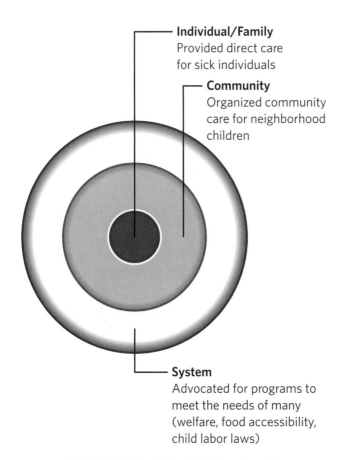

**Individual/Family**
Provided direct care for sick individuals

**Community**
Organized community care for neighborhood children

**System**
Advocated for programs to meet the needs of many (welfare, food accessibility, child labor laws)

**FIGURE 4.1** How Lillian Wald Practiced the Individual/Community/System Approach to Healthcare

*Elizabeth looks at the faxed pertussis report she has been given on 11-year-old Billy Johnson. Information includes Billy's birth date, address, phone number, and laboratory results, which are positive for pertussis. Next, Elizabeth looks up Billy in the computerized state immunization registry. She sees that he was vaccinated with five doses of DTaP vaccine, the last of which was administered at 5 years of age. Elizabeth recognizes that the immunity provided by the vaccine has possibly waned.*

### Activity

Reflect on the following questions:

■ What has Elizabeth discovered so far?

■ What are her next steps?

## Understands the Relationships Between Risk and Protective Factors, and Health Issues

No better classic example of understanding the relationship between a risk factor and a health issue exists than that of John Snow in mid-1800s London (Alfred, 2009). For unknown reasons, many people in London began to suffer and die as a result of cholera. People were fleeing the city because of fear, and without a known cause, they had little confidence that the disease could be stopped or prevented. John Snow created a map that began to identify where the deaths from cholera were occurring across London. This now-famous map (see Figure 4.2) yielded some clues for Snow, because he managed to visualize the areas where the deaths were most heavily concentrated. He suspected a water source, so to prohibit people from accessing this source of "risk," he removed the water pump handle:

> **1854:** Physician John Snow convinces a London local council to remove the handle from a pump in Soho. A deadly cholera epidemic in the neighborhood comes to an end immediately, though perhaps serendipitously. Snow maps the outbreak to prove his point… and launches modern epidemiology (Alfred, 2009, p. 1).

In the 21st century, PHNs continue to solve mysteries in identifying and eliminating health risks, and although conditions have improved in many parts of the world, reducing the risks from unsanitary conditions, these improvements are not universal. Consider the following observation:

> The 2010 cholera epidemic in Haiti (and the 2017 cholera outbreak that persists in Yemen) reminds us that cholera remains a deadly disease, not all that different from the time of John Snow. While Snow debated the appropriateness of the germ theory versus the miasmatic theory for the cause of the disease, current scientists are focusing on different, but related, hypotheses (University of California, Los Angeles [UCLA], 2010, p. 1).

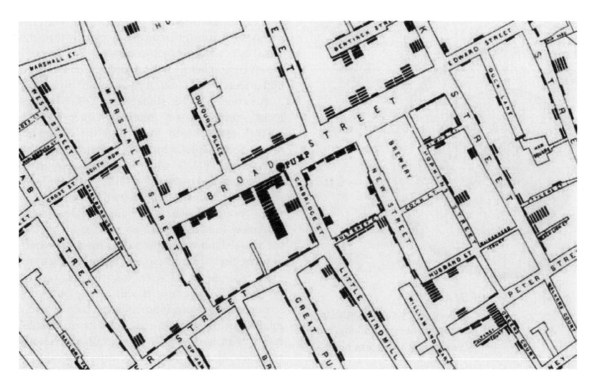

**FIGURE 4.2**  A Map Detailing Cholera Deaths in 1800s London; the Beginning of Epidemiology
*Source:* Alfred, 2009

Indeed, it is true that more than a century since Snow's solved mystery, PHNs continue to seek clear answers and solutions regarding the risks and diseases that are present in public health settings across the globe. In the United States, PHNs face complex challenges in meeting the needs of individuals, families, communities, and populations. Nurses need to identify risk and protective factors at multiple influencing levels. For example, a nurse might be working with a child recently diagnosed with asthma. The nurse needs to identify risk factors in the family environment that might be triggers for asthma episodes. Similarly, the nurse needs to assess for protective factors in the family, such as parental commitment to preventing episodes, which is an important asset the nurse can support with education and related tools. The nurse might want to go further and explore the neighborhood environment, including collaborating with school personnel, for possible risks or protections influencing the child.

It can take time to carefully and thoroughly assess risk and protective factors using a strengths-based approach. Usually, the time is well spent because the PHN will have a very clear picture of available assets as well as deficits to address when intervening on a particular health issue. Doing this proactively is a critical part of health promotion. Conducting assessments of risk and protective factors after a health issue has become apparent is important to minimize the effect of the health problem and to encourage positive intervention results. PHNs continually reassess for risk and protective factors, because these factors can be temporal; one day a risk might exist (e.g., lack of health insurance coverage), but the following week the family might have new health insurance coverage. PHNs commit to efforts that routinely assess, intervene, evaluate, and reassess.

A PHN also stays informed about emerging diseases and pandemic threats. For example, during 2015 pertussis cases decreased by 37% compared with 2014. See Table 4.2 for states that had the highest reported rates of pertussis in 2015. The majority of deaths continue to occur among infants younger than 3 months of age, and the incidence rate of pertussis among infants exceeds that of all other age groups. The Centers for Disease Control again observed increased rates in adolescents ages 13–15 as well as in 16-year-olds. In the case of pertussis, the PHN would recognize pertussis vaccination as a protective factor. Lack of vaccination, waning immunity from vaccination, and posing immune-compromising conditions would be risk factors.

*Elizabeth prepares to call Billy's parents. She places the protocol nearby and has her report form ready. Billy's mother answers the phone, and Elizabeth introduces herself as a PHN who works with infectious diseases. She explains how she has obtained a pertussis report on Billy and inquires whether his mother has about 15 minutes to speak with her. Billy's mother states that she operates an in-home daycare, but most of the children have not yet arrived.*

*Elizabeth mentally notes this information about the daycare and then explains that the purpose of the call is to identify what can be done to prevent the spread of the disease. Elizabeth starts with what she thinks is the most logical question—when did this cough start? Billy's mother recalls that he started coughing on September 17 and had a paroxysmal cough without a whooping sound. He occasionally coughed so hard that he vomited. About 1 week before his cough started, he had a low-grade fever and a runny nose.*

*Because his cough was not getting any better, his mother brought Billy to the clinic on September 26. Billy did not have pneumonia or any other complications of pertussis. He was given azithromycin antibiotic and is now on his third day of a 5-day course of treatment. Elizabeth jots down a note that states the period of infectivity started about September 10, or about a week before the cough started.*

*Next Elizabeth asks how many other family members are in the home. Billy lives with his parents and has no siblings. Neither parent has been coughing. Elizabeth discusses with his mother the public health recommendation that other household members take a preventive course of antibiotics. She agrees to call the clinic for prescriptions.*

**TABLE 4.2  States With Incidence of Pertussis the Same or Higher Than the National Incidence During 2015, Which Is 6.5/100,000 Persons**

| Nebraska | 27.2 | Oregon | 14.6 | Minnesota | 10.9 |
|---|---|---|---|---|---|
| Montana | 22.3 | Kansas | 14.5 | California | 9.2 |
| Maine | 21.1 | Alaska | 14.2 | Arizona | 8.5 |
| Washington | 19.3 | Wisconsin | 13.1 | Vermont | 7.8 |
| Colorado | 16.7 | Idaho | 11.7 | Pennsylvania | 6.9 |
| Utah | 16.6 | New Mexico | 11.6 | | |

*Source:* 2015 Final Pertussis Surveillance Report, Centers for Disease Control and Prevention [CDC], 2015

*To further assess for close contacts, Elizabeth asks questions about Billy's school. Billy told his mother "a lot of kids" were coughing in his classroom. Elizabeth states that she will talk to the school nurse about sending a notification letter to the parents of the students in Billy's classroom; Elizabeth is careful to inform the mother that Billy will not be identified in the letter. Elizabeth explains that she will also be working with the school to identify children who sit adjacent to Billy, as they might also need preventive antibiotics.* **"**

## Obtains and Interprets Information Regarding Risks and Benefits to the Community

PHNs need to know how to find and use data. Data drive so much of what PHNs do. In fact, PHNs determine health priorities by using data to identify key problem areas or concerns. PHNs also use data to evaluate whether interventions or programs are successful in reducing the risks or health problems in a local community. Unfortunately, data are not always easy to interpret or understand; data are often presented in such formats as tables, figures or graphs, or raw numbers. They might be posed as percentages or risk ratios. Although in-depth knowledge of data, formulas, and calculations is not necessary for entry-level PHNs, some awareness of how to read data and data types is useful.

### Data Trend in a Graph

Often, data are presented over time by using graphs to show what is happening in a community with respect to a particular health problem or population trend. For example,

a PHN might be interested in exploring trends related to tuberculosis cases in the community over the past 5 years—that is, the nurse is doing surveillance of TB in the jurisdiction (see Figure 4.3). The data in a graph form provide a snapshot of how the number of cases is increasing, maintaining, or decreasing. In the tuberculosis example, it is apparent that active TB cases are progressively increasing, whereas latent TB cases can dramatically decrease, increase, and then stabilize. This information might lead the PHN to ask questions about pulmonary versus nonpulmonary TB or population changes in the community and explore specific intervention strategies to reduce the number of active TB cases over the next few years.

 **Healthy People** **2020** **healthypeople.gov** The Healthy People 2020 website offers opportunities to explore the uses of data in public health. On the website, click "Data Search." From here, you can do a data search on a public health topic of interest to you. Select the health topic and then limit your search by a variety of factors, such as sex, age, race/ethnicity, and geographic location. The results are presented using the Healthy People 2020 indicators (goals/markers) and show trends over the past few years. What do you observe in the data you explore? How might these data be useful to a PHN engaged in health promotion?

### Data Trend per 100,000 in a Graph

Similarly, a PHN might examine the trend of chlamydia cases over a period of five years. Rather than looking at the raw number of cases (as in the tuberculosis example), the PHN might prefer to examine the rate of cases, which is always based on a ratio or number of cases per 100,000 persons. The raw case number in the tuberculosis example does not give a picture of how serious the problem is,

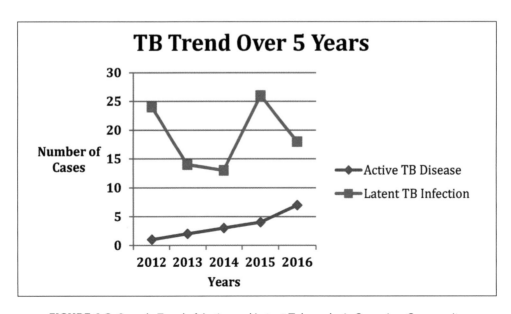

**FIGURE 4.3** Sample Trend of Active and Latent Tuberculosis Cases in a Community

because the graph does not indicate how many people are in the community. For example, if the community population count were 100 and there were 50 cases of latent TB, the PHN would be much more concerned than if there were 50 cases in a community population of 100,000. In the chlamydia example, the rate of cases appears to be increasing, from around 340 per 100,000 in year 1 to nearly 428 per 100,000 in year 5 (see Figure 4.4). This increase is concerning by itself, but the PHN might want to compare the rate in one community with the rate in another community. Comparing rates in different communities or populations provides the PHN with perspective about the relative severity of the disease incidence or prevalence and helps determine how to prioritize efforts to prevent the spread of chlamydia.

Evidence Example 4.2 discusses using data regarding incidence rates to identify a problem and evaluate the impact of a system-wide intervention—in this case the rate of tuberculosis among correctional system inmates.

## Data Comparison Between State and National Sources

Comparing health and disease trends across communities can be challenging and create turmoil if it is not done carefully. No community wants to appear worse than another when it comes to a health problem or condition. On the other hand, if resources are scarce, a community might want to justify acquiring greater access to available resources. Careful comparison of data within and across communities is vital to ensure that public health priorities are appropriate and that the chosen resource allocation is warranted. Comparison is useful because it can bring understanding of the severity or scope of a problem, especially if policymakers are unaware of the problem or not convinced that it requires attention.

### EVIDENCE EXAMPLE 4.2
**Use of Epidemiological Tuberculosis Data to Inform a New York State Corrections Intervention**

In a study addressing tuberculosis, data were used to inform strategies to prevent increases of tuberculosis among inmates in the New York State Corrections system (Klopf, 1998). Data indicated that the incidence of tuberculosis had increased over a 6-year period from 43 per 100,000 to 225 per 100,000, a serious problem that warranted intervention. Collaboratively, people from corrections, the local department of health, and the parole division developed a comprehensive TB control program that focused on the prevention and containment of disease. Importantly, they implemented a nurse-led case management program, using infection control nurses to carefully monitor and intervene on active and suspected TB cases. The program was truly comprehensive, including policies, development of a TB registry, surveillance, detection, and case management involving preventive and directly observed therapy among the inmates. The staff and inmates received education regarding testing, diagnoses, disease process, and treatment. It is believed that this comprehensive program contributed to the reduced incidence of TB. Six years later, the rate decreased from 225 per 100,000 to 61 per 100,000—a 73% reduction! The data informed the need for an intervention that relied heavily on nurses. The data also demonstrated, in part, the impact of the intervention program, showing a significant reduction in the new cases of TB among New York's inmates.

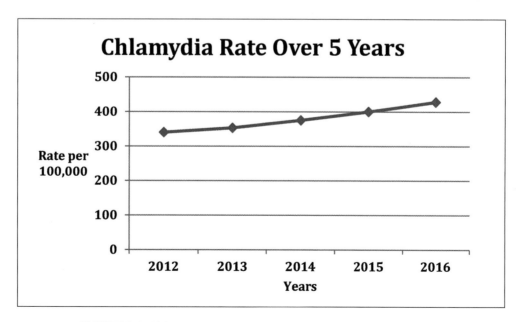

**FIGURE 4.4**  Chlamydia Example of Case Rate per 100,000 Over 5 Years

## EVIDENCE EXAMPLE 4.3
### Comparing Virtual and Outpatient Tuberculosis Clinic Models of Care

In a recent study, the use of a virtual public health clinic was compared with a traditional outpatient clinic for managing tuberculosis in a Canadian province (Long, Heffernan, Gao, Egedahl, & Talbot, 2015). The TB prevention and care model was delivered through one virtual and two outpatient clinics, which were subsequently assessed on 28 performance indicators. Overall, one clinic type did not demonstrate superiority to the other, which is promising for virtual or tele-health models of healthcare delivery and management for challenging public health concerns such as TB.

A good example of this scenario is Lyme disease, which is contracted through exposure to ticks. Lyme disease cases between 1996 and 2016 have varied from 252 to 1,431 cases in Minnesota and have steadily increased since 2002 (see Figure 4.5). However, without being able to compare these numbers to those of another state, it is difficult to determine whether the problem is serious or relatively consistent with national trends. The PHN investigating this issue might look beyond state-level data to what is occurring nationally. Review of national data provided by the CDC demonstrates that Minnesota has one of the highest density areas of Lyme disease, second only to states along the East Coast (see Figure 4.6). The data in Figure 4.6 are from a Geographic Information System (GIS) wherein a dot is placed within the county of residence for each confirmed case of Lyme disease. GIS is an example of a mapping tool that PHNs may use for surveillance. (See "Innovative Data Collection: Maps and Apps," for more GIS information.) These data would support efforts by PHNs to bring attention to the problem and to invest in preventive messages for Minnesotans regarding the spread of Lyme disease.

Often data are not easily and perfectly comparable between sources due to different years of reported data or different timeframes, and it's good to note when discrepancies exist. In Figures 4.5 and 4.6, both MDH and CDC data are reported for 2015, which offers a useful comparison. An effective PHN tries to find the most comparable data possible but does point out discrepancies when comparisons are made between incomparable data. Using data that are not a perfect match is not wrong, but these differences must be identified so that people can make informed decisions based on the existing data. It might not be true that people can make data say exactly what they want them to say, but it certainly is possible to inadvertently or purposefully present data in ways that might not be entirely accurate. Therefore, PHNs need to spend time practicing how to present data in meaningful, representative ways, and, equally vital, they need to have the ability to interpret and critique any data that are presented to them.

## Data Comparison Between National and Global Sources

To understand the context from which a client originates, a PHN may be interested in disease incidence in other parts of the world. The earlier PHN who graphed active TB cases against latent TB cases may have found increasing numbers of families from several parts of the world now living in her community. Reviewing information from the World Health Organization (WHO) will inform her of the distribution of TB elsewhere. This information can then be applied to determine communicable disease risk related to immigration patterns in her community.

## Data as Population Trends

Equally valuable are data that demonstrate population trends. These are most commonly presented in the form of a population pyramid, which at a glance provides a picture of population growth (see Figure 4.7). In this figure, the age distribution of people in the U.S. is portrayed. Compared with other years, one can visually see changing trends in population age distribution. This could be valuable to determining priorities for PHN interventions, particularly

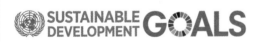

**Addressing Asthma to Improve Health in Cities**

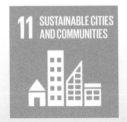

**GOAL 11** Nurses are on the front line globally for addressing asthma, which is the most common chronic condition among children that can have long-term consequences when left undiagnosed and undertreated. Nurses in Iceland and the United States developed an International School Nurse Care Coordination Model that informs strategies addressing asthma at both the student and the school levels, including symptom management, care coordination within and outside the school setting, and broader educational strategies (Garwick et al., 2015). Collaborative efforts such as this offer promise of achieving this SDG by recognizing where global challenges might be met with similar strategic models.

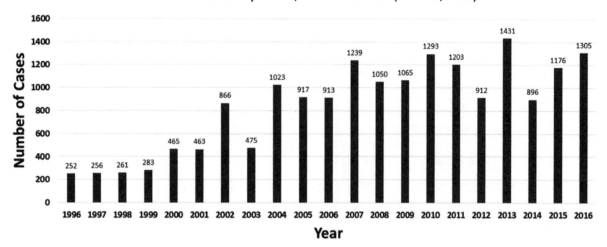

## Reported Cases of Lyme Disease in Minnesota by Year, 1996–2016 (*n* = 17,744)

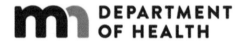

**FIGURE 4.5** Reported Cases of Lyme Disease in Minnesota, 1996–2016 (*n* = 17,744)
*Source:* Minnesota Department of Health [MDH], 2016

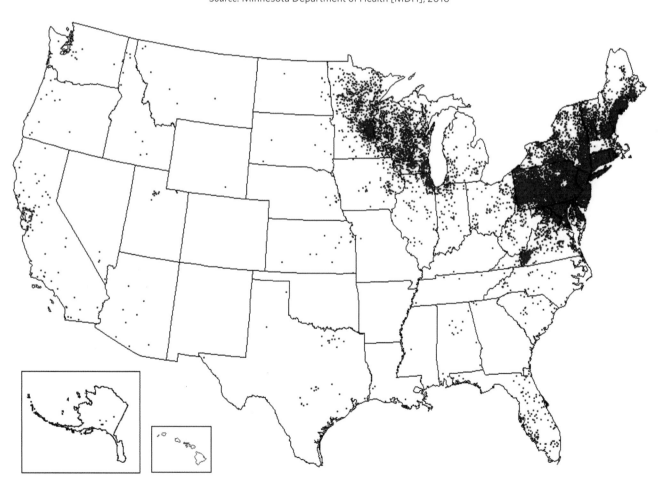

**FIGURE 4.6** Reported Cases of Lyme Disease—United States, 2016
*Source:* Centers for Disease Control and Prevention [CDC], 2016

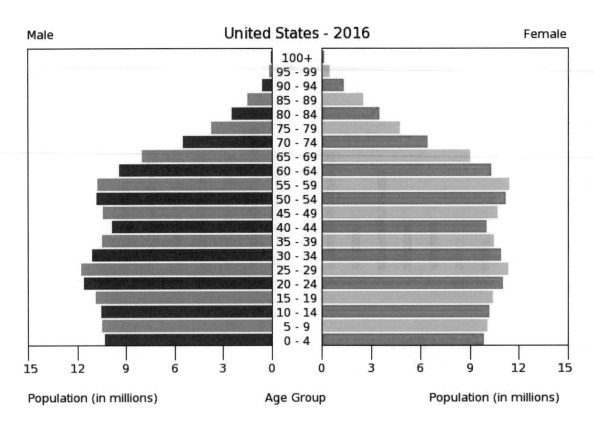

**FIGURE 4.7** Population Pyramid of United States—2016
*Source:* Central Intelligence Agency: *The World Factbook, 2016*

when resources are limited. Population data are important because they offer a glimpse into the big picture of how people are distributed, but the data by themselves might not be sufficient to guide intervention decisions or justify program budget priorities.

## Data as Risk Ratios and Odds Ratios

Another very common tool used to examine the data regarding risks and health outcomes is a 2×2 table (see Table 4.3). This table aids in understanding how a disease is distributed in a population based on the presence or absence of a risk factor. From this table, a PHN can calculate the rate of disease in each group; the risk ratio (RR: the rate of disease for those with the risk behavior divided by the rate of disease for those without the risk behavior); and the odds ratio (OR), which is regularly used to describe the likelihood of contracting a disease for someone with the risk factor compared to someone without. In the example shown in Table 4.3, the rate of disease for the "Yes" risk behavior group is 0.75 (75/100), and the rate of disease for the "No" risk behavior group is 0.02 (2/100). Already a relationship between the risk behavior and the disease seems obvious given the raw rates (0.75 versus 0.02). Taking this a step further, you can calculate the RR (0.75/0.02 = 37.5). PHNs do not often use the RR by itself, but it is an important calculation for those who might

be interested in more in-depth statistical comparisons and analysis, such as chi-square analysis. PHNs might not routinely calculate these numbers, but they often read and analyze research that includes reported rates, risk ratios, odds ratios, chi-squares, and levels of significance (i.e., $p < .001$ or $p < .05$). It is beyond the scope of this book to completely explain how to calculate each of these, but it is useful for PHNs to have an awareness of what the numbers mean and how to appropriately interpret them.

Table 4.3 shows an example of data used to calculate odds and an OR. This ratio is useful in identifying the odds of contracting the disease, given the presence or absence of a risk factor. The formula for calculating the OR is (a/c) / (b/d) = ad/bc. Specifically, the odds of contracting the disease in the presence of the risk factor is calculated by dividing the number of people with the disease and the risk by the number of people without the disease but with the risk (i.e., 75/25, or 3). Similarly, the odds of contracting the disease but not having the risk factor can be calculated 2/98, or 0.0204. The OR is calculated by dividing the odds with the risk factor by the odds without the risk factor (3/0.0204), or 147. In this example, someone with the risk factor is 147 times more likely to contract the disease than someone without the risk factor. A PHN with this information needs to make decisions on how to act based on many factors. For example, even though the OR is so high, the disease might not be life threatening, or the risk factor might not be common. The risk factor might easily be eliminated with an intervention, or the risk factor might not be easily identified, making it difficult to intervene. PHNs need to consider numerous factors when data are interpreted and then acted upon. PHNs have an important role in helping interpret data so that they are not used inappropriately to justify action or inaction.

## TABLE 4.3 Association Between Risk Factor and Disease

| Disease | | | |
|---|---|---|---|
| **Risk Factor** | **Yes** | **No** | **Total** |
| **Yes** | a | c | a + c |
| **No** | b | d | b + d |
| **Total** | a + b | c + d | a + b + c + d |

| Disease | | | |
|---|---|---|---|
| **Risk Factor** | **Yes** | **No** | **Total** |
| **Yes** | 75 | 25 | 100 |
| **No** | 2 | 98 | 100 |
| **Total** | 77 | 123 | 200 |

## Innovative Data Collection: Examples of Maps and Apps

Data are typically collected through surveillance systems at the local, state, or national levels. Sometimes healthcare professionals provide the data, and other times individuals, families, or communities are surveyed. PHNs need to be aware of the variety of tools used to collect epidemiological data, because they might participate in data collection, interpretation, or dissemination. A Geographic Information System (GIS) is an example of a tool growing in popularity in the field of public health. Technological advances make it possible for local PHNs (and the general public) to access GIS data and contribute to mapping efforts readily via smartphones, tablets, and laptops.

GIS tools can yield data useful to a neighborhood, community, state, or country in advancing public health priorities. The *County Health Rankings & Roadmaps* provide an annual check-up of the health of each county in the U.S. (County Health Rankings & Roadmaps, 2012). This publication shows that some places are doing very well, while others have room for improvement. Figure 4.8 shows maps that provide insights about health outcomes and health factors in Minnesota, with healthier counties depicted in lighter colors. See Figure 4.8, County Health Rankings & Roadmaps; and Figure 4.9, a sample interactive GIS map from the California Department of Public Health that addresses nutrition, from www.cnngis.org.

2018 Health Outcomes: Minnesota

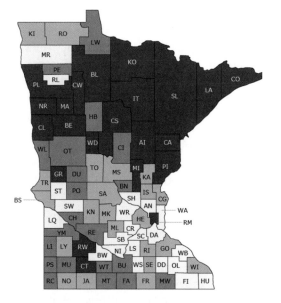

2018 Health Factors: Minnesota

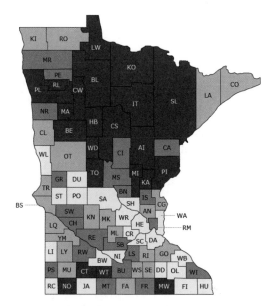

**FIGURE 4.8** County Health Rankings & Roadmaps: Minnesota
*Source:* County Health Rankings & Roadmaps, 2018

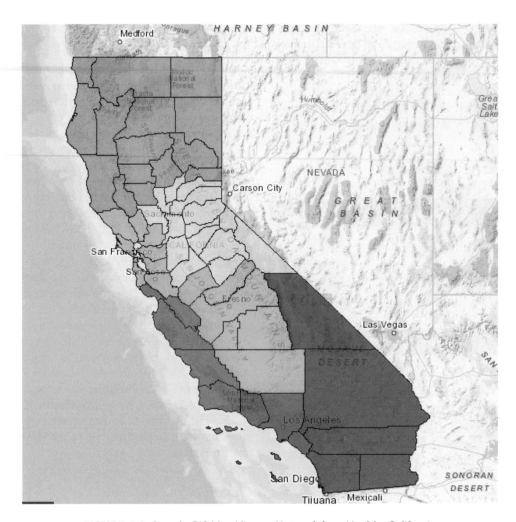

**FIGURE 4.9** Sample GIS Map Viewer: Network for a Healthy California

GIS data are also being used to carefully examine community-level assets and risks related to public health problems such as obesity prevention. For example, GIS data can aid in understanding how communities compare in terms of access to full-scale grocery stores, corner supermarkets, gas stations, and liquor stores. Additionally, GIS data can indicate the location of parks and transpose (e.g., overlay) violent crime data, which might provide insights into why youth in certain neighborhoods are reporting higher levels of physical activity than youth in other neighborhoods.

In emergency situations, GIS programs are playing a crucial role. In Haiti in 2010, a GIS program was used within the first few hours after the earthquake to update a baseline map of Haiti. People on the ground used OpenStreetMap, a GIS crowdsourced mapping program, to modify the existing map in real time, thereby facilitating rescue efforts. The pre-earthquake terrain maps that existed were not very helpful, but the real-time maps provided valuable support to search-and-rescue teams. Since then, the use of GIS to map disaster events and response has dramatically increased. Consider just a few of the following GIS resources that were available and used in 2017 to aid in addressing hurricanes (Harvey, Irma, Matthew, and others):

- Federal Emergency Management Agency (FEMA) Geoplatform (at http://fema.maps.arcgis.com/home/index.html) provides geospatial data and analytics for emergency management (see also www.geoplatform.gov)

- FEMA Geospatial Coordination Mapping and Data (see https://data.femadata.com/NationalDisasters/HurricaneHarvey/Documents/Geospatial%20Coordination%20Call%20Notes/ for Hurricane Harvey examples)

- American Red Cross Online Mapping provides information about open shelters and ongoing storm data (see http://arc-nhq-gis.maps.arcgis.com/home/index.html)

- National Oceanic and Atmospheric Administration NowCOAST provides real-time coastal observations, warnings, and forecasts (see https://nowcoast.noaa.gov/)

- Ushahidi crowdsource mapping was used to aid in response and recovery efforts (see https://irmamiami.ushahidi.io/views/map) including oil spill tracking after Hurricane Harvey (see https://skytruth.ushahidi.io/views/map)

## EVIDENCE EXAMPLE 4.4
### Using Big Data to Inform PHN Home Visiting Interventions

There is so much data generated in every home visit, and over time and across visits, the data repository grows and becomes a valuable source of broad information. PHNs have traditionally provided the data, offering rich charting and thorough details for each home visit, but now PHNs are using these data to understand patterns and inform interventions to a much greater extent. Monsen et al. (2017) analyzed data from 4,263 women who had received home visits, examining social and behavioral determinants of health as well as outcomes following the home visits. Analyses demonstrated that minority women showed greater improvements following the interventions and revealed the value of using big data to begin to unravel intervention elements and intervention outcomes.

## EVIDENCE EXAMPLE 4.5
### Screening for Neurodevelopmental Delays in Four Communities in Mexico and Cuba

Cuban and Mexican PHNs used a newly developed computerized evaluation instrument to assess and compare the prevalence of neurodevelopmental problems in three areas: language/communication, psychomotor, and hearing/vision (Guadarrama-Celaya et al., 2012). Four hundred children ages 1 to 5 years were screened using the Neuropediatric Development (NPED) screening tool in urban and suburban cities in Cuba and Mexico. Results demonstrated failures in all communities (e.g., 2.3% vision, 16.5% language) and differences by country (e.g., higher failures rate for hearing in Cuban communities). Results also demonstrated successful use of this computerized Spanish-language tool for broad community assessment of key neurodevelopmental problems among children at important stages of development. This tool can facilitate earlier identification and intervention so that long-term neurodevelopmental problems can be avoided as children develop.

Mapping is also being used to monitor and visualize outbreaks across the globe (see http://www.healthmap.org/en/) and can be valuable historically to review an outbreak, such as the 2014 Ebola outbreak (see https://www.cdc.gov/vhf/ebola/outbreaks/2014-west-africa/distribution-map.html). The data behind the mapping are useful not only in the real-time incidents that require response and intervention, but also in the future, as scientists use data to develop algorithms that could help to predict future outbreaks. With public health professionals questioning when, not if, the next worldwide outbreak or pandemic threat might occur, the ability to see and process a large amount of real-time data, and historic data, is very important.

Consider learning about the Global Health Security Agenda (see https://www.ghsagenda.org/) to "advance a world safe and secure from infectious disease threats, to bring together nations from all over the world to make new, concrete commitments, and to elevate global health security as a national leaders-level priority" (Global Health Security Agenda [GHSA], 2017, para. 1). This initiative is extensive, promoting efforts that engage global partners, local government, universities, those already in the workforce, and those who are about to graduate and enter the public health workforce as public health nurses, veterinarians, and environmental health professionals. Examples of these initiatives are found online: One Health Workforce at https://medium.com/one-health-workforce and PREDICT at http://www.vetmed.ucdavis.edu/ohi/predict/.

In addition to broad use of mapping data in public health, there are real-time data collection strategies being used to more quickly and more thoroughly understand public health problems and to more efficiently deliver public health interventions. Consider the extensive and overwhelming availability of smartphone apps designed to help individuals manage their health, quit an unhealthy behavior, begin a healthy one, and track every step along the way. Visit an app store and do a search for a common public health challenge you might address as a PHN working with individuals or families. You will find dozens, if not hundreds, of possible tools. Of value are articles that summarize the benefits and challenges of these apps, as well as websites that offer rankings and scores to help potential users consider the right app for them. An example is provided for mental health apps at https://adaa.org/finding-help/mobile-apps. Not every situation warrants use of an app (or a map), and it is really important for PHNs to understand this. Just because a technological tool exists does not inherently mean it should be used. PHNs need to consider the challenge being addressed, the stakeholders, the benefits or challenges associated with the technological solution, and then make an informed decision about using it.

## Applies an Epidemiological Framework When Assessing and Intervening With Communities, Systems, Individuals, and Families

How a PHN comes to understand a problem and its possible causes and solutions is somewhat dependent on the framework that the PHN uses. The *epidemiological triangle* has traditionally been used to understand disease transmission. This triangle consists of identifying a host system affected by the condition, an agent that causes the condition, and the environment that contributes to the condition. Host considerations include genetics; inherent characteristics, such as age and gender; acquired characteristics, such as immune status; and lifestyle factors. Agents are typically categorized as infectious, chemical, or physical agents. Environmental factors might include a variety of physical, social, and economic factors. Interactions between these three elements of the triangle are examined to determine how diseases are transmitted and how intervention strategies can be targeted to stop or prevent transmission of the health conditions. Using influenza as an example of the three triangle components, the host would be the individual susceptible to the flu, the agent is the influenza virus, and the environment might be the physical apartment that is overcrowded and underheated (Clark, 2008).

This model has been adapted to consider more complex scenarios that might be contributing to disease or illness (see Figure 4.10). It is an important adaptation, because for most health problems that PHNs address, the contributing factors are complex and multifaceted. Illnesses result not merely from a simple transmission in the right time and place but also because of factors not easily controlled or resolved (e.g., poverty, inadequate housing, food shortages).

For many in public health, complex contributing factors to poor health or well-being have been informed by such models as the web of causation. The name itself implies greater complexity than the epidemiological triangle, yet this model is also not perfect. For example, imagine a spider web (where the name is drawn from) and how you might use the web design to identify all the factors influencing the center of the web (i.e., the disease, such as cardiovascular disease or asthma, or the social health problem, such as teen pregnancy). After you have drawn the web, you are faced with a dilemma—specifically, which related thread to address first. How do you decide whether to prioritize a biological-related factor or a social-based factor? The web might help identify numerous potential causes, contributors, and influences, yet the model by itself does not yield readily apparent strategies or solutions. More than 10 years ago, Nancy Krieger (1997) identified these criticisms of the web framework and proposed an ecosocial framework for developing epidemiological theories about public health problems and possible solutions. The central question answered using an ecosocial framework is, "Who and what is responsible for population patterns of health, disease, and well-being, as manifested in present, past, and changing social inequalities in health?" (Krieger, 2001a, p. 694).

A shift in thinking about traditional epidemiology models has occurred, with growing recognition of the importance of social epidemiology, the field that acknowledges and seeks to address the complex combination of biological and social factors influencing health and well-being. Social epidemiology was initially defined in the 1950s but has in more recent decades grown in popularity and use among public health professionals (Krieger, 2001b, 2012). PHNs need to be aware of the trends in public health as well as the theories that guide understanding of the "risk-asset-problem-intervention" relationships in public health.

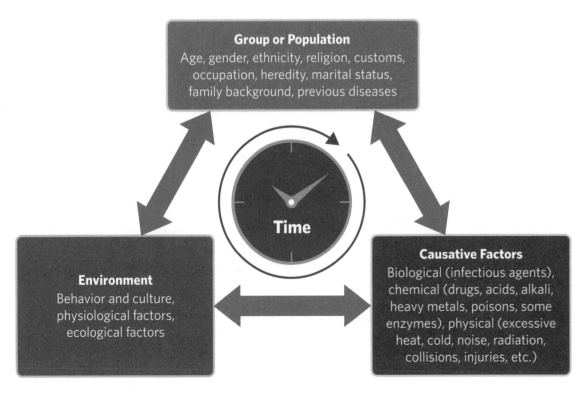

**FIGURE 4.10** Epidemiological Triangle in the 21st Century
*Source: Merrill, 2017, p. 11*

## THEORY APPLICATION
### Ecosocial Theory

Krieger's ecosocial theory offers an integrated framework that considers pathways of public health problems in the context of life course (e.g., from infancy to older adulthood), and ecological layers (e.g., individual, family, community, system, etc.). Critical to the theory is the explanatory manner in which complex, intersectional risks and protections can be considered when examining a public health or social problem (see Krieger, 2012, p. 938, for a modeling of the framework applied to racism, for example). Krieger states that the ecosocial theory is a tool that:

> fosters analysis of current and changing population patterns of health, disease, and well-being in relation to each level of biological, ecological and social organization (e.g., cell, organ, organism/individual, family, community, population, society, ecosystem) as manifested at each and every scale, whether relatively small and fast (e.g., enzyme catalysis) or relatively large and slow (e.g., infection and renewal of the pool of susceptible for a specified infectious disease) (Krieger, 2001b, p. 671).

Nursing practice should always be informed by theory. It is relatively easy in nursing practice to get caught up in the tasks one has to do and to forget, at times, to take a step back, reflect, and consider why something is being done a certain way or why certain events are occurring. Theories are always advancing, and an effective PHN strives not only to use theory but also to keep up with theoretical ideas that guide and inform practice and the care of individuals, families, communities, and populations. Epidemiology is an ideal example of the value and importance of theory as a guide for understanding and intervening in extremely complex societal health problems and conditions.

Another important theoretical framework in public health that PHNs should be aware of is referred to as *life course epidemiology*. Historically, as the focus of epidemiology shifted from infectious disease to chronic illness in the mid–20th century, new and expanded paradigms emerged to better recognize and understand the antecedents and causes of chronic diseases. Consider adverse childhood experiences (ACEs); these are now commonly understood as important life events that can have physical and mental health effects that persist into adulthood (Felitti et al., 1998). ACEs include a range of experiences, but most common are those that children experience directly (e.g., sexual abuse, emotional abuse, physical abuse), and through exposure in the home (e.g., parental substance use or incarceration, parental mental health problems, parental abuse, parental divorce or separation). Numerous studies since the original ACEs Study conducted by the CDC and Kaiser

Permanente (see https://www.cdc.gov/violenceprevention/acestudy/index.html) have been done, showing the strong—and in some cases, predictive—relationship between exposure to these risks in childhood and poor outcomes in young adulthood and adulthood (Holman et al., 2016; Wolff, Baglivio, & Piquero, 2015).

The life course perspective views health not in stages separate from each other (infancy, early childhood, adolescence, adulthood) but as a continuum. As Krieger (2001a, p. 695) describes, "Life course perspective refers to how health status at any given age, for a given birth cohort, reflects not only contemporary conditions but embodiment of prior living circumstances." A classic life course study was the research on the effects of the 1944–1945 Dutch famine that linked malnutrition with subsequent effects on human development and mental performance (Stein, Susser, Saenger, & Marolla, 1975). Throughout the life course continuum, biological, behavioral, environmental, psychological, and social factors dynamically interact, contributing to one's health. As Matthias Richter (2010, p. 458) summarizes, "This perspective was truly helpful to contribute to a better understanding of biological, behavioural and social influences—from gestation to death—for health as well as health inequalities."

> ❝ *The next area for Elizabeth to assess for close contacts is the in-home daycare. Billy's mother states that they have a split-entry home and that the lower level is for the licensed daycare. On a normal day, she has five children who stay until 5:30 p.m. In addition, a set of 1-year-old twin girls stay until approximately 11:00 p.m. Billy's mother indicates that since Billy has been ill, he has stayed only on the upper level, away from most of the lower-level childcare children. However, the situation with the twins is different: Billy eats supper with them and plays with them until bedtime. The twins have been exposed to pertussis and, according to the definition in the protocol, are considered face-to-face contacts.*
>
> *Elizabeth asks whether the twins' parents have been told about Billy's pertussis. The mother states that she has not told them because she is concerned about losing her clients and income. Elizabeth explains that the public health recommendation is that the twins receive preventive antibiotics because of their close contact with Billy. Billy's mother agrees to notify the twins' parents by passing out to all parents a standardized notification letter from the PHN.* ❞

Public health nursing is grounded in the science of epidemiology. On numerous levels, epidemiological data help describe the scope of a problem, prioritize intervention strategies, and evaluate outcomes or trends over time. Data are presented and collected using many different formats; nurses need the skills to interpret and critique these data, regardless of how they are presented. PHNs also use epidemiological theories to inform actions and priorities for addressing public health problems. PHNs need to use and contribute to the development of theories that recognize the social complexities influencing public health problems in the 21st century.

## Ethical Considerations

As seen in the narrative woven throughout this chapter, the daycare provider was concerned about a loss of income and her reputation as a provider. Many times, PHNs confront challenging situations in their practice. For example, reporting a nuisance house situation to the city building inspector might prompt the eviction of a renter or harassment from a landlord. Although they are trying to protect children living in less than desirable circumstances, PHNs' actions might have unintended consequences for entire families.

Similarly, interventions focused on reducing the exposure to lead paint in older homes might be embarrassing or financially difficult. Although the health department might offer a free home/environmental inspection for the detection of lead paint, this activity might force families to temporarily leave their homes, which some may perceive as an invasion of privacy. Moving in with relatives for a day might be embarrassing for some; for others, staying in a hotel might be beyond the family budget. Some health departments offer a free service to abate lead in a home if the family has not done so. Although this solution is helpful in covering up a lead source, the repainting services are often spotty and unsightly in appearance. The benefits of reducing lead exposure to children must be weighed against the other consequences for the family. See Table 4.4 for ethical perspectives and applications relevant to epidemiological principles in public health nursing.

**TABLE 4.4  Ethical Action in Using Epidemiological Principles in Public Health Nursing**

| Ethical Perspective | Application |
|---|---|
| Rule Ethics (principles) | ■ PHNs should use epidemiology to assess and develop interventions that promote beneficence.<br>■ PHNs can support the autonomy of those they are working with, even when uncomfortable changes are needed to minimize the spread of disease. |
| Virtue Ethics (character) | ■ PHNs need to demonstrate respect for individuals, families, and communities when suggesting promotion or prevention strategies; this can be challenging but necessary, especially when some might refuse to adhere to the actions being recommended.<br>■ PHNs should be persistent in understanding the complexity of factors contributing to a problem so that potential solutions are comprehensive and yield lasting changes. |
| Feminist Ethics (reducing oppression) | ■ PHNs can advocate for system-level changes that promote the well-being of those who often feel they have no voice (e.g., tenants who are unable to ask a landlord to maintain heat levels during the winter).<br>■ PHNs should explore societal changes that can improve the underlying environment for people, such as increasing the minimum-wage law so that families have additional resources to sustain and promote health. |

## KEY POINTS

- Epidemiology is an important foundation to the work of PHNs.
- There is a growing shift from traditional epidemiological models toward more complex models that consider social influences on health, such as a social epidemiological model.
- Epidemiological data, including prevalence and incidence data, help set national and local public health priorities.
- PHNs can and should use epidemiological data to advocate for health promotion priorities in their areas of influence.

## REFLECTIVE PRACTICE

Investigating outbreak possibilities can be challenging, but it can also present opportunities to practice great communication skills. Elizabeth handled a situation that could have been extremely difficult in a professional, thoughtful manner. She asked the right questions and managed to express concern rather than judgment. By building a good relationship right away, Elizabeth received honest responses from the childcare provider, and together they determined who had been exposed and an appropriate course of action.

1. What do you imagine will be some follow-up steps that Elizabeth will take in this situation?

2. How can Elizabeth be a resource for the childcare provider if her clients grow angry when they are informed about the possible exposure?

3. Who might be additional partners to Elizabeth within the health department as she follows this case until it is resolved?

4. How might Elizabeth address an ethical issue, such as whether some of the exposed refuse preventive treatment?

5. How will Elizabeth know whether this case investigation has been successful? What will be important for Elizabeth to document?

6. How will the numbers that Elizabeth has collected as part of this investigation be useful to others at her local health department? At the state level? At the national level?

7. How might Elizabeth use each of the Cornerstones of Public Health Nursing (see Chapter 1) in this case investigation?

## APPLICATION OF EVIDENCE

1. What are some ways you can use the ecosocial theory to examine contributing and influencing factors on complex public health problems in the United States in the 21st century, such as obesity or the opioid epidemic?

2. Examine the different types of data presented in this chapter (e.g., rates, maps) and identify when you might use one type of data more than another type.

3. As a PHN working in a community, identify three to five sources of state- or federal-level data you would want to use in demonstrating how your community issues compare to others.

## References

Alfred, R. (2009). Sept. 8, 1854: Pump shutdown stops London cholera outbreak. Retrieved from http://www.wired.com/thisdayintech/2009/09/0908london-cholera-pump/

Centers for Disease Control and Prevention. (2001). Updated guidelines for evaluating public health surveillance systems: Recommendations from the Guidelines Working Group. *MMWR, 50*(RR13), 1–35. Retrieved from http://www.cdc.gov/mmwr/preview/mmwrhtml/rr5013a1.htm

Centers for Disease Control and Prevention. (2015). 2015 Final Pertussis Surveillance Report. Retrieved from https://www.cdc.gov/pertussis/downloads/pertuss-surv-report-2015.pdf

Centers for Disease Control and Prevention. (2016). Lyme disease maps. Reported cases of Lyme disease by state or locality, 2005–2015. Retrieved from https://www.cdc.gov/lyme/stats/maps.html

Central Intelligence Agency: *The world factbook.* (2016). North America: United States. Retrieved from https://www.cia.gov/library/publications/resources/the-world-factbook/geos/us.html

Clark, M. (2008). *Community health nursing: Advocacy for population health* (5th ed.). Upper Saddle River, NJ: Pearson Education.

County Health Rankings & Roadmaps. (2012). Minnesota. University of Wisconsin Population Health Institute. Retrieved from http://www.countyhealthrankings.org/app/minnesota/2018/overview

Earl, C. (2009). Medical history and epidemiology: Their contribution to the development of public health nursing. *Nursing Outlook, 57*(5), 257–265.

Felitti, V. J., Anda, R. F., Nordenberg, D., Williamson, D. F., Spitz, A. M., Edwards, V., & Koss, M. P. (1998). Relationship of childhood abuse and household dysfunction to many of the leading causes of death in adults: The Adverse Childhood Experiences (ACE) study. *American Journal of Preventive Medicine, 14*(4), 245–258.

Friis, R. H. (2018). *Epidemiology 101* (2nd ed.). Burlington, MA: Jones & Bartlett

Garwick, A. W., Svavarsdóttir, E. K., Seppelt, A. M., Looman, W. S., Anderson, L. S., & Örlygsdóttir, B. (2015). Development of an International School Nurse Asthma Care Coordination Model. *Journal of Advanced Nursing, 71*(3), 535–546.

Global Health Security Agenda. (2017). About. Retrieved from https://www.ghsagenda.org/about

Guadarrama-Celaya, F., Otero-Ojeda, G. A., Pliego-Rivero, F. B., Porcayo-Mercado, M., Ricardo-Garcell, J., & Perez-Abalo, M. C. (2012). Screening of neurodevelopmental delays in four communities of Mexico and Cuba. *Public Health Nursing, 29*(2), 105–115.

Henry Street Consortium. (2017). *Entry-level population-based public health nursing competencies.* St. Paul, MN: Author. Retrieved from http://www.henrystreetconsortium.org

Holman, D., Ports, K., Buchanan, N., Hawkins, N., Merrick, M., Metzler, M., & Trivers, K. (2016). The association between adverse childhood experiences and risk of cancer in adulthood: A systematic review of the literature. *Pediatrics, 138*(Suppl. 1), S81–S91.

Klopf, L. (1998). Tuberculosis control in the New York State Department of Correctional Services: A case management approach. *American Journal of Infection Control, 26*(5), 534–538.

Krieger, N. (1997). Epidemiology and the web of causation: Has anyone seen the spider? *Social Science and Medicine, 39*(7), 887–903.

Krieger, N. (2001a). A glossary for social epidemiology. *Journal of Epidemiology and Community Health, 55*(10), 693–700.

Krieger, N. (2001b). Theories for social epidemiology in the 21st century: An ecosocial perspective. *International Journal of Epidemiology, 30*(4), 668–677.

Krieger, N. (2012). Methods for the scientific study of discrimination and health: An ecosocial approach. *American Journal of Public Health, 102*(5), 936–945.

Kuh, D., Ben-Shlomo, Y., Lynch, J., Hallqvist, J., & Power, C. (2003). Life course epidemiology. *Journal of Epidemiology and Community Health, 57*(10), 778–783.

Le, C. T. (2001). *Health and numbers: A problem-based introduction to biostatistics* (2nd ed.). New York, NY: Wiley-Liss.

Lind, C., & Smith, D. (2008). Analyzing the state of community health nursing: Advancing from deficit to strengths-based practice using appreciative inquiry. *Advances in Nursing Science, 31*(1), 28–41.

Long, R., Heffernan, C., Gao, Z., Egedahl, M. L., & Talbot, J. (2015). Do "virtual" and "outpatient" public health tuberculosis clinics perform equally well? A program-wide evaluation in Alberta, Canada. *PLoS ONE, 10*(12), e0144784. doi:10.1371/journal.pone.0144784

Merrill, R. M. (2017). *Introduction to epidemiology* (7th ed.). Sudbury, MA: Jones and Bartlett.

Minnesota Department of Health. (2016). Reported cases of Lyme disease in Minnesota by year, 1996–2015. Retrieved from http://www.health.state.mn.us/divs/idepc/diseases/lyme/casesyear.pdf

Monsen, K. A., Brandt, J. K., Brueshoff, B. L., Chi, C., Mathiason, M. A., Swenson, S. M., & Thorson, D. R. (2017). Social determinants and health disparities associated with outcomes of women of childbearing age who receive public health nurse home visiting services. *Journal of Obstetric, Gynecologic, and Neonatal Nursing, 46*, 292–303.

Richter, M. (2010). It does take two to tango! On the need for theory in research on the social determinants of health. *International Journal of Public Health, 55*, 457–458.

Stein, Z., Susser, M., Saenger, G., & Marolla, F. (1975). *Famine and human development: The Dutch hunger winter of 1944–45.* New York, NY: Oxford University Press.

University of California, Los Angeles. (2010). John Snow. Retrieved from http://www.ph.ucla.edu/epi/snow.html

Valanis, B. (1999). *Epidemiology in health care* (3rd ed.). Stamford, CT: Appleton and Lange.

Wolff, K., Baglivio, M., & Piquero, A. (2015). The relationship between adverse childhood experiences and recidivism in a sample of juvenile offenders in community-based treatment. *International Journal of Offender Therapy and Comparative Criminology, 61*(11), 1210–1242.

# CHAPTER 5

# COMPETENCY #3

## Utilizes the Principles and Science of Environmental Health to Promote Safe and Sustainable Environments for Individuals/Families, Systems, and Communities

■ **Patricia M. Schoon**
*with Noreen Kleinfehn-Wald, Carolyn M. Porta, and Stacie O'Leary*

*Jeff, Gena, Max, and Dana are working with Candace, the school nurse, at an environmental magnet elementary school. Candace tells them that she has documented an increase in asthma attacks and asthma-related absences since the beginning of the flu season a month ago. She asks the students to do an assessment, kind of like a modified community assessment, to identify the potential causes of the increased incidence. The students are having a meeting to discuss how to organize their assessment.*

*Jeff states, "I think we need to research all of the causes of asthma and asthma attacks and what might place these students at risk for increased attacks."*

*Gena responds, "This is going to be complicated. My niece has asthma and my sister is always looking for asthma triggers. My sister also recently met with the school nurse to develop an asthma action plan to use at school. There are so many risk factors."*

*Dana comments, "I don't know much about environmental health. I think I want to do some reading about what it is and what environmental health has to do with nursing."*

*Max responds, "I agree with Dana. When I think of environmental health and nursing I think of how we dispose of hazardous waste materials in the hospital. There is also the climate change issue, but I don't know what this has to do with nursing. I need to figure out where asthma triggers fit in all of this."*

*Gena reflects, "Besides this community assessment, we are all making home visits with a public health nurse [PHN]. Maybe some of what we learn will help us with our assessment of the families we are visiting and with the interventions we do with our PHN preceptors."*

*The students review the environmental health PHN competencies they will be developing as they complete this project. Jeff starts a to-do list and writes a list of definitions the group will need as they research their topic from an environmental perspective.*

---

**JEFF'S NOTEBOOK**

**COMPETENCY #3** Utilizes the Principles and Science of Environmental Health to Promote Safe and Sustainable Environments for Individuals/Families, Systems, and Communities

A. Promotes environments that facilitate holistic well-being and health, healing, and healthy lifestyles for individuals/families, systems, and communities

   1) Assesses environmental risk factors and protective factors for individuals/families, systems, and communities

   2) Engages in actions to reduce environmental risk factors and strengthen protective factors for individuals/families, systems, and communities

   3) Takes actions to reduce and manage harmful waste products from individuals/families, systems, and communities

   4) Evaluates the outcomes of actions to promote healthy environments

*(continues)*

## JEFF'S NOTEBOOK
### COMPETENCY #3 (continued)

B. Seeks to protect individuals/families, systems, and communities from environmental hazards

1) Educates individuals, families, systems, and communities about environmental hazards and harmful lifestyle factors

2) Recommends modifications in home, neighborhood, workplace, and community environments to increase safety for individuals and families across the life span

3) Supports right-to-know legislation and regulations that protect and inform the public about hazardous products

C. Considers the diverse values, beliefs, cultures, and circumstances of individuals/families and populations when recommending and implementing healthy environmental interventions

1) Is attentive to diverse lifestyle factors and assesses potential health and safety risks related to them

2) Accepts and supports diversity in environmental lifestyle factors

3) Makes referrals when appropriate to governmental agencies when harmful environmental lifestyle factors place children and vulnerable adults at risk

D. Promotes stewardship of the environment at local, national, and international levels

1) Advocates for sustainable natural and built environments

2) Advocates for environmental justice for vulnerable and under-represented populations

3) Supports policies that promote safe and sustainable natural and built environments and water and food systems

*Source:* Henry Street Consortium, 2017

### USEFUL DEFINITIONS

**Built Environment:** Includes products, structures, buildings, or transportation created or modified by human beings.

**Environment:** "Reflects the aggregate of those external conditions and influences affecting the life and development of an organism... physical, chemical, biological, and social factors that affect the health status of people" (Merrill, 2017, p. 214); "factors external to the human or animal that cause or allow transmission" (p. 8).

**Environmental Health:** "Environmental health comprises those aspects of human health, including quality of life, that are determined by physical, chemical, biological, social, and psychosocial factors in the environment. It also refers to the theory and practice of assessing, correcting, controlling, and preventing those factors in the environment that can potentially affect adversely the health of present and future generations."—draft definition developed at a WHO consultation in Sofia, Bulgaria, 1993 (U.S. Department of Health and Human Services [U.S. DHHS] Environmental Health Policy Committee, Risk Communication and Education Subcommittee, 1998).

**Environmental Stewardship:** The responsibility for environmental quality shared by all those whose actions affect the environment (Environmental Protection Agency Environmental Action Council, 2005).

**Exposure:** A three-phase process: "1) contact is between a target and one or more agents in the same environment; 2) agent accesses target by one or more routes of entry; and 3) the agent enters the target by crossing a barrier or boundary" (Thompson & Schwartz Barcott, 2017, p. 1315).

**Hazard:** Ability of an environmental agent to do harm.

**Natural Environment:** Includes the physical environment (e.g., air, water, land, soil, plants, weather, climate) and biological and chemical entities that exist in the environment.

**Planetary Health:** The achievement of the highest attainable standard of health, well-being, and equity worldwide through judicious attention to the human systems—political, economic, and social—that shape the future of humanity, and the Earth's natural systems that define the safe environmental limits within which humanity can flourish. Planetary health is the health of human civilization and the state of the natural systems on which it depends (Lancet Commission, 2015; Whitmee et al., 2015).

**Precautionary Principle:** When an activity raises threats of harm to human health or the environment, precautionary measures should be taken even if some cause and effect relationships are not fully established scientifically. In this context, the proponent of an activity, rather than the public, should bear the burden of proof (Chaudry, 2008).

**Risk:** The likelihood of harm occurring once an individual is exposed to a hazard (United Nations [UN], 2015).

**Social Environment:** Social interactions, behaviors, norms, institutions, and access to healthcare.

**Sustainable Community:** A sustainable community is one that is economically, environmentally, and socially healthy and resilient. It meets challenges through integrated solutions, rather than through fragmented approaches that meet one of those goals at the expense of the others (Institute for Sustainable Communities, n.d.).

# What Is Environmental Health?

When you think of the environment, what comes to your mind? The first things that probably come to mind are the physical locations in which you spend your daily life, such as your home, neighborhood, parks, and open green spaces. When you consider the health of the environment, you must pay attention to both the seen (e.g., air, water, land) and the unseen (e.g., microscopic pollutants) as well as the social factors, including individual and societal behaviors, that shape the world. A holistic definition of environmental health would include physical, chemical, biological, social, and behavioral factors that influence the environment. A thorough understanding of environmental health requires looking beyond the factors that compose "environment" and determining whether it is healthy or unhealthy. You need to also carefully consider the interactive effects, and you need to further analyze the role of human behavior and response to the environment that is consequently shaping the world and impacting health.

## Challenges of Environmental Health

In this chapter, you will read about both the immediate and the long-term challenges of environmental health, ranging from the hazards and exposures that you encounter on a daily basis to the broader encompassing global challenges of climate change. Public health nurses (PHNs) give attention to the immediate environmental risks faced by individuals, families, and communities, such as the availability of clean water, healthy food, and safe home and community environments. In many parts of the world there are threats to health related to the presence and disposal of biological and chemical hazards. These environmental challenges to health are substantial and necessitate action to mitigate them and promote health and well-being. Exposure to environmental hazards poses significant threats to health that include acute illness, infectious and chronic diseases, and premature deaths (i.e., those occurring before expected life span). The impact of environmental hazards on mortality and morbidity is referred to as the global disease burden, as illustrated in the following quotation:

> Twenty-three percent of global deaths and 22% of global disability adjusted life years were attributable to environmental risks in 2012... The global disease burden attributable to the environment is now dominated by noncommunicable diseases. Susceptible ages are children under five and adults between 50 and 75 years (Prüss-Ustün et al., 2017).

Responses to environmental health challenges involve efforts to eliminate or weaken the hazard, reduce the potential for exposure to the hazard, and mitigate the effects of the exposure.

## History of U.S. Environmental Health Movement

The contemporary environmental health movement in the United States began with the 1962 publication of the book *Silent Spring*, written by Rachel Carson, a marine biologist. She published her research on chemical pesticides, which resulted in the government banning the agricultural pesticide DDT, a synthetic aromatic hydrocarbon (U.S. Fish and Wildlife Service, 2012).

From 1942 to 1953, a chemical company dumped chemical hazardous waste into Love Canal, an aborted Niagara River canal project that ran through a 15-acre working-class neighborhood (Kleiman, 2017). In the 1970s, investigative reporters revealed a cluster of illnesses including epilepsy, asthma, migraines, and nephrosis, as well as abnormally high rates of birth defects and miscarriages occurring in families that lived near Love Canal. Contaminated water was found in the basements and yards of residents as well as in the school playground built over the canal. Activist women, mostly mothers in the Love Canal neighborhood, tried to get the New York State government to take action, but it did not. Between 1978 and 1981, 939 families were relocated by the federal government. This tragedy mobilized concerned citizens nationwide to lobby Congress to act to make businesses responsible for cleanup of toxic waste dumps that they created. In 1980, Congress passed The Superfund Bill (i.e., Comprehensive Environmental Response, Compensation, and Liability Act). These citizen actions were the beginning of a grassroots environmental movement that continues to the present day.

# Environmental Health— At the Core of Nursing Practice

PHNs are concerned about how the environment affects individuals, families, and the community/society at large. They consider the ongoing interactions between their clients and the environment and the cumulative effects of environmental hazards on health status. PHNs assess both the protective and the risk factors of the natural and the built physical environment and take actions to reduce environmental risk factors to improve the health status of individuals, families, and communities.

Since the time of Florence Nightingale, nurses have identified the relationship between the environment and health outcomes. In *Notes on Nursing,* Nightingale lists five things that must be present to have a healthy home; although generated in the 19th century, they remain relevant to the 21st century: pure air, pure water, efficient drainage, cleanliness, and light (Nightingale, 1860). Nightingale was responsible for applying principles of cleanliness in the care of the injured during war, which likely resulted in numerous saved lives.

Clara Barton, trained as a teacher and not a nurse, provided nursing care to Union soldiers during the Civil War and was officially named head nurse for one of General Benjamin Butler's units in 1864. Her experience in the Civil War began her long history of helping those in need in times of conflict and disaster. Barton was instrumental in starting the American Red Cross in 1881 and was president of the Red Cross until 1904. She then started National First Aid Association of America; the organization's priority was emergency preparedness (Michaels, 2015).

Years later, Lillian Wald, recognized as the first public health nurse in the U.S., worked to improve horrifically overcrowded and infested housing conditions in New York City. She believed that the crowded and dismal living conditions of immigrants and children on the Lower East Side of New York resulted in poor health outcomes and began providing nursing services in peoples' homes. She used her societal position to lobby for safe spaces for children to play in New York City, and helped to establish the first parks and playgrounds for children in the 20th century (Filiaci, n.d.). Wald founded the Henry Street Settlement in 1893 and led that organization until 1933, providing health and social services to people who suffered health consequences for the environmental health condition of their place of residence (Henry Street Settlement, 2017).

The Institute of Medicine's (IOM) 1995 landmark publication, *Nursing, Health, and the Environment,* addressed environmental health as a core function of nursing practice in all clinical practice areas and not just the province of nurses who specialize in environmental health (IOM, 1995). The IOM also identified the importance of using the population-based public health nursing approach for environmental health issues and the need to prepare more nurses at the baccalaureate level so that the nursing profession would have greater capacity to address the environmental health concerns of populations as well as individuals. In 2007, the American Nurses Association (ANA), recognizing the importance of environmental health as a core component of the scope of practice of professional nursing, published the *ANA's Principles of Environmental Health for Nursing Practice with Implementation Strategies* (see Table 5.1).

A coalition of U.S.-based nurses created the Alliance of Nurses for Healthy Environments (ANHE) in 2008 (ANHE, 2017). This alliance has published standards for environmental health nursing, developed an online free eBook, *Environmental Health in Nursing* (2016), maintains a listing of environmental hazards (see https://envirn.org/) and has

## TABLE 5.1 ANA's Principles of Environmental Health for Nursing Practice

1. Knowledge of environmental health concepts is essential to nursing practice.

2. The Precautionary Principle guides nurses in their practice to use products and practices that do not harm human health or the environment and to take preventive action in the face of uncertainty.

3. Nurses have a right to work in an environment that is safe and healthy.

4. Healthy environments are sustained through multidisciplinary collaboration.

5. Choices of materials, products, technology, and practices in the environment that impact nursing practice are based on the best evidence available.

6. Approaches to promoting a healthy environment respect the diverse values, beliefs, cultures, and circumstances of patients and their families.

7. Nurses participate in assessing the quality of the environment in which they practice and live.

8. Nurses, other health care workers, patients, and communities have the right to know relevant and timely information about the potentially harmful products, chemicals, pollutants, and hazards to which they are exposed.

9. Nurses participate in research of best practices that promote a safe and healthy environment.

10. Nurses must be supported in advocating for and implementing environmental health principles in nursing practice.

*Source:* ANA, 2007, p. 16

### TABLE 5.2 Top Ten Reasons That Nurses and Environmental Health Go Together

- Nurses provide healing and safe environments for people.
- Nurses are trusted sources of information.
- Nurses are the largest healthcare occupation.
- Nurses work with persons from a variety of cultures.
- Nurses effect decisions in their own homes, work settings, and communities.
- Nurses are good sources of information for policymakers.
- Nurses translate scientific health literature to make it understandable.
- Nurses with advanced degrees are engaged in research about the environment and health.
- Health organizations recognize nurses' roles in environmental health.
- Nursing education and standards of nursing practice require that nurses know how to reduce exposures to environmental health hazards.

*Source:* ANHE, 2016, p. 2

workgroups for education, research, practice, and policy/advocacy. ANHE has identified ten reasons why it is important and appropriate for nurses to be involved in environmental health (see Table 5.2).

## The Precautionary Principle

PHNs take actions to prevent harm to their clients. However, the cause-effect relationship between some environmental hazards or potential hazards is not always clear. PHNs use the Precautionary Principle to guide their actions in protecting themselves and their families, clients, and community. The following definition provides guidelines for applying the Precautionary Principle to nursing actions.

> When an activity raises threats of harm to human health or the environment, precautionary measures should be taken even if some cause and effect relationships are not fully established scientifically. In this context the proponent of an activity, rather than the public, should bear the burden of proof. The process of applying the Precautionary Principle must be open, informed, and democratic and must include potentially affected parties. It must also involve an examination of the full range of alternatives, including no action (Science and Environmental Health Network, 1998).

Using the Precautionary Principle makes good sense. Start by considering what you can do in your home, neighborhood, and workplace to reduce exposure to hazards. You can also look at correlation and make common sense

decisions about actions you should take. For example, long before the causal relationship between the ultraviolet rays of the sun and skin cancer was known, people took precautions about time spent in the sun to avoid sunburn. The acronym ACT serves as a critical-thinking approach to known and potential environmental hazards, including those that pose both immediate and long-term actual and potential risks:

**A. Assessment:** Assess environmental hazards and health risks.

**C. Critical thinking:** Reflect on the consequences of these risks and how best to mitigate or eliminate them in the short and long term. Consider the sustainability of interventions and the evidence base for their likely success.

**T. Take Actions:** Know best practices to reduce environmental hazards and risks, and apply them. Consider PHN interventions at the individual/family, community, and systems levels of PHN practice.

## Environmental Health— The Role of the PHN

The role of the PHN in environmental health is dependent in part on the employment location of the PHN, the structure of the public health agency, and existing laws and regulations. Some agencies include an environment health section, and some employ a single environmental health specialist or a sanitarian. Agencies provide services for building code compliance, solid waste disposal, and hazardous waste removal. If there is a sanitarian on staff, the PHN may serve as a consultant to the sanitarian or work with those cases that need long-term follow-up due to a medical or health impact. In agencies where there is not a sanitarian, PHNs may do the environmental risk assessment themselves.

PHNs often collaborate with human service providers working in child protection or with vulnerable adults. The PHN might accompany a social worker to a home to assess safety conditions or might request a social worker to intervene after doing an initial home visit. Family lifestyle patterns are diverse, so it is important to consider whether the differences in conditions are benign or harmful to family members. The PHN might need to make a determination as to whether the conditions are significant enough to warrant removal or temporary relocation of an individual. The PHN may also be involved in a plan to improve the livability of a dwelling. Some environmental situations, such as hoarding, can be very complex and could involve social workers, mental health professionals, law enforcement, and others to address the situation.

Existing laws and ordinances greatly shape the role of the PHN in addressing environmental hazards or risks. For example, a state law or local ordinance may designate a public health inspection. If such is the case, then there is usually a process to give legal orders to abate a situation, and a process to follow in the event the property owner does not comply. The PHN may be involved in tracking the progress made or consulting with the local court system if there is noncompliance. Some states legally designate local public health to be the final authority on cleanup of methamphetamine houses (homes that have been contaminated because of the presence of a meth lab). Often public health nurses need to be fluent on issues related to lease agreements, tenant rights, and accessing low-cost legal assistance as they provide counsel to vulnerable clients.

Nurses also need to advocate with medical providers and insurance companies to provide equipment that reduces the risks of those with chronic disease who are exposed to environmental hazards in the home. For example, home care nurses who have clients with respiratory conditions may need to advocate for air purifiers to improve the quality of indoor air. PHNs may also be the advocate for those living in sub-standard housing or in areas where there are significant outdoor environmental hazards. There is a known disparity in the availability of healthy homes and healthy living environments, which has a disparate impact on the poor and minorities (U.S. DHHS, 2009). PHNs may need to advocate with policymakers to improve the opportunities for disadvantaged populations to have access to healthy homes and neighborhoods.

*Jeff and Max have been thinking about the role of the nurse in environmental health. They feel overwhelmed. They talk with Gena and Dana, who have just made their first home visit with a public health nurse. Dana made a home visit to a young woman who is pregnant and was worried about environmental exposures she might have had that could harm her baby. During a visit to a young family with a child with asthma, Gena found out that the family has bedbugs.*

*Dana reflects, "What we are learning in our home visiting experiences about environmental health can help us determine what environmental factors we need to consider when looking for the causes of increased asthma attacks. I think we need to look at the physical environment both at home and at school to see what the risks are. Let's focus on the students' homes and their families. We need to look for the asthma triggers."*

*Gena reminds them, "We also need to think about the school environment—both the physical and the social aspects. We need to find out what the school staff know about asthma triggers and what they are doing that protects the children with asthma."*

*Max states, "I am going to research environmental asthma triggers."*

*Jeff responds, "We need to find more resources."*

### Online Activity

Help Max and Jeff research environmental asthma triggers. Here are a few online resources for you to use. Refer to the information on the following websites and make a list of environmental asthma triggers.

- Environmental Health in Nursing, an open-source textbook, written by members of the Alliance of Nurses for Healthy Environments at https://envirn.org/wp-content/uploads/2017/03/Environmental-Health-in-Nursing.pdf
- Environmental Triggers of Asthma at https://www.atsdr.cdc.gov/csem/csem.asp?csem=32&po=6
- Asthma and Allergies and Their Environmental Triggers at https://kids.niehs.nih.gov/topics/pollution/asthma-and-allergies/index.htm
- Childhood Asthma at http://asthmaandallergies.org/asthma-allergies/childhood-asthma/

## Individual/Family Level of Practice

This section focuses on identifying key environmental hazards that have a direct effect on individuals and families and strategies for how to prevent or mitigate the exposures and their effects. A few hazards often encountered by PHNs in their personal lives and daily work are discussed. Five common types of environmental hazards are found in the home, in the workplace, and in schools:

- **Chemical:** Medications; illegal drugs; pesticides; formaldehyde (found in almost all new products containing glue); volatile organic compounds (VOCs) found in household products such as paints, varnishes, wax, mothballs, many cleaning and disinfecting products, personal hygiene products, and cosmetics; and industrial chemicals used in cars and in the workplace
- **Physical:** Radon, radiation, weather, sound, vibration, impact
- **Mechanical:** Pressure, ergonomics, confined space, repetitive motion
- **Biological:** Bacteria, viruses, parasites, mold, allergens, pet dander
- **Sociocultural:** Violence and war, interpersonal abuse, institutionalized racism

The impact of the exposure to human beings and animals is often multifaceted and might have immediate, short-term, or long-term influence. The three-phase process of exposure includes: 1) exposure of the target host with one or more environmental agents; 2) ability of the agent to access one or more routes of entry in the target host; and, 3) entry of the agent into the target host by crossing a barrier or boundary (Thompson & Schwartz Barcott, 2017, p. 1315).

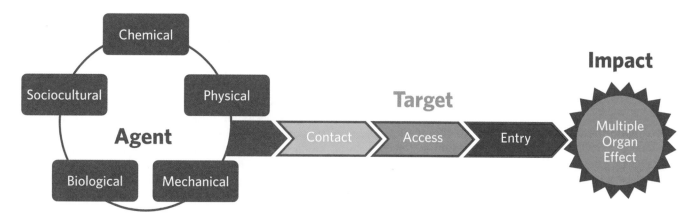

**FIGURE 5.1** Process of Exposure and Impact

Figure 5.1 illustrates the process of exposure, access, and the potential impact on multiple organs in the body of the host. The impact to the host organs may be short-term, long-term, or delayed.

### Online Activity

PHNs must continually update their knowledge about environmental hazards, their impact on health, and interventions to reduce exposures and to respond to exposures. Read more about:

- **VOCs** at https://www.epa.gov/indoor-air-quality-iaq/volatile-organic-compounds-impact-indoor-air-quality

- **Formaldehyde** at https://www.epa.gov/formaldehyde/facts-about-formaldehyde

- **Mothballs** at http://npic.orst.edu/ingred/ptype/mothball/health.html

1. What information did you learn that you could share with families to help reduce their chemical exposure?

2. How would you provide technical information about chemicals in words understandable to diverse audiences?

## Exposure Over the Life Span

There are "critical windows of vulnerability" across the life span, including pregnancy, fetal development, early childhood, and adolescent development. Exposure to toxic chemicals during fetal development and early childhood can lead to deficits later in life (ANHE, 2016; Sanchez, Hu, Litman, & Tellez-Rojo, 2011). In a study by Sutton and colleagues, all the pregnant women tested were found to have hazardous chemicals in their bloodstream including lead, mercury, toluene, perchlorate, bisphenol A (BPA), phthalates, pesticides, perfluorochemicals (PFCs), polychlorinated biphenyls

(PCBs), and polybrominated diphenyl ethers (PBDEs) (Sutton et al., 2012). Many chemicals cross the placental barrier. Toxic chemical exposure during pregnancy may result in increased poor birth outcomes (e.g., preterm birth, low birth weight, birth defects); increased rates of autism; and poor outcomes into adulthood including chronic diseases, cancer, obesity, and decreased life expectancy. Preconception exposure may also result in declines in both male and female fertility and fecundity (Sutton et al., 2012).

Exposure to common household products such as plastic food containers and water bottles can leak phthalates (man-made chemicals used to make plastics harder or more flexible) into food and water, causing endocrine system damage that is especially harmful to children and pregnant women (National Scientific Council on the Developing Child, 2006; World Health Organization [WHO], 2011). Heavy metals such as lead, mercury, manganese, and organophosphates (OPs) are common ingredients in insecticides and cause damage to fetuses and young children. These chemicals inhibit brain architecture and development and can result in cognitive and behavioral deficits both early and later in life. One in six children in industrialized countries are reported to have neurodevelopmental disorders, and it is estimated that 5% to 20% of these are caused by toxic environmental exposures (Thompson & Schwartz Barcott, 2017).

Children's health problems resulting from everyday exposure to contaminated water, poor sanitation, inadequate food supply resulting in malnutrition, indoor smoke, disease vectors such as mosquitoes, and unsafe use of chemicals and waste disposal have been identified as among the highest environmental burden of disease worldwide (WHO, 2011, 2017). Children, particularly young children, can often be found playing on the floor and on the ground outside; they touch, taste, and inhale a variety of potentially toxic substances. They are exposed to potentially toxic indoor air in schools and toxins brought home from work by adults (ANHE, 2016). WHO (2017) has identified seven areas of environmental threats to children in both developing and advanced industrialized countries:

- **Chemical hazards:** Exposure to both the "old" and "new" chemicals, of *anthropogenic* (results of human actions on nature) and natural origin, present in the places where children spend time.

- **Air pollution (indoor and outdoor):** Exposure to ozone, $SO_2$, $NO_2$, sulfate particles (a major fraction of the particle burden in urban air), carbon soot, polycyclic aromatic hydrocarbons, carbon monoxide, and tobacco smoke are some typical air contaminants known to affect morbidity and mortality. Indoor air pollution from use of biomass fuel in developing countries is a major public health problem, as it contributes heavily to the mortality of children under 5 years of age.

- **Household water insecurity:** Although in developing countries the main concern is microbiological contamination, a number of water pollutants have a tremendous impact on public health, including arsenic, lead, fluoride, and pesticides.

- **Poor hygiene and sanitation:** These hinder the maintenance of clean environments—the washing, cleaning, and removal of chemicals, dirt, and pollutants.

- **Disease vectors:** The use of pesticides to combat malaria, dengue, and other vector-borne diseases increases the risk of children's exposure to these products.

- **Injuries and accidents:** Poisoning, both intentional and nonintentional due to toxicants (e.g., a child drinking poisonous household chemicals stored in bottles previously used for beverages).

- **Emerging issues:** Climate change, depletion of the ozone layer, the potential risk posed by electromagnetic fields and by chemicals that persist in the environment (persistent organic pollutants [POPs]).

Older adults, for different reasons than children, are also more vulnerable to environmental hazard exposure (Geller, 2010). Reasons for this vulnerability include reduced immune and metabolic system functions, decreased pharmacokinetic function, reduced nutrition, physical trauma, and the presence of chronic diseases. Older adults have already experienced multiple exposures over their life span. Their age, sex, culture, socioeconomic status, potential social isolation, and place of residence can also play a role in the extent of the exposures and subsequent impacts on health and well-being. Older adults are at high risk primarily for cardiac, respiratory, and mental health conditions due to extreme weather events; they also have the highest mortality rate from these events (Leyva, Beamon, & Davidson, 2017).

# Environmental Hazards in the Home Environment

Environmental hazards exist in the home, neighborhood, workplace, school, and the larger community. PHNs who make home visits, or work in schools or in occupational settings, need to assess the home for existing and potential environmental hazards and work with their clients to reduce them. PHNs must also be aware of the potential environmental causes of signs and symptoms that individuals and families are experiencing.

Identifying the effects of the exposure is much easier to do than identifying the exposure and its source, particularly if the exposure was distant from the person's home or distant in time of exposure. Figure 5.2 demonstrates multiple stages from source to exposure to disease.

## Everyday Lifestyle Exposures

Exposure to volatile organic compounds (VOCs) occurs in the home environment and other environments where you spend your everyday life. The majority of chemicals in the marketplace have had no testing as to their safety, so specific levels of exposure and risk have not been identified (Sutton et al., 2012). However, you may not assume that there is any safe level of exposure. The Precautionary Principle applies when considering use of chemicals in your everyday life, such as infant skincare products and antimicrobial cleaning products. Human beings and animals are exposed to environmental hazards across the life span. However, hazards differ in their level of risk and impact based on age, ethnicity, and social conditions such as poverty. Exposure to environmental hazards is cumulative over the life span (see Chapter 4). The hazard level (i.e., how harmful is the agent) and the number of exposures results in the level of risk to an individual (UN, 2015).

It is important for PHNs to understand the risks and levels of those risks that their clients experience. Common chemicals found in the home, which pose a significant threat to individuals and families, are presented in Table 5.3.

Air pollution occurs in outside air (ambient air) and indoor air. Each home has its own unique cluster of indoor air pollutants. The cumulative effect of noise exposure has resulted in approximately 26 million Americans with noise-induced hearing loss that is usually permanent (Plotnick, 2017). Noise-induced hearing loss (NIHL) is preventable (WHO, 2015b). Table 5.4 outlines common causes of indoor air pollution and their effects.

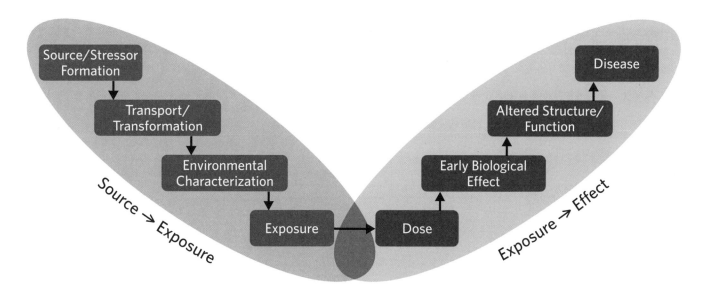

The environmental public health continuum describes the pathway from the formation or release of pollutants through to effects on human populations.

**FIGURE 5.2**  Environmental Public Health Exposure Continuum
*Source:* Geller, 2010, p. 11

## TABLE 5.3  Common Household Chemicals

| Chemical | Where It's Found |
| --- | --- |
| Pesticides | Mosquito sprays, other insect repellents, and anti-microbial sanitizers. Low-dose single exposure to pesticides is not fatal; continuous exposure over time can lead to diseases affecting the nervous and reproductive systems and your kidneys and cause cancer. |
| Phthalates and PVC (polyvinyl chloride) | Often used as construction materials and found in plastic products. When PVC is burned, it releases dioxin—one of the most toxic substances known. PVC is found in window blinds, flooring, vinyl shower curtains, baby toys, cosmetics, and most of the plastic products used at home. |
| Parabens | Used as a preservative in cosmetics, skincare products, pharmaceutical products, and as food additives. Parabens may cause breast cancer, decreased male fertility, and endocrine problems. |
| Bisphenol A (BPA) | Chemical found in hard plastics and in the coatings of food and drink cans and in the majority of everyday products (e.g., baby bottles, water bottles, dental fillings, household electronics, and many more). BPA is an endocrine disruptor and can interfere in the behavior of hormones. It causes reproductive disorders, male impotence, heart disease, and asthma. It affects the quality of a woman's eggs and can cause breast cancer. A Centers for Disease Control and Prevention (CDC) study showed that 95% of human adult urine samples and 93% of children's urine samples had Bisphenol A. |
| Ammonia | Popular cleaning product. Direct exposure to ammonia can irritate eyes and lungs, and in direct contact with the skin can cause burns or rashes. When mixed with bleach or other chlorine products, it can produce deadly chloramine gas. |

*Source:* The World Counts, 2014

**TABLE 5.4  Indoor Air Pollution**

| Airborne Pollutant | Impacts on Health |
| --- | --- |
| Cockroaches and dust mites, which produce allergens | Respiratory problems, exacerbation of asthma |
| Pet dander, saliva, skin flakes, feathers, and urine | Respiratory problems, allergies, asthma exacerbation, eye irritation, skin rashes |
| Crowded and humid environments, which increase spread of bacteria and viruses | Respiratory problems, exacerbation of asthma |
| Mold | Allergies; asthma; irritation to eyes, nose, throat, lungs, skin |
| Cleaning supplies/household products, some containing volatile organic compounds (VOCs) | Respiratory problems, exacerbation of asthma, headaches |
| Scents and perfumes from personal cosmetics, soaps, air fresheners (VOCs) | Respiratory problems, allergies, skin rashes, exacerbation of asthma |
| Building and paint products, carpets (may contain asbestos, lead, formaldehyde, VOCs, other chemicals) | Respiratory problems, coughing, shortness of breath, fatigue, nausea, headaches, cancer |
| Lead (paint before 1978, contaminated soil, dust, workplace exposure brought home) | Cognitive and behavioral problems; affects all body systems, leading to chronic disease and death |
| Wood smoke (indoor and outdoor) | Coughing, wheezing, asthma attacks, heart attacks, lung cancer, and premature death |
| Second-hand smoke—no safe level<br><br>More than 24 million, or about 37% of children in the U.S., have been exposed to secondhand smoke | 7,330 deaths from lung cancer and 33,950 deaths from heart disease<br><br>150,000 to 300,000 lower respiratory tract infections occur annually in infants and children under 18 months of age, resulting in between 7,500 and 15,000 hospitalizations<br><br>430 sudden infant death syndrome (SIDS) deaths in the U.S. annually |
| Asbestos fibers in building materials in older buildings | Asbestosis (scarring of lungs)<br><br>Lung cancer |
| Radon—naturally occurring gas present in unsafe levels in 1/15 U.S. homes.<br><br>The Midwest has the highest rates of radon in the home; 1/3 of the homes in Minnesota likely have enough radon to cause significant health risks with long-term exposure (http://mn-radon.info/MN_general.html) | Second-greatest cause of lung cancer |
| Carbon monoxide (colorless odorless gas produced when fuel is burned) from stoves, fireplaces, space heaters, lawnmowers, gas stoves, grills, power tools, automobile exhaust | Flu-like symptoms, nausea, dizziness, weakness, headache, disorientation, impaired vision and coordination, depression, anxiety, death |
| Ambient noise/noise pollution<br><br>Eighty-five decibels are considered the highest safe exposure level up to a maximum of 8 hours | 12.5% of 6- to 19-year-olds (6.8 million) and 16.8% of 12- to 19-year-olds (5 million) in the U.S. have documented evidence of elevated hearing thresholds directly attributed to noise exposure |

*Sources:* American Academy of Allergy, Asthma, & Immunology, 2018; American Lung Association, 2017; Cantley et al., 2015; Dangerous Decibels, 2018; National Institute on Deafness and Other Communication Disorders (NIDCD), 2017; Potera, 2011; WHO, 2016

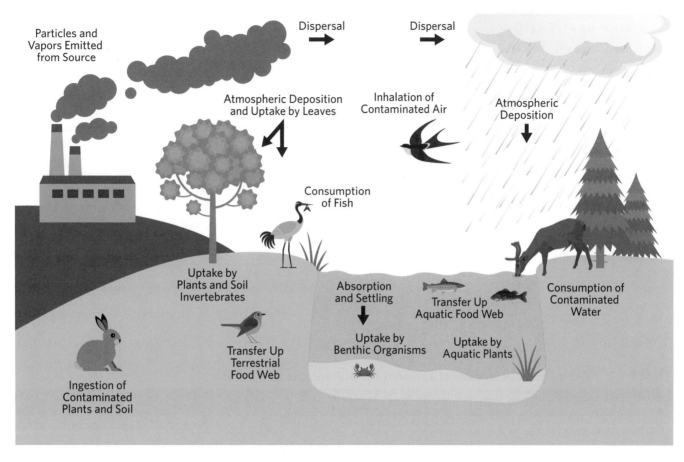

**FIGURE 5.3** Multimodal Air Pollution Pathways
*Source:* EPA, n.d.

It is important for PHNs to have access to online, digital, and paper resources to use in health teaching and referral interventions. Some environmental health hazard resources that may be helpful in working with families or communities include:

■ **Hazardous Air Pollutants** at https://www.epa.gov/haps

■ **Water Topics** at https://www.epa.gov/environmental-topics/water-topics

■ **Water Pollution** at https://www.nrdc.org/issues/water-pollution

■ **Causes and Effects of Water Pollution** at http://www.gogreenacademy.com/causes-and-effects-of-water-pollution/

■ **Sources and Impacts of Contaminants in Soils** at http://cwmi.css.cornell.edu/sourcesandimpacts.pdf

■ **Biological Hazards** at https://www.ccohs.ca/oshanswers/biol_hazards/

■ **Chemical Hazards and Toxic Substances in the Workplace** at https://www.osha.gov/SLTC/hazardoustoxicsubstances/index.html

■ **Radiation Protection** at https://www.epa.gov/radiation

While focusing on air pollution, it is important to note that some pollutants such as mercury may be transported by multiple pathways including air, water, soil, vegetation, and animals (Environmental Protection Agency [EPA], n.d.). Besides inhalation, exposure may occur through direct contact with the skin and ingestion into the gastrointestinal track. This multiexposure pathway model is illustrated in Figure 5.3.

## Assessing for Environmental Exposure

PHNs are often confronted with individuals and families with new or chronic signs and symptoms or diseases such as cancer that have no identified cause. Because environmental hazards and pollutants are so closely linked to health status, it is important for PHNs to carry out a comprehensive assessment to evaluate the potential environmental causes of individual and family signs and symptoms to determine if and what environmental exposures are causing the current health problem. Table 5.5 outlines the IPREPARE tool (Paranzino, Butterfield, Nastoff, & Ranger, 2005), which includes assessment components as well as actions that are needed, such as emergency or nonemergency referrals, health education, and environmental hazard reduction.

## THEORY APPLICATION

### Children's Exposure to Radon and Secondhand Smoke in the Home Environment and Lung Cancer Prevention

There were 224,390 new cases of lung cancer in the United States in 2015. The leading cause of lung cancer is firsthand smoke followed by radon and secondhand smoke (SHS). Exposure to both radon and tobacco smoke in the home environment increases the risk for lung cancer. Radon, present throughout the United States, is responsible for approximately 21,800 lung cancer deaths annually. Children are especially vulnerable to the synergistic effects of exposure to both SHS and radon. It is important for parents to be aware of this heightened risk for their children. A study using McBride's Teachable Moment Model (TM) was carried out to determine whether having young children living in the home motivated adults to acquire skills when presented with specific teachable moments. The teachable moments studied were: lung cancer worry and lung cancer risk (a member of the household was a smoker, or there was a history of lung cancer in the family), synergistic risk (awareness of risk of daily exposure to SHS and radon), and health-related self-concept (health-enhancing behaviors, intentions, attitudes, and self-efficacy). Having children in the home was not found to be a significant predictor of any of these teachable moments. This finding suggested that there is a critical need to raise awareness of parents about the home environmental risk of SHS and radon to their children. Public health nurses were identified as key professionals in the home environment who could work with parents to increase their awareness of the synergistic risk of SHS and radon and assist parents in acquiring the resources needed to improve the safety of the home environment for their children (Huntington-Moskos, Rayens, Wiggins, & Hahn, 2016).

## TABLE 5.5 CDC's Environmental Assessment for Individuals and Families

| I-PREPARE | Assessment and Interventions |
| --- | --- |
| I – Investigate Potential Exposure | Exposure history of family members (i.e., recent signs and/or symptoms or pattern of illness experienced after exposure to chemicals, pesticide, other environmental factors). Improvement to health when away from home or work. |
| P – Present Work | Environmental hazards and toxins and exposure history at work or school |
| R – Residence | Potential toxic exposures at home, drinking water, home building materials, chemicals stored at home |
| E – Environmental Concerns | Environmental concerns in neighborhood: water, air, soil, farms, and industries |
| P – Past Work | Environmental hazards and toxins and exposure history at work or school |
| A – Activities | Family activities at home and in community with potential exposures to biological or chemical agents that could be toxic, alternative medications and treatments, recent travel |
| R – Referrals and Resources | Referral to primary care provider or emergency assistance<br>■ Local health department, environmental health agency, poison control<br>■ Agency for Toxic Substances and Disease Registry<br>■ Association of Occupational and Environmental Clinics<br>■ Material Safety Data Sheets (MSDS)<br>■ Occupational Safety and Health Administration<br>■ U.S. Environmental Protection Agency |
| E – Educate | Education and educational materials to reduce risk of exposure, mitigate environmental hazards, take steps after exposure |

*Source:* Modified from Paranzino et al., 2005

## Activity

Candace, Dana, Jeff, and Max are working on modifying the IPREPARE assessment tool. How would you modify it?

■ Do you think this tool would be useful for assessing the increase in asthma attacks in the school setting?

■ How would you modify the tool?

■ Who would you interview with the tool: the students, parents, or school staff?

---

" *Jeff, Max, Dana, and Gena meet to plan their environmental assessment to identify the causes of the increase in asthma attacks and absences in students with asthma. They discuss assessing the presence of asthma triggers and whether there had been any recent changes in the asthma triggers in the home and school environment.*

*Dana says, "I recently researched asthma triggers. Here is the list of what I found: tobacco smoke and smoke from burning wood and grass, outdoor air pollution, dust mites, cockroaches and their droppings, furry pets, mold, some food and food additives, some medications, scents and fragrances, cold dry air, and high humidity—it seems like everything kids are exposed to!"*

*Jeff adds, "I found that exercise, recent respiratory illnesses, and emotions that cause hyperventilation can also cause asthma attacks. We really need to find out what has changed recently for these students." Both students reported they got their information from a CDC\* website at https:// www.cdc.gov/asthma/triggers.html.*

*Max asks, "What if I modify the IPREPARE assessment that we learned about in class and then we can use it to interview the students with asthma and their parents to see what has changed in the students' environment here at school and at home?"*

*Gena adds, "We also need to interview the teachers and Candace to see what might have changed at school. Candace told me that there can be hidden allergens at school like latex in the gloves, dust on the iPads, plants in the classroom, and foods brought in from home. Let's schedule a meeting with Candace and the principal to see if we can develop a survey and do the interviews."*

*The students meet with Candace, who suggests the steps they might take to start gathering data. They could look at attendance data on individual students and review the notes the nurse had entered into the students' records as to why the students were absent. Some parents may not realize why their child had asthma or had an asthma attack, so the school nurse usually asked the parents about the child's symptoms. Candace thinks that a short survey can be sent home to parents whose children either had asthma or have been absent in the last month. She says the survey can be sent in both English and Spanish. Candace agrees to ask parents who she will talk with in the next few weeks if they would be willing to fill out the survey.*

*Jeff asks, "Would it be useful for us to develop a handout on asthma triggers and how to reduce asthma triggers at home?"*

*Candace answers, "That would be a good idea. You might also want to include information on how to manage asthma attacks at home and when to follow up with a visit to a medical provider. I have some parents who do not have a primary care provider or do not go to follow-up visits and may not use their children's inhalers correctly. I have a few suggestions about online resources you can use, and you can probably look for others as needed. I can have these handouts translated into Spanish if you do not find any in Spanish."*

*Max adds, "We should also do a walk-through of the school to identify asthma triggers and maybe survey the staff about what they have noticed when students have asthma attacks. Jeff, could you help me with that?"*

*Jeff responds, "Sure. We need to check out the animals in the classrooms and the rest of the school. What about assessing the outside environment for asthma triggers?"*

*Dana says, "Gena and I will do that. We have already done a windshield survey. We still need to look up the air quality index for the area. We can observe students during gym class and when they are outside for recess and see if any of them have difficulty breathing when exercising."*

*Candace responds, "We need to get the principal's permission to do the walkabout in the school, staff survey, and observation of the students. Your assessment results and handouts will really help me and the staff."*

*Jeff found some good online resources the students used for the survey and for the handouts.* "
\*CDC, 2012

---

## Activity

These are the following resources that Jeff found on childhood asthma management and the environment.

■ **Asthma Home Environment Checklist**
https://www.epa.gov/asthma/
asthma-home-environment-checklist

■ **Asthma-Friendly Child Care Checklist**
http://asthmaandallergies.org/asthma-allergies/
childcare-asthma-checklist/

■ **IGGY and the Inhalers**
https://iggyandtheinhalers.com/

1. How would you use the Asthma Home Environmental Checklist with a family whose child was recently diagnosed with asthma?

2. If you had to make a one-page handout for children ages 8–10, what would you include from these resources?

## Activity

A 65-year-old woman with a full-body skin rash that had persisted for 30 years was presented at Dermatology Grand Rounds in a Midwestern hospital. The head dermatologist reviewed all the medical interventions that were tried and failed. A nurse practitioner attending Grand Rounds asked the woman, "Do you take showers or tub baths?" When the woman replied that she always took tub baths, the nurse practitioner asked a second question, "Do you put anything in your bath water?" The woman replied, "Yes, I have put Lysol in my bathwater ever since the birth of my last child. My obstetrician told me to clean the tub with Lysol, so I figured that bathing in it would also be a good idea."

Discuss:

1.  What did you learn from this case study about human health and environmental risks?

2.  Is it possible that besides a skin rash, the Lysol might have been absorbed through the skin and caused any other body system damage?

3.  What did you learn about the health information people need to protect themselves from environmental hazards?

4.  What PHN interventions might you provide as follow-up to this woman?

## Healthy Homes

The health and safety of families in their home environment is influenced by more than environmental pollution. Other environmental factors include how the home was designed, constructed, and maintained; the presence or absence of safety devices (e.g., smoke detectors, radon detectors, safe water temperature for bathing, etc.); and the behaviors of those who live in the home (Surgeon General, 2009). In 2009, the Surgeon General instituted a policy for the development and maintenance of healthy homes. A healthy home checklist as well as a pictograph of the checklist was published (see Figure 5.4).

*Dana accompanies Laura, her PHN preceptor, in staffing an environmental health information table at the Women Infants and Children (WIC) office. Because it will soon be summer and there are many good fishing lakes in the area, the chosen topic is fish consumption. Laura presents the standard teaching material from the state health department on methylmercury content in fish, limiting fish consumption during pregnancy, and what is known about the fish populations and mercury in local lakes.*

*One visitor to the table is a woman who already had three spontaneous miscarriages. On her fourth pregnancy, she states she wants as many safeguards as possible, and inquires about other environmental hazards. Laura and the woman discuss reading product labels on oil-based paints, solvents, pesticides, insect repellants, and insecticides. Dana has recently read about green cleaning and so with Laura's permission, Dana and the woman discuss using nontoxic cleaners such as baking soda and vinegar in the home. They also discuss food preparation and the importance of washing fruits and vegetables well to reduce pesticide residue.*

*On the way back to the office, Dana asks Laura if there is science-based evidence on how women can protect themselves during preconception. Laura said there is not a lot of information, but it is best to assume that there is no safe chemical exposure, so it is best to avoid as many chemicals as possible. Dana notes that this was the Precautionary Principle at work again.*

### 🌐 Online Activity

Safety starts in your own home with your own family. Once you safety-proof your own home, you will be better able to help others safety-proof their homes. You will know what is possible and differentiate the real from the ideal. In your own home you still use the same critical thinking skills that you use as a nurse, assessing your home for potential environmental hazards. Use ACT to assess for actual and potential hazards, keeping the Precautionary Principle in mind.

**A Assessment:** Make a list of all the household products and personal care products that are used in your home. Review the listed ingredients, which may or may not be a complete list. Research the products on the Internet to identify the chemical and biological components that are hazardous to your health. Access websites such as the American Lung Association at http://www.lung.org/our-initiatives/healthy-air/indoor/indoor-air-pollutants/.

**C Critical Thinking:** Consider options to improve the safety of your home and your family members. Review the *Ten Environmental Hazards You Can Live Without* at http://www.chaa.org/EarthDayCheckList.pdf. Make a list of options you are willing to take. Review best practices at sites such as Minnesota Healthy Homes at http://www.health.state.mn.us/topics/healthyhomes/.

**T Take Actions** to improve the safety of your home and your family members. Use green cleaning approaches by avoiding antibacterial soaps and cleaners, and consider using homemade cleaning products (Lawler, 2016).

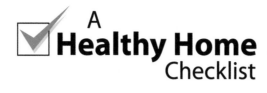

# A
# Healthy Home
## Checklist

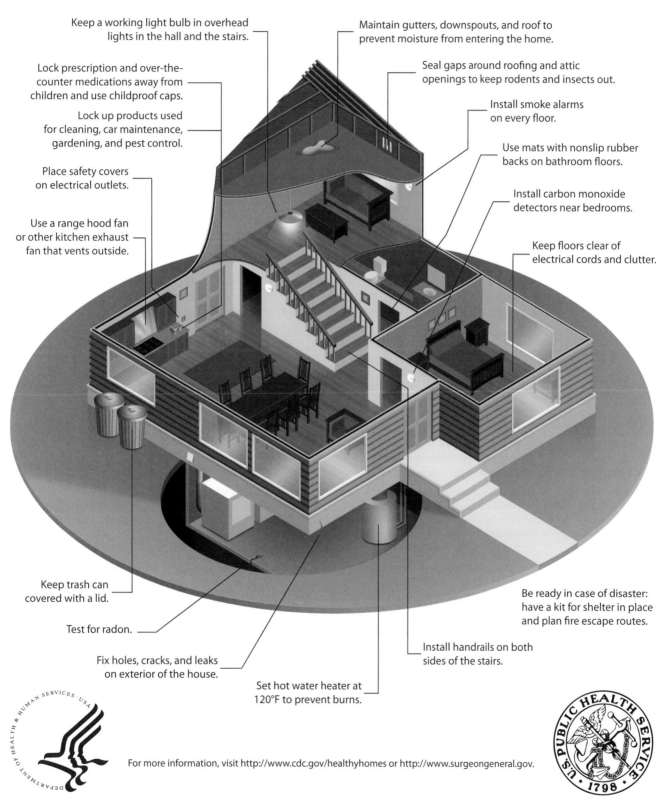

Keep a working light bulb in overhead lights in the hall and the stairs.

Maintain gutters, downspouts, and roof to prevent moisture from entering the home.

Lock prescription and over-the-counter medications away from children and use childproof caps.

Seal gaps around roofing and attic openings to keep rodents and insects out.

Lock up products used for cleaning, car maintenance, gardening, and pest control.

Install smoke alarms on every floor.

Place safety covers on electrical outlets.

Use mats with nonslip rubber backs on bathroom floors.

Use a range hood fan or other kitchen exhaust fan that vents outside.

Install carbon monoxide detectors near bedrooms.

Keep floors clear of electrical cords and clutter.

Keep trash can covered with a lid.

Be ready in case of disaster: have a kit for shelter in place and plan fire escape routes.

Test for radon.

Install handrails on both sides of the stairs.

Fix holes, cracks, and leaks on exterior of the house.

Set hot water heater at 120°F to prevent burns.

For more information, visit http://www.cdc.gov/healthyhomes or http://www.surgeongeneral.gov.

**FIGURE 5.4**  Surgeon General's Healthy Home Checklist
*Source:* Surgeon General, 2009

## Home and Neighborhood Environment

Many home safety tools on the Internet may be used by the PHN or family. The ages of family members as well as their health status should be considered when selecting a tool to use. Sometimes a family has a specific concern such as fire safety, or home safety for toddlers, or fall risks for the elderly. Your agency or nursing instructor may have tools for you to use for specific family needs. A few tools from credible sources are listed in Table 5.6.

It is also important to consider the safety of the neighborhood. A walkability survey would be useful to look for both protective factors such as sidewalks, curb cuts, and lighting and risk factors such as lack of stop signs, heavy traffic, litter, and water hazards (see Chapter 3).

### TABLE 5.6  Home Safety Assessment Tools

| | |
|---|---|
| Fire Prevention | ▪ **U.S. Fire Administration, Home Safety Checklist**<br>https://www.usfa.fema.gov/downloads/pdf/home_safety_checklist.pdf<br>▪ **American Red Cross, Fire Safety Checklist**<br>http://www.redcross.org/images/MEDIA_CustomProductCatalog/m4340073_FireSafety.pdf<br>▪ **Safe Kids Worldwide, Fire Safety:** Safety tips for fire and other hazards for different age groups of children<br>https://www.safekids.org/fire |
| Child Safety | ▪ **Kids Health Household Safety Checklists:** kitchen; bedroom; outdoor; floors, walls, furniture; electrical; bath, garage, laundry<br>http://kidshealth.org/en/parents/household-checklist.html<br>▪ **Safe Kids Worldwide, Home Safety:** multiple online environmental education resource<br>https://www.safekids.org/safetytips/field_venues/home?gclid=EAIaIQobChMIk4D90bWU2AIVQrnACh2N0gJXEAAYAiAAEgLXmfD_BwE<br>▪ **American Academy of Pediatrics, Home Safety Checklist and Education**<br>http://www.pediatricspec.com/resources/HomeSafety.pdf |
| Vulnerable Adult | ▪ **AARP Caregiving Checklist**<br>https://assets.aarp.org/external_sites/caregiving/checklists/checklist_homeSafety.html<br>▪ **CDC Home Fall Prevention Checklist for Older Adults**<br>https://www.cdc.gov/steadi/pdf/check_for_safety_brochure-a.pdf<br>▪ **Home Safety Checklist from California Department of Aging**, Senior Housing Information and Support Center, adapted from Home Safety Summary Checklist developed by CHIPPS<br>http://www.qualitycares.com/wp-content/uploads/2017/02/home_safety_checklist.pdf<br>▪ **National Council on Aging, Home Fall Prevention Checklist for Older Adults**<br>https://www.ncoa.org/resources/check-for-safety-a-home-fall-prevention-checklist-for-older-adults/ |
| General Tools | ▪ **Home Safety Smartcheck:** home maintenance, child safety, adult safety, emergency<br>http://www.homesafetysmartcheck.com/home-safety-checklists_5143_ct.aspx<br>▪ **National Safety Council, Top Causes of Unintentional Injury and Death in Homes and Communities**<br>http://www.nsc.org/learn/safety-knowledge/Pages/safety-at-home.aspx?gclid=EAIaIQobChMIk4D90bWU2AIVQrnACh2N0gJXEAAYASAAEgJh0fD_BwE<br>▪ **Electrical Safety Foundation International**—multiple education and safety tools including workplace<br>http://www.esfi.org/about-us<br>▪ **Surgeon General—A Healthy Home Checklist**<br>https://www.surgeongeneral.gov/library/calls/checklist.pdf |
| Disaster Preparedness | ▪ **Ready.gov, Building a Disaster Preparedness Kit**<br>https://www.ready.gov/build-a-kit#<br>▪ **Federal Emergency Management Agency, Basic Preparedness:** 34-page document with lists and tools<br>https://www.fema.gov/media-library-data/20130726-1549-20490-2111/basic_preparedness.pdf<br>▪ **American Red Cross, Make a Plan,** guidelines, checklist, English and Spanish<br>http://www.redcross.org/get-help/how-to-prepare-for-emergencies/make-a-plan |

Max and Jeff are talking about their home visiting experiences.

Max recounts, "Last week I made a home visit with Laura, my PHN preceptor, to Rose, an older woman who had called the county public health agency to find out if there was any available assistance for someone with bedbugs. During a phone call before the visit Laura found out that Rose is a disabled 75-year-old woman with limited financial means who lives alone and is estranged from her husband and son. Rose got bedbugs from a neighbor's home and has had trouble getting rid of them because she has trouble seeing them due to her poor vision. Rose has edematous legs due to mild kidney failure. To make it worse, the bugs are biting Rose's swollen legs."

Jeff says, "Rose's apartment's bedbug infestation certainly fits what we have been reading about how older adults may be more vulnerable to environmental hazards. Is she able to keep her house clean?"

Max responds, "The house is clean and tidy with very little furniture. Rose is sleeping in a broken-down lounge chair rather than her bed, which is infested. However, we found that the chair is also infested. Laura and I assessed Rose's legs and found that she had 3+ nonpitting edema in both legs, and three superficial half-inch ulcers near the ankles from the bites. The bites really bother her. I helped Laura apply dressings to the ulcers and wrap Rose's legs with ace wraps. Laura suggested Rose purchase a mattress cover and return to sleeping in bed. But Rose does not have enough money for a mattress cover or for bedbug treatment."

Jeff comments, "That is really a lot of problems. What did you do next?"

Max says, "Laura asked me to research effective bedbug treatments, and I found that thermal treatment is best practice. Bedbugs and eggs die within 90 minutes at 118°F (48°C) or immediately at 122°F (50°C). I helped Laura contact community safety net organizations and donors to find funds for the heat treatment, a mattress pad, and a new lounge chair. Laura contacted a local exterminator who uses heat treatment and got a reduced rate for the client. We are going to make a home visit tomorrow and see if the heat treatment worked and change the ankle ulcer dressings. Hopefully we won't see any new bedbug bites."

Jeff reflects, "I never thought about the problems bedbugs could cause. I talked with Gena yesterday and she told me that one of the students with asthma exacerbations has bedbugs at home and that the bedbugs could be an asthma trigger. Gena said she read that in a scientific journal from Australia.* I guess bedbugs are everywhere! The student's parents were not sure how to get rid of them. I will have to tell Gena about the heat treatment."

Max responds, "I will get you the information for the exterminator who uses the heat treatment.

Max continues, "One thing that Laura mentioned was that on our next visit we should probably do a home safety assessment. Laura noticed that Rose was somewhat unsteady on her feet and that she seemed to have some difficulty preparing her meals. Rose wants to continue to live in her own home. Laura gave me a Home Safety Checklist that she downloaded from the California Department of Aging** to review before our visit. We can use the checklist to identify Rose's strengths, needs, and risks. We might be able to help Rose make a few changes to make her home safer. Laura said that after we complete the home safety assessment and determine if Rose needs help with her basic activities of daily living, she will refer her for an assessment to determine if Rose is eligible for home care services. Jeff, I know that you are going to make a home visit to an 80-year-old man who lives alone. If you want to use the checklist, here is the website address: http://www.qualitycares.com/wp-content/uploads/2017/02/home_safety_checklist.pdf."

*Doggett, Dwyer, Peñas, & Russell, 2012; ** California Department of Aging, 2017

## Community Level of Practice

All nurses, not just PHNs, are expected to integrate environmental health concerns into their nursing practice. Consider that the people you care for in all clinical settings have experienced or will experience exposures to a variety of environmental hazards at home, at work, at school, and throughout the community. Although you can provide health education to individuals and families to help them reduce their exposures or take actions to mitigate the impact of these exposures, this does not reduce the hazards in the environment. Therefore, you need to consider how you might advocate for safe communities in which you and your patients live. In order to do this, you will need to become knowledgeable about the existing and potential environmental hazards in your community. You will need to understand how these hazards will affect the natural environment and the citizens of the community as well as the vulnerable populations who are most at risk. You will need to know who has the power and authority to make decisions about the environmental health of your community, and how to work with these stakeholders. It is important to know how you as a citizen and as a health professional can influence the decision-makers in your community to advocate for a safe community environment.

Evidence Example 5.1 tells about how the children in Flint, Michigan, were vulnerable to lead poisoning due to their living conditions and the poor decisions made by governmental policy makers that led to tragic unanticipated consequences.

The children of Flint, Michigan, were vulnerable for three reasons: their age, the socioeconomic status of their families, and the place in which they lived. Environmental hazards are experienced inequitably when you consider place-based and individual-level psychosocial stressors. Morello-Frosch and Shenassa (2006) propose a holistic conceptual framework that demonstrates the interconnection of environmental hazard exposures, place-based stressors, and individual-level psychosocial stressors. They believe that the combination of hazards such as air pollution, housing and neighborhood quality, and poverty concentration interact with individual stressors that result in increased physiologic degradation and health outcomes such as chronic disease and poor birth outcomes (see Figure 5.5). This environmental "riskscape" of social inequalities, place-based stressors, and individual stressors results in increased vulnerability to environmental hazards such as indoor secondhand smoke and outdoor air pollution and leads to decreased health outcomes.

An evolving area of environmental science focuses on the *exposome*—the totality of exposures from external environment and biological responses throughout a lifetime, including lifestyle. Researchers have studied the cumulative impact on biophysical health using biomarkers (Dennis et al., 2016, p. 1504; Niedzwiecki & Miller, 2016). For example, the exposure to the sociocultural hazard of traumatic experiences during childhood (i.e., adverse childhood experiences; see Chapter 4) has persistent effects throughout the life span, some that will not become evident until adulthood.

Human beings have the ability to regulate internal physiological responses to physical and psychosocial stressors. This response is known as *allostasis*. When individuals experience multiple environmental hazard stressors, allostasis occurs. Over time, the cumulative effect on the body is *allostatic load* (Morello-Frosch & Shenassa, 2006). At-risk individuals and at-risk populations may have an increased allostatic load (see Figure 5.5).

It is important that PHNs assess the environment in which they and their clients live from a holistic perspective, considering the added risk of environmental inequalities.

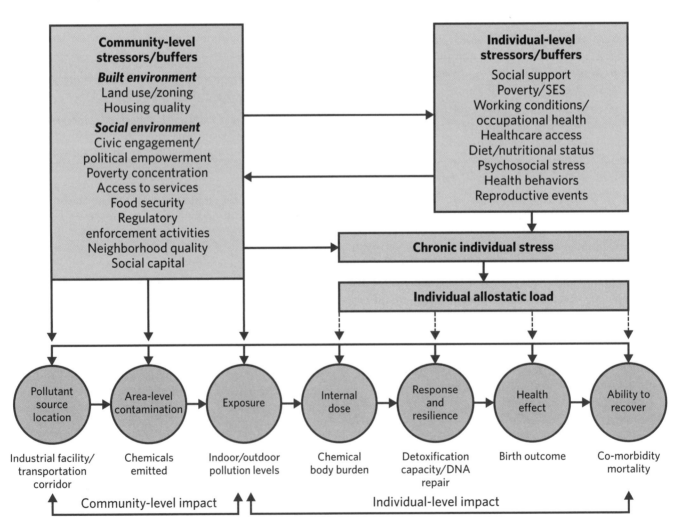

**FIGURE 5.5** Morello-Frosch & Shenassa's Environmental "Riskscape"
*Source:* Morello-Frosch & Shenassa, 2006, p. 1151

## EVIDENCE EXAMPLE 5.1

### Flint, Michigan, Lead Poisoning

The residents of Flint, Michigan, were poisoned by their own water supply in 2014 when water from the Flint River rather than Lake Huron began to flow into the pipes that supplied water to their homes (Bellinger, 2016). The decision was made by a state-appointed emergency manager, not local officials. Corrosion-control treatments for lead pipes carrying water required by the EPA and the Lead and Copper Rule (it regulates the amount of lead and copper that may be in drinking water) were discontinued, and the water from the Flint River became 19 times as corrosive as the water from Lake Huron. The corrosion in the pipes leached lead into the water. Forty percent of families in Flint, Michigan, lived below the poverty line. Lead levels in the water in six of the nine city wards, mainly those with the highest levels of poverty, became extremely toxic. The blood lead concentration in children above the reference value of 5 $ug$ per deciliter rose from 2.4% to 4.9% from 2013 to 2015 and from 4.0% up to 10.6% in children living in neighborhoods that had the greatest contamination of lead in the water. No lead level is considered safe. "The burden of childhood lead poisoning has always weighed most heavily on populations that are politically and economically disenfranchised" (Bellinger, 2016, p. 1102).

# Community Environmental Assessment

PHNs who work for county and state agencies take part in periodic community assessments that usually include information on the health status of residents, a comparative analysis of sub-population health status and identification of health disparities and public health priorities. It is important that PHNs collaborating with interdisciplinary teams also assess the environmental health of their communities and how exposure to environmental hazards affects health outcomes of the population, particularly populations most at risk, including pregnant women, infants and young children, older adults, and those with chronic diseases.

In addition, it is important to consider the cumulative impact of repeated exposures to multiple hazards over a lifetime and the physiological and psychological impact of these exposures. Individual human, organizational, and societal actions or inactions that increase human exposure to environmental toxins must also be assessed. Table 5.7 outlines the components that could be included in a holistic environmental health assessment of the community in which you live and work.

If a population within the community is experiencing signs and symptoms that could have an environmental

**TABLE 5.7 Environmental Health Community Assessment by Health Determinant Categories**

| Biological Health Determinants | Behavioral Health Determinants |
|---|---|
| **Populations At-Risk** | **Exposure History of Environmental Toxins** |
| ▪ Preconception | ▪ Type of hazard |
| ▪ Pregnant women and girls | ▪ Type of exposure |
| ▪ Fetuses and newborns | ▪ Populations exposed |
| ▪ Infants and young children | ▪ Frequency and duration |
| ▪ School-age children and adolescents | ▪ Location/place |
| ▪ Workers in high-risk, high-exposure jobs | ▪ Occupation and business related |
| ▪ Individuals with chronic disease or immunosuppressed | |
| ▪ Individuals with life-long exposures | |
| ▪ Older adults | |
| ▪ Indigenous people living on the land | |

| Physical Environmental Health Determinants | Social Environmental Health Determinants & Social Actions |
|---|---|
| **Environmental Toxins in Natural Environment** | **Socio-Cultural Environmental Hazards** |
| ▪ Air | ▪ Interpersonal violence and abuse |
| ▪ Water | ▪ Conflict and war |
| ▪ Earth | ▪ "Riskscape" of social inequality |
| ▪ Biozone | |
| **Environmental Toxins in Built Environment** | **Institutional and Societal Response Patterns** |
| ▪ Chemical | ▪ Lack of knowledge or scientific evidence |
| ▪ Physical | ▪ Denial of knowledge or science |
| ▪ Mechanical | ▪ Collective social actions or lack thereof |
| ▪ Biological | ▪ Regulations and laws: protective, weak, or absent |

cause, an IPREPARE assessment could also be conducted by interviewing a sub-group of the population. The PHNs could work with a public health epidemiologist to identify a survey method that would provide an accurate picture of the population's exposure history.

*Gena reports, "Max and Jeff just finished analyzing the family IPREPARE surveys with the school nurse. They found that some of the parents reported more dust in their homes because they were keeping their windows open more. They said they would vacuum more often and maybe close the windows when it was windy. Two families noticed more insects in their apartments and were going to ask the apartment manager for assistance getting rid of them. The school nurse is going to refer those families to the county public health nurse who works in the Asthma Program."*

*Max stresses, "We also need to consider what environmental factors outside of the school and the families' homes might have caused the increase in the asthma attacks."*

*Gena responds, "When Dana and I did our windshield survey, we noticed that there are some really big smokestacks in some of the local factories. I should also check on wood smoke pollution. Air pollution is an asthma trigger. I am going to check online with the state Pollution Control Agency and find out if the air quality index has increased and if it is toxic.*

*Later that day Gena reports, "Yesterday the ozone level was moderate, which is okay, but the particle level was reported as unhealthy for sensitive individuals. So, I looked at the reports for the last six months. The particle level was moderate six months ago. Something changed. I am going to call my mother. She works for the city, and maybe she can find out what has changed.*

*One week later Gena reports, "My mother said that some of the air pollution regulations for industries that use a lot of fossil fuels were eliminated or weakened by the state legislature several months ago. The air quality has fluctuated a lot since then depending on what the local industries are doing."*

Poor ambient (outdoor) air quality is a global environmental health issue that results in increased morbidity and mortality. In 2014, WHO reported that 92% of the world population lived in places that did not meet the WHO air quality guidelines and that outdoor air pollution caused an estimated 3 million premature deaths in 2012 (WHO, 2016). Although 88% of these deaths occurred in the Western Pacific and Southeast Asian regions, all nurses should be aware of the air quality in their communities and its impact on individual and population health.

Dana and Gena meet with their nursing instructor and Candace, the school nurse, to identify a list of possible actions they might take to try to convince the community to reverse the increased outdoor air pollution that could be contributing to the increase in asthma attacks (community level of practice). Their list included actions that could be taken using public health nursing interventions.

■ **Social marketing:** Create a brochure about the increased air pollution in the community and send it home in the students' backpacks.

■ **Collaboration:** Work with the county environmental health specialist and epidemiologist to develop a county health department handout on air pollution, asthma, and respiratory illnesses.

■ **Policy development:** Meet with legislators to discuss the increase in air pollution in their community and give the legislators the health department handout.

■ **Community organizing:** Encourage the school Parent-Teacher Organization to mobilize the parents, their families, neighbors, and friends to encourage their city, county, and state elected officials to take actions to reduce the increased air pollution.

What actions might you take if you were Dana or Gena?

## Climate Change

To discuss climate change, it is important to understand the differences between weather, climate, global warming, and climate change. The National Aeronautics and Space Administration (NASA, 2018) defines and contrasts the phenomena:

■ *Weather* refers to atmospheric conditions that occur locally over short periods of time—from minutes to hours or days. Familiar examples include rain, snow, clouds, winds, floods, or thunderstorms. Weather is local and short-term.

■ *Climate* refers to the long-term regional or even global average of temperature, humidity, and rainfall patterns over seasons, years, or decades. Climate is global and long-term.

■ *Global warming* refers to the upward temperature trend across the entire earth since the early 20th century, and most notably since the late 1970s, due to the increase in fossil fuel emissions since the industrial revolution. Worldwide since 1880, the average surface temperature has gone up by about 0.8°C (1.4°F), relative to the mid-20th-century baseline established between 1951 and 1980.

■ *Climate change* refers to a broad range of global phenomena created predominantly by burning fossil fuels, which add heat-trapping gases to the earth's atmosphere. These phenomena include the increased temperature trends described by global warming, but also encompass changes such as sea level rise; ice mass loss in Greenland, Antarctica, the Arctic, and mountain glaciers worldwide; shifts in flower/plant blooming; and extreme weather events.

Climate change is a significant cause of disruption of both the ecosystem and societal systems. The scientific consensus is that climate change over the last 60 years is primarily a response to human actions and that those who contribute the least to climate change disproportionately experience the consequences of climate change (Nicholas & Breakey, 2017; U.S. Global Change Research Program, 2014a, 2014b).

Mitigation efforts are inadequate. Fossil fuels are the primary environmental hazard endangering the earth (Hellerstedt, 2017). Burning fossil fuels results in increased carbon dioxide in the atmosphere. The global concentration of carbon dioxide in the atmosphere reached 400 ppm in 2013, the highest concentration ever. A limit of 350 ppm is believed to be necessary to prevent dangerous climate change. The temperature of the earth is now 1.8 degrees Celsius higher than the temperature of the preindustrial era; an increase of 2 degrees is considered catastrophic to sea levels, food production, biodiversity, and water supplies. Without significant reduction of carbon dioxide in the atmosphere, the temperature of the Earth is expected to rise 3.7 to 4.8 degrees Celsius by the end of the 21st century. The harm to both the ecosystem and the social system and to humans is an ongoing phenomenon (Ocko, 2016; see Figure 5.6). Global effects of climate change include rising seas, extreme weather and weather pattern changes, decreased air quality, reduced reliability of water quality and supply, disruptions to agriculture, increased inability of the ecosystem to restore itself, and reduced health outcomes experienced at higher rates by vulnerable populations.

Although nearly all scientists agree that the actions of human beings are a major cause of climate change, many people still do not believe or concur with this knowledge (ProCon.org, 2017). Read *Is Human Activity Primarily Responsible for Global Climate Change?* (http://climat-echange.procon.org) to review the arguments for and against human actions as the cause of climate change. Many would argue, however, that even if someone does not believe climate change is *caused* by human actions, the prudent thing is to *act* in a manner that mitigates the potential causes of

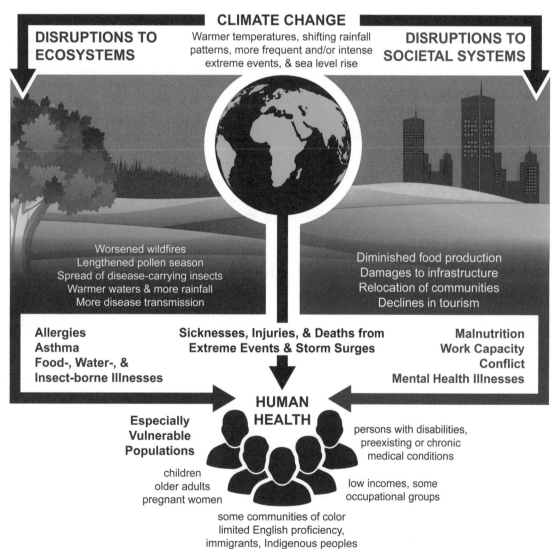

**FIGURE 5.6** The Impacts of Climate Change on Human Health
*Source:* Ilissa Ocko, Environmental Defense Fund, 2016. http://blogs.edf.org/climate411/2016/04/05/
the-impacts-of-climate-change-on-human-health-a-sobering-new-report/

climate change. It is hard to argue with the benefits of protecting natural green spaces. The Precautionary Principle applies to actions everyone can take to protect the earth.

The long-term environmental hazards are much more complex, difficult to confront, and sometimes not as visible. The Lancet Commission (Whitmee et al., 2015) postulates that the "far-reaching changes to the structure and function of the Earth's natural systems are not only a threat to human health but that these changes have been caused by humankind" (p. 1974). Human health is threatened by extensive environmental changes in the air, water, land, and entire ecosystem. The Commission identified three challenges and failures that need to be addressed to provide for a sustainable environment:

■ **Imagination challenges:** Understanding what is being done to the environment and the significant harm that is occurring.

■ **Knowledge failures:** Knowing what the drivers of environmental change are and how to combat them.

■ **Implementation failures:** Lack of governmental and institutional actions to address environmental threats and change.

The Lancet's 2017 evaluation of progress toward its 2015 policy recommendations identified progress in the majority of the 10 policies (Watts et al., 2017, pp. 1–3):

1. Investment in climate change and research

2. Scale-up financing for climate-resilient health systems

3. Phase out coal-fired power

4. Encourage city-level low carbon transmission

5. Rapidly expand access to renewable energy

6. Agree on and implement an international treaty that facilitates transition to low-carbon economy

7. Develop an independent collaboration to provide expertise in implementing policies that mitigate climate change, promote public health, and monitor progress

In their recent review of the health of the environment, Watts et al. (2017) conclude that:

■ The human symptoms of climate change are unequivocal and potentially irreversible, affecting the health of populations around the world.

■ The delayed response to climate change over the past 25 years has jeopardized human life and livelihoods; however, over the last 5 years there has been an accelerated response.

■ The voice of health professionals is driving the current response to climate change.

**Activity**

Reflect on the climate change challenges of imagination, knowledge, and implementation that you have observed.

■ What challenges have you noted in your community, your employment setting, and the healthcare setting?

■ What actions need to be taken to change these failures into successes?

■ Do you have a role to play in confronting these challenges?

## Role of Nursing

Nursing is an evidence-based profession. As such, you must pay attention to the evidence and respond in kind. Climate change is not only real, it has a disparate impact on certain populations.

Climate change results in health disparities as those most powerless and disenfranchised experience a disproportionate share of the burdens of climate change. Women, girls, those who live in poverty, and those who live in developing countries are most at risk for the consequences of climate change. The Mary Robinson Foundation-Climate Justice (MRFCJ) has identified seven principles of climate justice that are consistent with the ethical principles of the nursing profession (MRFCJ, 2015; Nicholas & Breakey, 2017):

■ **Principle 1:** Respect and protect human rights

■ **Principle 2:** Support the right to development

■ **Principle 3:** Share benefits and burdens equitably

■ **Principle 4:** Ensure that decisions on climate change are participatory, transparent, and accountable

■ **Principle 5:** Highlight gender equality and equity

■ **Principle 6:** Harness the transformative power of education for climate stewardship

■ **Principle 7:** Use effective partnerships to secure climate justice

Nurses are recognized for taking leadership in the management and mitigation of the health consequences of climate change at national and international levels. An example of this leadership occurred when members of ANHE were invited to the White House to discuss their role in these efforts (Angelini, 2017). ANHE is an excellent role model for environmental stewardship. The International Council of Nurses (ICN) believes that nurses should play both a strategic and an operational role in mitigating the effects of climate change on health (ICN, 2011).

Nurses will be on the front lines caring for those experiencing the health consequences of climate change, and nurses have a powerful voice that needs to be heard and can truly make a difference (Angelini, 2017, p. 83).

The traditional planning and response pattern to an environmental disaster has three phases: prevention, mitigation (weaken the impact), and restoration (rebuild infrastructure and improve quality of life). Climate change is an ongoing disaster that has occurred and is occurring. Human society is now in the mitigation and restoration phases of this worldwide disaster. While public health nursing focuses on primary prevention, when it comes to climate change, PHNs will need to focus on secondary and tertiary prevention strategies at the community level of practice.

## Communities Working Together

Communities need to work together to provide for sustainable environments now and in the future. Sustainable communities are those that are healthy and resilient economically, environmentally, and socially. Community members work together to find integrated solutions to community problems, using resources to meet immediate needs with the knowledge that resources need to be conserved for future generations. Elements of a sustainable community include safe and healthy housing, transportation that does not add to environmental pollution, access to healthy food, and social and economic opportunities for its citizens (ANHE, 2016).

As individual communities strive toward the creation of sustainable communities, the global community needs to work toward the goal of planetary health, achieving the highest attainable standard of health, well-being, and equity worldwide. The Lancet Commission on Planetary Health claims that this goal will be achieved only if serious attention is paid to the political, economic, and social human systems that shape the future of the earth and humanity (Whitmee et al., 2015).

### 🌐 Online Activity

Identify one to two environmental hazards or areas in your community that could be improved to create a healthier community environment. Visit the interactive website of the Agency for Toxic Substances and Disease Registry (ATSDR) at https://www.atsdr.cdc.gov/sites/brownfields/actionmodeltoolkit/ (ATSDR, n.d.). The ATSDR has created a toolkit (ATSDR Action Model Toolkit) to help citizens improve the health of the community environment. View the videos and review the steps of the toolkit. Identify an action plan for one environmental hazard that you have identified in your community.

---

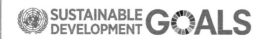

**World Toilet Day**

**6 CLEAN WATER AND SANITATION**

**GOAL 6** Today, 2.5 billion people (about a third of the world's population) around the world live with unsafe sanitation, and an estimated 801,000 children younger than 5 years of age die from diarrhea each year, mostly in developing countries (CDC, 2016).

The UN and the Water Environment Federation (WEF) (https://www.wef.org/) sponsor a World Toilet Day each year on November 19.

#### World Toilet Day—Time for Action

World Toilet Day is on November 19—a day inspiring action to help address our global sanitation crisis and recognize the incredible strides that sanitation has made for public health. WEF members have the technical expertise and passion to help the 2.5 billion people living without a household toilet that disposes of their waste safely. And to quote Amina J. Mohammed, deputy secretary-general of the United Nations, "We've got the tools, let's make it happen." UN-Water's theme for World Toilet Day 2017 was wastewater, and related Sustainable Development Goals include universal access to a safely managed household toilet by 2030, making sanitation central to eradicating extreme poverty. A variety of materials, messages, and tools to help educate about human waste and what can be done about it can be found at World Toilet Day, and WEF members are encouraged to participate.

To complement the UN's wastewater theme, WEF has assembled and distributed resources to help member associations and members communicate the importance of protecting our water infrastructure and systems via proper disposal of waste and appropriate flushables (pee, paper, and poo). Go to the World Toilet Day website (http://www.worldtoiletday.info/) for that package including resources for social media. Also, WEF's line of public education bill stuffers for water quality professionals now includes *Let's Talk Toilets* (https://www.e-wef.org/Default.aspx?TabID=251&productId=59910777), which highlights the importance of what should and should not be flushed. Working together, we can act to raise awareness about the importance and value of toilets to a healthy, sustainable global environment.

*Source:* Modified from Water Environment Federation Blog, 2017

## Environmental Stewardship

*Environmental stewardship* is defined as individuals taking responsibility for their own choices in their personal, occupational, and community activities (EPA, 2005). It involves taking responsibility for environmental quality in all aspects of your life. Environmental stewardship may also extend to governance and be viewed as a responsibility of both the public and the private sectors. To achieve a sustainable environment that is healthy and equitable and reduces the global environmental disease burden, multiple intersecting actions need to occur: focusing on primary prevention, ongoing environmental risk analysis, managing current and emerging environmental risks, and intersectoral collaboration at local, national, and global levels (Prüss-Ustün et al., 2016).

There are many organizations with an environmental stewardship mission. Three nonprofit organizations that have a global focus include:

- The **Planetary Health Alliance,** funded by the Rockefeller Foundation, is a consortium of over 70 dedicated universities, NGOs, government entities, research institutes, and other partners around the world committed to advancing planetary health. The organization works to build a rigorous evidence base that may be used by decision-makers to create policy solutions for planetary health (Planetary Health Alliance, 2017).

- The **Environmental Defense Fund** is a worldwide nonprofit that focuses on climate change, expanding sustainable ocean fishing, increasing resilience of ecosystems, and reducing human exposure to pollutants (Environmental Defense Fund, 2017).

- **Women's Earth Alliance** (WEA) empowers women to protect the earth. The WEA has implemented women's environmental and entrepreneurship projects in 18 countries for safe water, clean energy, regenerative farming, women's land rights, and other projects (WEA, 2016).

Nurses with a holistic approach to health are environmental stewards. PHNs, because of their population social justice perspectives and their positions in the community as advocates for the health of individuals, families and entire communities are viewed as ideal advocates to address the challenges of climate change at the local, state, federal, and international levels (Anderko, 2017). You might research an organization in your own community that supports environmental stewardship at the local level and consider supporting or joining it.

## Systems Level of Practice

PHNs interact with many different community systems (i.e., institutions) that affect the environment and the lives of the people who live in the community. The healthcare system, as well as educational, business, transportation, governmental, and recreational systems, are key community systems that influence environmental health. All nurses who work within systems that impact the health of the environment are responsible for taking actions to reduce both environmental hazards and exposure to the environmental hazards.

The healthcare system has a significant impact on environmental health. A major environmental hazard in healthcare is waste and its impact on humans and the environment. Healthcare waste may be divided into eight areas: infectious, pathological, sharps, chemicals, pharmaceuticals, genotoxic, radioactive, and nonhazardous. High-income countries produce the most waste—an average of 0.5 kg per bed per day—while low-income countries produce only about 0.2 kg. About 15% of the waste is hazardous. Home-care waste also has a significant impact on the environment (WHO, 2015a).

Nurses are at high risk for exposure to hazardous waste and are in key positions to reduce both hazardous and nonhazardous waste (Schenk, Butterfield, Postma, Barbosa-Leiker, & Corbett, 2015). The International Council of Nursing (ICN) published three position statements on the role of the nurse in environmental health: the role of the nurse in addressing environmental health risks and lifestyle behaviors that impact health status (2011); the role of the nurse in managing and reducing healthcare waste (2010); and the ethical, moral, and legal responsibility for nurses and all stakeholders to provide for a safe working environment (2017). ICN believes that nurses should be directly involved in the decision-making process about purchase of disposable products, the disposal of these products, and the use of safe products. They should use the Precautionary Principle when making decisions about product acquisition, use, and disposal, and they should take actions to increase use of recycling. ICN stresses that nurses need ongoing education about how their work impacts the environment and the safety of healthcare staff and patients.

Many organizations within healthcare are advocates for healthy environments and take positions and actions in the areas of education, research, and practice. Nurses play a significant role in healthcare stewardship. The following sections discuss the organizations that provide significant healthcare stewardship.

**Alliance of Nurses for Healthy Environments (ANHE)**
https://envirn.org/

ANHE is a group of nurse educators in academic and practice settings who support environmental nursing education at the undergraduate and graduate levels and are involved in education and research and have published a free online textbook on Environmental Health. ANHE also collaborates with other organizations to advocate for climate change remediation.

**Children's Environmental Health Network (CEHN)**
http://cehn.org/

CEHN is a national multidisciplinary organization whose mission is to protect the developing child from environmental health hazards and promote a healthier environment. CEHN goals are to promote the development of sound public health and child-focused national policy; stimulate prevention-oriented research; educate health professionals, policymakers, and community members in preventive strategies; and elevate public awareness of environmental hazards to children.

**Health Care Without Harm—U.S. and Canada**
https://noharm-uscanada.org/content/us-canada/about-us

Health Care Without Harm, with its partners around the world, shares a vision of a healthcare sector that does no harm, and instead promotes the health of people and the environment. The organization is working to implement ecologically sound and healthy alternatives to healthcare practices that pollute the environment and contribute to disease.

**Practice Greenhealth**
https://practicegreenhealth.org/about/history

In 1998, the American Hospital Association and the U.S. Environmental Protection Agency signed a landmark agreement to advance pollution-prevention efforts in United States healthcare facilities. This agreement became the cornerstone of the Hospitals for a Healthy Environment (H2E) program and called for virtual elimination of mercury waste; reduction of the healthcare sector's total waste volume; chemical waste minimization; and educational and information-sharing activities focused on pollution prevention and toxics minimization. In 2008, H2E changed its name to Practice Greenhealth and updated its mission.

Practice Greenhealth is a nonprofit membership organization grounded on the principles of positive environmental stewardship and best practices in healthcare to create sustainable healthcare with better, safer, greener workplaces and communities. Its goals are to prevent and reduce waste in the healthcare sector; achieve carbon neutrality in healthcare; reduce energy and water usage; build, renovate, and purchase responsibly; demonstrate mission through respectful work environments; engage communities on environmental sustainability in design, construction, and operations; lead the way in responsible buildings and operations; increase recycling programs; and phase out hazardous substances and toxic chemicals.

*Jeff, Gena, Max, and Dana now understand how the educational system impacts the health of its students. Their particular concern is how the school environment could be affecting the health of the children with asthma. They observe students in the classroom and outside at recess and during physical education classes, interview the school staff, review the policies and procedures of the environmental magnet school, and assess the built environment of the school building. Jeff and Gena report the potential risk factors they found for the increase in asthma attacks to Candace, the school nurse, and the principal. They compiled all their information into a table.*

Table 5.8 outlines the protective and risk factors that students with asthma face at the magnet school.

*Dana and Max identify the immediate priorities:*

- *Educate school staff on asthma triggers in the school environment and how to reduce asthma triggers.*

- *Remove the birds from the two classrooms and replace them with animals that do not shed dander.*

- *Create a policy for all student asthma attacks to be reported to the school nurse.*

- *Pursue options to replace cleaning products with VOCs to green cleaning products.*

*Dana explains, "The Precautionary Principle should be used because VOCs might be serving as asthma triggers for some of the students. I found a good handout, Controlling Asthma in Schools, from the CDC that could be used in policy discussions with school administration.*

*The principal and the school nurse agree with these recommendations. They also discuss the potential for addressing the air quality issue with the school board and other elected officials. Candace, the school nurse, is going to take the concerns to the Student Parent Advisory Committee, the local public health department, and the pediatrician who consults with the school district to see what other collaborative actions might be taken.*

**TABLE 5.8 Protective Factors and Risk Factors for Students With Asthma at Environmental Magnet School**

| Biological Health Determinants | Behavioral Health Determinants |
|---|---|
| ▪ **Risk factor:** All students enrolled in the school were in age range consistent with the most common developmental stage of onset.<br><br>▪ **Risk factor:** Students with asthma had more episodes of breathing difficulties when outside, during running activities in the gym, and in classrooms with pets that shed dander.<br><br>▪ **Risk factor:** Several students who did not have a diagnosis of asthma were observed having breathing difficulties when outside and involved in running activities. | ▪ **Protective factor:** Teachers reported that students were able to independently use their inhalers.<br><br>▪ **Protective factor:** All students with asthma had inhalers either with them or in the health office.<br><br>▪ **Protective factor:** Students who carried inhalers with them used them as needed and did not go to the health office.<br><br>▪ **Risk factor:** All students with asthma were housed in classrooms with pets that shed pet dander.<br><br>▪ **Risk factor:** Some students did not have inhalers with them; inhalers were in the health office. |
| **Physical Environmental Health Determinants** | **Social Environmental/Social Actions Health Determinants** |
| ▪ **Protective factor:** The school building was clean with little dust and no mold found in classrooms, gym, or the lunch room.<br><br>▪ **Risk factor:** A change in the ambient air (outdoor) air quality index measurement showed an increase in particles from moderate to unhealthy over the past 6 months.<br><br>▪ **Risk factor:** Birds were recently added to two classrooms; students with asthma have had a recent increase in their asthma attacks.<br><br>▪ **Potential risk factor:** Cleaning products with VOCs are in use. | ▪ **Protective factor:** The school nurse has action plans for all students with asthma.<br><br>▪ **Risk factor:** Staff reported they were unaware of which pets shed dander; they were not aware that bird feathers shed dander. They did not know how to reduce asthma triggers in their classrooms.<br><br>▪ **Risk factor:** Staff did not report asthma attacks to the school nurse if the attacks were resolved with use of an inhaler. |

**Online Activity**

Review the information on the following websites. How would you determine if all of the asthma triggers identified and all of the interventions discussed are based on scientific evidence? How might the Precautionary Principle guide you in making decisions where the evidence might be inconclusive? What policy and procedure recommendations might you make to the school board?

▪ Controlling Asthma in School (CDC, n.d.) at https://www.cdc.gov/asthma/pdfs/schools_fact_sheet.pdf

▪ Managing Asthma in the School Environment at https://www.epa.gov/iaq-schools/managing-asthma-school-environment

## Ethical Considerations

As a nurse, you are in a critical position to make a difference in the environmental health of your community and of the people you encounter in the healthcare system. Nurses care for individuals from birth to death in all clinical settings where healthcare is provided. Nurses are considered the final protective barrier between individuals and their physical and social environments within the healthcare system and within the community. This chapter presented an overview of how environmental hazards affect individuals, families, and entire communities. The degradation of the environment is a global problem with both global and local consequences. You might be overwhelmed when considering all the actions that need to be taken to protect people from the environment and the environment from people.

So, be *glocal*—think global, act local. Identify the major environmental hazards that you, your family, your patients/clients, and your community are exposed to on a daily basis. Choose one hazard for action. Use the ACT process to acquire the needed knowledge, consider your options for improving environmental health and the health of your patients, and take actions to do so. Consider what a difference you can make. The ethical principles in Table 5.9 provide a guide for your actions.

**TABLE 5.9 Ethical Action in Environmental Health**

| Ethical Perspective | Application |
|---|---|
| Rule ethics (principles) | ▪ Adhere to existing environmental health regulations that protect the environment and protect humans and animals from exposure to environmental triggers.<br>▪ Follow procedures for safe disposal of hazardous waste materials.<br>▪ Apply scientific evidence and best-practice evidence related to environmental health to nursing practice in all settings. |
| Virtue ethics (character) | ▪ Apply the Precautionary Principle when a cause-effect relationship is thought to exist but has not been fully documented in scientific literature.<br>▪ Tell the truth about climate change and the impact of industrial and healthcare toxic waste materials. Take responsibility for your own actions in creating excess healthcare waste or disposal of toxic healthcare waste. |
| Feminist ethics (reducing oppression) | ▪ Advocate for policies that address the existence of climate change and how to mitigate the effects of climate change.<br>▪ Advocate for the protection of vulnerable individuals and populations from environmental hazards.<br>▪ Take action in your daily nursing practice to safeguard patients/clients from exposure to environmental hazards. |

Table based on work by Racher, 2007, and Volbrecht, 2002

## KEY POINTS

- Environmental health should be part of the core of nursing practice.
- A holistic definition of environmental health includes physical, chemical, biological, social, and behavioral factors that influence the environment.
- Environmental health affects human health, and human actions affect environmental health.
- Exposure to environmental hazards occurs on a daily basis at home, at work, at school, and in the community.
- Environmental hazard exposure at any point in your life may negatively affect the rest of your life and health.

- The Precautionary Principle serves as a guide in making decisions about exposure to environmental hazards.
- Environmental hazards affect vulnerable populations disproportionately.
- Climate change has occurred and is having a negative impact on the environment and on all forms of life.
- Stewardship of the environment is the responsibility of everyone.
- PHNs respond to environmental health hazards and issues at all three levels of PHN practice.

## REFLECTIVE PRACTICE

Jeff returned to the county public health agency to spend another day with Laura, his PHN preceptor. Laura's supervisor asked her if she could create an Environmental Health Resource and Referral List based on the environmental and nuisance phone calls that PHNs in her department had received over the past 2 months. Laura did a content analysis of caller issues and created a table with call volume, the PHN interventions used, and resources (see Table 5.10).

Laura created a reference sheet, listing phone numbers to request an inspection or to make a referral. She asked Jeff if he would work on developing a list of web-based resources

for the environmental health problems identified by callers. Because Jeff only has a day to work on this project, he needs to prioritize the environmental health issues he would research.

■ Based on the content analysis that Laura completed, what would Jeff identify as his environmental health priorities?

■ What other members of the interprofessional public health team might Jeff consult with to find resources?

■ What resources in this chapter might Jeff want to include in his list of web-based resources?

**TABLE 5.10  Content Analysis of Environmental Health Issues Calls to PHN**

| Client Problem | Call Volume | Intervention & Resource |
| --- | --- | --- |
| Mold in rental unit exacerbating asthma | 10 | *Health Teaching* – EPA website |
| Home remoleling project causing elevated blood lead level | 1 | *Health Teaching* – state health department resources; *Referral* for 3-month follow-up blood draw |
| Discovery of asbestos in newly purchased home | 1 | *Health Teaching* – state health department resources; *Referral* to certified removal service |
| Complaint of cockroaches at the store of an apple orchard | 1 | *Policy Enforcement* – Report to state health department for inspection |
| Request for radon testing | 3 | *Health Education* – state health department; *Referral* for testing kits |
| Report of food poisoning from restaurant | 5 – single episode | *Health Event and Disease Investigation* – Report to state health department for restaurant inspection |
| Mold present in condemned house next door | 1 | *Health Teaching* – EPA website; *Referral* to city hall |
| Contact dermatitis from chlorinated hot tub at local hotel | 1 | *Referral* – primary care provider; *Health Event and Disease Investigation* – Report to state health department for hotel inspection |
| Traveler complained of bedbugs in local hotel | 1 | *Health Teaching* – local health department website; *Health Event and Disease Investigation* – Report to state health department for hotel inspection |

## APPLICATION OF EVIDENCE

1. What have you learned about environmental hazards in the home environment that might lead to a change in your behavior to improve the environmental health of your home?

2. What have you learned about environmental health hazards and patterns of exposure that can help you in providing nursing care to vulnerable populations?

3. What can you do in your nursing practice to reduce the amount of healthcare waste and the disposal of toxic healthcare waste?

4. What chronic health conditions may be a result of exposure to environmental hazards?

5. How could you become involved in environmental stewardship?

# References

Agency for Toxic Substances and Disease Registry. (n.d.). *ATSDR Action Model Toolkit*. Retrieved from https://www.atsdr.cdc.gov/sites/brownfields/actionmodeltoolkit/

Alliance of Nurses for Healthy Environments. (2016). *Environmental health in nursing*. Retrieved from https://envirn.org/wp-content/uploads/2017/03/Environmental-Health-in-Nursing.pdf

Alliance of Nurses for Healthy Environments. (2017). *The history of ANHE*. Retrieved from https://envirn.org/about/

American Academy of Allergy, Asthma, & Immunology. (2018). Pet allergy. Retrieved from http://www.aaaai.org/conditions-and-treatments/allergies/pet-allergy

American Lung Association. (2017). Indoor air pollutants and health. Retrieved from http://www.lung.org/our-initiatives/healthy-air/indoor/indoor-air-pollutants/

American Nurses Association. (2007). *ANA's principles of environmental health for nursing practice with implementation strategies*. Retrieved from https://www.nursingworld.org/~4af4f2/globalassets/docs/ana/ethics/principles-of-environmental-health-online_final.pdf

Anderko, L. (2017). Climate change and public health: Nurses can make a difference. *Public Health Nursing, 34*(2), 99–100. doi:10.1111/phn.12316

Angelini, K. (2017). Climate change, health, and the role of nurses. *Nursing for Women's Health, 21*(2), 79–83.

Bellinger, D. C. (2016). Lead contamination in Flint—An abject failure to protect public health. *The New England Journal of Medicine, 374*(12), 1101–1103. doi:10.1056/NEJMp1601013

California Department of Aging, Senior Housing Information and Support Center. (2017). *Home safety checklist*. Retrieved from http://www.qualitycares.com/wp-content/uploads/2017/02/home_safety_checklist.pdf

Cantley, L. F., Galusha, D., Cullen, M. R., Dixon-Ernst, C., Rabinowitz, P. M., & Neitzel, R. L. (2015). Association between ambient noise exposure, hearing acuity, and risk of acute occupational injury. *Scandinavian Journal of Work, Environment & Health, 41*(1), 75–83. doi:10.5271/sjweh.3450.

Centers for Disease Control and Prevention. (n.d.). *Controlling asthma in schools: Success of CDC's National Asthma Control Program*. Retrieved from https://www.cdc.gov/asthma/pdfs/schools_fact_sheet.pdf

Centers for Disease Control and Prevention. (2012). Common asthma triggers. Retrieved from https://www.cdc.gov/asthma/triggers.html

Centers for Disease Control and Prevention. (2016). Global water, sanitation, and hygiene (WASH). Retrieved from https://www.cdc.gov/healthywater/global/wash_statistics.html

Chaudry, R. V. (2008). The precautionary principle, public health, and public health nursing. *Public Health Nursing, 25*(3), 261–268. doi:10.1111/j.1525-1446.2008.00703.x

Dangerous Decibels. (2018). Noise-induced hearing loss can be prevented. Retrieved from http://dangerousdecibels.org/

Dennis, K. K., Auerbach, S. S., Balshaw, D. M., Cui, Y., Fallin, M. D., Smith, M. T., … Miller, G. W. (2016). The importance of the biological impact of exposure to the concept of the exposome. *Environmental Health Perspectives, 124*(10), 1504–1510. Retrieved from http://dx.doi.org/10.1289/EHP140

Doggett, S. L., Dwyer, D. E., Peñas, P. F., & Russell, R. C. (2012). Bed bugs: Clinical relevance and control options. *Clinical Microbiology Reviews, 25*(1), 164–192. Retrieved from http://doi.org/10.1128/CMR.05015-11

Environmental Defense Fund. (2017). Our work. Retrieved from https://www.edf.org/our-work

Environmental Protection Agency. (n.d.). Multimedia fate and transport modeling–overview. Retrieved from https://www.epa.gov/fera/multimedia-fate-and-transport-modeling-overview

Environmental Protection Agency Innovation Action Council. (2005). *Everyday choices: Opportunities for environmental stewardship*. Retrieved from https://archive.epa.gov/stewardship/web/pdf/rpt2admin.pdf

Filiaci, A. M. (n.d.). *Lillian Wald—Public health progressive*. Retrieved from http://www.lillianwald.com/

Geller, A. M. (2010). The susceptibility of older adults to environmental hazards. *Journal of the American Society on Aging, 33*(4), 10–18.

Hellerstedt, W. L. (2017). Climate change is happening and it demands a public health response. *Climate Change and Public Health, Spring 2017,* 1–7. Retrieved from https://www.researchgate.net/publication/317569526_Climate_Change_and_Public_Health

Henry Street Consortium. (2017). *Entry-level population-based public health nursing competencies*. St. Paul, MN: Author. Retrieved from www.henrystreetconsortium.org

Henry Street Settlement. (2017). Lillian Wald. Retrieved from https://www.henrystreet.org/about/our-history/lillian-wald/

Huntington-Moskos, L., Rayens, M. K., Wiggins, A., & Hahn, E. J. (2016). Radon, secondhand smoke, and children in the home: Creating a teachable moment for lung cancer prevention. *Public Health Nursing, 33*(6), 529–538. doi:10.1111/phn.12283

Institute for Sustainable Communities. (n.d.). Definition of sustainable community. Retrieved from http://www.iscvt.org/impact/definition-sustainable-community/

Institute of Medicine. (1995). *Nursing, health, and the environment*. Washington, DC: National Academies Press. Retrieved from https://www.nap.edu/download/4986

International Council of Nurses. (2010). *Healthcare waste: Role of nurses and nursing*. [Position statement]. Retrieved from http://www.icn.ch/images/stories/documents/publications/position_statements/E07_Medical_Waste.pdf

International Council of Nurses. (2011). *Reducing environmental and lifestyle related health risks*. [Position statement]. Retrieved from https://noharm-uscanada.org/sites/default/files/documents-files/455/Reducing_Env_Health_Hazards.pdf

International Council of Nurses. (2017). *Occupational health and safety for nurses*. [Position statement]. Retrieved from http://www.icn.ch/images/stories/documents/publications/position_statements/ICN_PS_Occupational_health_and_safety.pdf

Kleiman, J. (2017). Love Canal: A brief history. Geneseo, NY: SUNY Geneseo. Retrieved from https://www.geneseo.edu/history/love_canal_history#

Lancet Commission. (2015). Planetary health. Retrieved from https://www.mailman.columbia.edu/research/urbanhealth-initiative/planetary-health

Lawler, K. (2016). Green cleaning in homes. In Alliance of Nurses for Healthy Environments (Ed.), *Environmental health in nursing* (pp. 82–85). Retrieved from https://envirn.org/wp-content/uploads/2017/03/Environmental-Health-in-Nursing.pdf

Leyva, E. W. A., Beamon, A., & Davidson, P. M. (2017). Health impact of climate change in older people: An integrative review and implications for nursing. *Journal of Nursing Scholarship, 49*(6), 670–678. doi:10.1111/jnu.12346

Mary Robinson Foundation – Climate Justice. (2015). Principles of climate justice. Retrieved from https://www.mrfcj.org/wp-content/uploads/2015/09/Principles-of-Climate-Justice.pdf

Merrill, R. M. (2017). *Introduction to epidemiology* (7th ed.). Sudbury, MA: Jones and Bartlett.

Michaels, D. (Ed.). (2015). Clara Barton. National Women's History Museum. Retrieved from https://www.womenshistory.org/education-resources/biographies/clara-barton

Morello-Frosch, R., & Shenassa, E. D. (2006). The environmental "riskscape" and social inequality: Implications for explaining maternal and child health disparities. *Environmental Health Perspectives, 114*(8), 1150–1153. doi:10.1289/ehp.8930

National Aeronautics and Space Administration. (2018). What's in a name? Weather, global warming and climate change. Retrieved from http://climate.nasa.gov/resources/global-warming/

National Institute on Deafness and Other Communication Disorders. (2017). Noise-induced hearing loss. Retrieved from https://www.nidcd.nih.gov/health/noise-induced-hearing-loss

National Scientific Council on the Developing Child. (2006). *Early exposure to toxic substances damages brain architecture: Working Paper No. 4.* Retrieved from https://46y5eh11fhgw3ve3ytpwxt9r-wpengine.netdna-ssl.com/wp-content/uploads/2006/05/Early_Exposure_Toxic_Substances_Brain_Architecture-.pdf

Nicholas, P. K., & Breakey, S. (2017). Climate change, climate justice, and environmental health: Implications for the nursing profession. *Journal of Nursing Scholarship, 49*(6), 606–616. doi:10.1111/jnu.12326

Niedzwiecki, M. M., & Miller, G. W. (2016). The exposome paradigm in human health: Lessons from the Emory Exposome Summer Course. *Environmental Health Perspectives, 125*(6). Retrieved from https://doi.org/10.1289/EHP1712

Nightingale, F. (1860). *Notes on nursing.* New York, NY: D. Appleton and Company. Retrieved from http://digital.library.upenn.edu/women/nightingale/nursing/nursing.html

Ocko, I. (2016). The impact of climate change on human health—A sobering new report. Environmental Defense Fund. Retrieved from http://blogs.edf.org/climate411/2016/04/05/the-impacts-of-climate-change-on-human-health-a-sobering-new-report/

Paranzino, G., Butterfield, P., Nastoff, T., & Ranger, C. (2005). I PREPARE: Development and clinical utility of an environmental exposure history. *AAOHN Journal, 53*(1), 37–42.

Planetary Health Alliance. (2017). Our mission. Retrieved from https://planetaryhealthalliance.org/our-mission

Plotnick, B. (2017). Noise-induced hearing loss (NIHL). Healthy Hearing. Retrieved from https://www.healthyhearing.com/help/hearing-loss/noise

Potera, C. (2011). INDOOR AIR QUALITY: Scented products emit a bouquet of VOCs. *Environmental Health Perspectives, 119*(1), A16. Retrieved from https://www.ncbi.nlm.nih.gov/pmc/articles/PMC3018511/

Pro.Con.org. (2017). Is human activity primarily responsible for global climate change? Retrieved from https://climatechange.procon.org/

Prüss-Ustün, A., Wolf, J., Corvalán, C., Neville, T., Bos, R., & Neira, M. (2016). *Preventing disease through healthy environments* (2nd ed.). World Health Organization. Retrieved from http://apps.who.int/iris/bitstream/10665/204585/1/9789241565196_eng.pdf?ua=1

Prüss-Ustün, A., Wolf, J., Corvalán, C., Neville, T., Bos, R., & Neira, M. (2017). Diseases due to unhealthy environments: An updated estimate of the global burden of disease attributable to environmental determinants of health. *Journal of Public Health, 39*(3), 464–465. Retrieved from https://academic.oup.com/jpubhealth/article/39/3/464/3003007

Racher, F. (2007). The evolution of ethics for community practice. *Journal of Community Health Nursing, 24*(1), 65–76.

Sanchez, B. N., Hu, H., Litman, H. J., & Tellez-Rojo, M. M. (2011). Statistical methods to study timing of vulnerability with sparsely sampled data on environmental toxicants. *Environmental Health Perspectives, 119,* 409–415. Retrieved from https://ehp.niehs.nih.gov/1002453/

Schenk, E., Butterfield, P., Postma, J., Barbosa-Leiker, C., & Corbett, C. (2015). Creating the Nurses' Environmental Awareness Tool (NEAT). *Workplace Health & Safety, 83*(9), 381–391. doi:10.1177/2165079915592071

Science and Environmental Health Network. (1998). Wingspread Conference on the precautionary principle. Retrieved from http://sehn.org/wingspread-conference-on-the-precautionary-principle/

Surgeon General. (2009). A healthy home checklist. From *The Surgeon General's call to action to promote healthy homes.* Retrieved from https://www.surgeongeneral.gov/library/calls/checklist.pdf

Sutton, P., Woodruff, T. J., Perron, J., Stotland, N., Conry, F. A., Miller, M. D., & Giudice, L. C. (2012). Toxic environmental chemicals: The role of reproductive health professionals in preventing harmful exposures. *American Journal of Obstetrics & Gynecology, 207*(3), 164–173. Retrieved from https://www.ncbi.nlm.nih.gov/pmc/articles/PMC4682569/pdf/nihms-364231.pdf

Thompson, M. R., & Schwartz Barcott, D. (2017). The concept of exposure in environmental health for nursing. *Journal of Advanced Nursing, 73*(6), 1315–1330. doi:10.1111/jan.13246

United Nations. (2015). *Globally Harmonized System of Classification and Labelling of Chemicals (GHS)* (6th ed.). Retrieved from https://www.unece.org/fileadmin/DAM/trans/danger/publi/ghs/ghs_rev06/English/ST-SG-AC10-30-Rev6e.pdf

U.S. Department of Health and Human Services. (2009). *The Surgeon General's call to action to promote healthy homes.* Retrieved from https://www.ncbi.nlm.nih.gov/books/NBK44192/pdf/Bookshelf_NBK44192.pdf

U.S. Department of Health and Human Services Environmental Health Policy Committee, Risk Communication and Education Subcommittee. (1998). An ensemble of definitions of environmental health. Retrieved from https://health.gov/environment/DefinitionsofEnvHealth/ehdef2.htm

U.S. Fish and Wildlife Service. (2012). Rachel Carson. Retrieved from https://www.fws.gov/refuge/Rachel_Carson/about/rachelcarson.html

U.S. Global Change Research Program. (2014a). *Climate change impacts in the United States: Highlights.* Retrieved from http://s3.amazonaws.com/nca2014/high/NCA3_Highlights_HighRes.pdf?download=1

U.S. Global Change Research Program. (2014b). *Climate science: Special report.* Retrieved from https://science2017.globalchange.gov/downloads/CSSR2017_FullReport.pdf

Volbrecht, R. M. (2002). *Nursing ethics: Communities in dialogue.* Upper Saddle River, NJ: Pearson/Prentice Hall.

Water Environment Federation. (2017). World Toilet Day [Blog post]. Retrieved from https://www.wef.org/

Watts, N., Amann, M., Ayeb-Karlsson, S., Belesova, K., Bouley, T., Boykoff, M., . . . Costello, A. (2017, October 30). The *Lancet* Countdown on health and climate change: From 25 years of inaction to a global transformation for public health. Retrieved from http://www.thelancet.com/journals/lancet/article/PIIS0140-6736(17)32464-9/fulltext

Whitmee, S., Haines, A., Beyrer, C., Boltz, F., Capon, A. G., de Souza Dias, B. F., … Yach, D. (2015). Safeguarding human health in the Anthropocene epoch: Report of the Rockefeller Foundation–*Lancet* Commission on planetary health. *The Lancet, 386*(10007), 1973–2028. Retrieved from http://www.thelancet.com/journals/lancet/article/PIIS0140-6736(15)60901-1/fulltext

Women's Earth Alliance. (2016). What we do. Retrieved from http://womensearthalliance.org/about-us/what-we-do/

The World Counts. (2014, May 19). A chemical world. Retrieved from http://www.theworldcounts.com/stories/Chemicals-Used-in-Daily-Life

World Health Organization. (2011). *Children and chemicals: Children's health and the environment* [WHO training package for the health sector]. Retrieved from http://www.who.int/ceh/capacity/chemicals.pdf

World Health Organization. (2015a). *Health-care waste* [Fact sheet]. Retrieved from http://www.who.int/mediacentre/factsheets/fs253/en/

World Health Organization. (2015b). *Make listening safe* [Brochure]. Retrieved from http://www.who.int/pbd/deafness/activities/MLS_Brochure_English_lowres_for_web.pdf

World Health Organization. (2016). *Ambient (outdoor) air quality and health* [Fact sheet]. Retrieved from http://www.who.int/mediacentre/factsheets/fs313/en/

World Health Organization. (2017). Children's environmental health—Environmental risks. Retrieved from http://www.who.int/ceh/risks/en/

# COMPETENCY #4

## Practices Within the Auspices of the Nurse Practice Act

■ **Marjorie A. Schaffer**

*with Jill Timm*

"*Jennifer, a public health nurse (PHN), has worked for the Weaver County Health Department for 10 years. Jennifer's first nursing position, after completing her bachelor of science in nursing (BSN) and passing nursing boards, was on a medical-surgical unit in a large metropolitan hospital. Since her public health experience in nursing school, she has been anxious to find a PHN position. She now works at a small local health department in the town of Aurora, the county seat of Weaver County.*

*Aurora is surrounded by an agricultural community. Corn, soybeans, and sugar beets are the major crops. Cattle are also raised in this area. The town of Aurora has a population of 15,000. German immigrants settled Aurora in the 1850s. Today, Aurora is a multicultural community. The racial makeup is 91% Caucasian, 2% African-American, 2% Hispanic or Latino, 1% Native American, 1% Asian, 1% Pacific Islander, and 1% other. The median income is $33,000.*

*Weaver County has a significant population of migrant workers from Mexico who provide a large portion of the workforce for many farms in the area and also provide the labor for a poultry-processing company located on the northern edge of the county. This processing company opened 10 years ago. The town has needed to learn to adapt to a new cultural group.*

*Sarah, a public health nursing student, has been assigned to work with Jennifer to complete her public health nursing field experience. She is excited to start this experience. Sarah is completing her undergraduate BSN degree at a university about 45 miles from Weaver County. She is familiar with Weaver County only through media reports regarding the difficult racial issues in the county over the past years. Sarah grew up in an urban area, where a variety of cultures and races were represented. She is Korean and was adopted into an American family as an infant. Sarah is eager to learn not only about the role of the PHN but also how the community environment affects the work of the Weaver County Public Health Department and its PHNs.*

*As Sarah has been reflecting on her public health nursing class, she remembers the three core functions of public health—assessment, policy development, and assurance. Along with this underlying framework, Sarah knows the importance of the Cornerstones of Public Health Nursing. She is particularly interested in learning about how independent nursing practice is carried out and how PHNs use the Public Health Intervention Wheel in Weaver County. Sarah will spend 5 weeks with Jennifer, learning as much as possible about public health nursing.*"

## SARAH'S NOTEBOOK

**COMPETENCY #4  Practices Within the Auspices of the Nurse Practice Act**

A. Understands the scope of nursing practice (independent nursing functions and delegated medical functions)

B. Establishes appropriate professional boundaries

C. Maintains confidentiality

D. Demonstrates ethical, legal, and professional accountability

E. Delegates and supervises other personnel

F. Understands the role of a public health nurse as described under public health nursing registration

G. Considers how to practice public health nursing in a variety of public and private healthcare settings

*Source:* Henry Street Consortium, 2017

### USEFUL DEFINITIONS

**Accountability:** "To be answerable to oneself and others for one's own choices, decisions and actions as measured against a standard" (American Nurses Association [ANA], 2015, p. 41).

**Assignment:** "Designating nursing activities or tasks to be performed by another nurse or unlicensed assistive person" (Minnesota Nurses Association, 2013, p. 10).

**Confidentiality:** Nondisclosure of health information that is considered to be private.

**Delegation:** "Transferring to a competent individual the authority to perform a selected nursing task in a selected situation" (Minnesota Nurses Association, 2013, p. 10).

**Independent Practice:** Professional decision-making guided by professional standards of the profession; scope of practice that includes independent functions might also be defined legally.

**Nurse Practice Act:** State statute that describes the practice of nursing; describes scope of professional nursing practice.

**Professional Boundaries:** "The spaces between the nurse's power and the patient's vulnerability. The power of the nurse comes from the nurse's professional position and access to sensitive personal information" (National Council of State Boards of Nursing, 2014).

**Public Health Nursing Registration:** Requirements for practicing public health nursing, which are not universal across all states.

**Reflective Supervision:** A supervisor-supervisee relationship that pays attention to the influence of relationships on other relationships, the parallel process, and empowers the supervisee to discover solutions/concepts through consciously using strategies that include active listening and waiting. The goal of reflective supervision is to support staff who then support families and create a more effective working relationship (Zero to Three, 2017).

**Supervision:** Guidance by an RN "consisting of the activities included in monitoring as well as establishing the initial direction, delegating, setting expectations, directing activities and courses of action, critical watching, overseeing, evaluating, and changing a course of action" (Minnesota Nurses Association, 2013, p. 10).

## Understanding Public Health Nursing Roles Ethically, Legally, and Professionally

This chapter discusses the Nurse Practice Act and how state legislation guides independent practice in public health nursing. Every state has its own Nurse Practice Act that lays out legal specifications for definitions, titles, licensing, and other parameters for the practice of nursing. Because much of public health nursing involves independent decision-making on the part of nurses and in collaboration with others, PHNs need to be aware of how the Nurse Practice Act for their state guides their professional role and defines professional accountability. Nurse Practice Acts also address the scope of practice for advanced practice registered nurses.

Each state has a board of nursing that develops guidelines through rules and regulations that go through a public review before they are enacted. The board of nursing also sets standards for prelicensure nursing education and clinical learning experiences, reviews complaints of misconduct, and follows up with any needed disciplinary action. Amber Zupancic-Albin, a nurse and lawyer, describes each state's Nurse Practice Act as "your nursing rulebook," which specifies rules for ethical and professional conduct for nurses. She represents nurses who are being investigated by the nursing board for a violation of the act. Zupancic-Albin identified five categories of common violations: failure to promote patient safety, dishonesty, controlled substances, improper supervision or delegation, and poor documentation and communication (Zupancic-Albin, 2017).

Although Nurse Practice Acts vary somewhat among states, they all include the following components (Russell, 2012, p. 37):

- Definitions
- Authority, power, and composition of the board of nursing
- Educational program standards
- Types of titles and licenses
- Protection of titles
- Requirements for licensure
- Grounds for disciplinary action, other violations, and possible remedies

States may revise their Nurse Practice Act based on new roles and expertise in the nursing profession. For example, Evidence Example 6.2 addresses the addition of holistic, complementary, and integrative therapies into the scope of practice.

When PHNs practice independently, they make decisions based on their own expert knowledge and skills, professional standards, and the best evidence that guides nursing practice. Independent practice in public health

---

**EVIDENCE EXAMPLE 6.1**

**Core Elements of U.S. Nurse Practice Acts**

Jarrin (2010) conducted an analysis of the core elements of Nurse Practice Acts in the United States for all 50 states and the District of Columbia. The researcher used qualitative analysis software to identify the major themes and frequency of occurrence in the Nurse Practice Acts (see Table 6.1).

**TABLE 6.1  Nurse Practice Act Themes**

| Theme | Percentage of Occurrence |
|---|---|
| Care in the context of nursing | 98% |
| Nursing process | 88% |
| Supervision or delegation of nursing | 82% |
| Executing the medical regimen | 73% |
| Health maintenance and prevention | 65% |
| Teaching nursing | 65% |

*Source:* Jarrin, 2010, p. 170

---

**EVIDENCE EXAMPLE 6.2**

**American Holistic Nurses Association Nurse Practice Act Summary**

The American Holistic Nurses Association is conducting a yearly analysis of Nurse Practice Acts about language changes that address holistic, complementary, or integrative therapies in the RN scope of practice. Four states (Illinois, Nevada, Oregon, and Texas) recognize holistic nursing as a specialty. Seventeen states include references and/or identify separate position statements on holistic or complementary health approaches (American Holistic Nurses Association, 2016).

---

settings differs from the experience of nurses in hospitals and other structured settings, in which medical orders are required for many nursing tasks. On some occasions in public health settings, a physician's order is needed for reimbursement from insurance, Medicare, or Medicaid for public health nursing services. Standing orders for vaccinations or condition-specific protocols also require physician oversight and review.

## What Is the Scope of Public Health Nursing Practice?

Chapter 1 explains that the scope of practice includes the boundaries of safe and ethical practice. The Public Health Intervention Wheel (see Chapter 2) describes what PHNs do and further explains activities that fall within the scope of public health nursing practice. In public health nursing, PHNs often collaborate with staff from different disciplines. It is important to clarify job descriptions and professional roles so that representatives from each discipline make the best use of their specific expertise as they work together on reaching a common goal.

**TABLE 6.2 Task Analysis of PHN Interventions**

| Task/Intervention | Frequency |
| --- | --- |
| Emergency preparedness | 100% |
| Health teaching to individuals and families | 100% |
| Receive and make referrals | 100% |
| Immunization clinics | 93% |
| Health promotion/prevention programs in the community | 88% |
| Case management | 88% |
| Facilitate vulnerable individuals' access to services | 87% |
| Work with groups related to public health issues | 87% |
| Home visits | 83% |
| Health teaching to groups | 82% |
| Work with vulnerable children and/or adults | 81% |
| Investigate disease and other health threats | 78% |
| Health screening | 78% |
| Educational classes, meetings, workshops for providers | 73% |
| Advocate for increased healthcare availability and access | 70% |
| Community organizing activities | 60% |
| Lead groups related to public health issues | 47% |

*Source:* Schaffer et al., 2015

In addition to PHNs, examples of other occupations in the public health workforce are clerical staff, health educators, nutritionists, epidemiologists, emergency preparedness staff, environmental health workers, information specialists, and public health physicians (Beck & Boulton, 2015). The Institute of Medicine (IOM) released a progress report on its 2010 seminal report on *The Future of Nursing: Leading Change, Advancing Health* that delineated the competencies and skills needed by nurses in order to be fully instrumental in influencing delivery of care in a rapidly changing healthcare environment. For PHNs, the development of skills and competencies in interprofessional collaboration and leadership is necessary for working with others to accomplish health system redesign that aims to provide quality, accessible, and affordable care (IOM, 2015).

A study on the work of PHNs (Schaffer, Keller, & Reckinger, 2015) demonstrated the breadth and consistency of public health nursing practice. Sixty PHNs, representing 28 states, completed two online surveys about their professional activities. Many of the activities implemented by the PHNs were consistent with the interventions from the Public Health Intervention Wheel and represent the scope of public health nursing practice. See Table 6.2 to find out which interventions PHNs in the study used most often.

In this same study, the PHNs were asked which activities they thought had the greatest impact on the health of the community. The activities they perceived to have the greatest impact were: "(1) childhood immunizations, (2) communicable disease (including tuberculosis and sexually transmitted infections), surveillance, education, and investigation, (3) maternal and child health-focused activities (early intervention and school readiness activities, prenatal and parenting education, case management of high-risk families, and growth and development follow-up), and (4) linking people to resources" (Schaffer et al., 2015, p. 716). When asked about how the lack of public health nursing services would affect the health of the community, they identified the following potential negative effects: (1) an increase in disease and health problems, (2) worse health related to no focus on prevention, 3) loss of services for vulnerable populations, (4) a negative impact on the public health system, and (5) negative effects for local health departments.

Study participants observed that PHNs are viewed as trustworthy, approachable, and holistic, which contributes to the public's confidence in recommendations made by PHNs. A PHN captured the important contribution of PHNs to the health of communities:

> While all aspects of public health are important, it is the nurse who pulls all the little pieces together. It is the nurse who looks at the big picture to ensure services are being received (p. 118).

## EVIDENCE EXAMPLE 6.3
### Independent Practice

A national sample of school nurses completed an electronic survey on their use of the public health interventions as defined in the Public Health Intervention Wheel. Screening, referral and follow-up, case management, and health teaching were the most frequently performed interventions. School nurses reported that they spent 65% of their time on individual-level interventions, 22% on community-level interventions, and 14% on systems-level interventions. Participants reported conducting activities consistent with the Public Health Intervention Wheel, although 67% of the participants were not familiar with the Wheel. The Public Health Intervention Wheel can be used by school nurses to guide their practice and explain to the school community what school nurses do. Understanding Wheel interventions at the three levels of practice will assist school nurses in improving the health status of a greater number of students at the population level (Schaffer, Anderson, & Rising, 2016).

In Hennepin County, Minnesota, the Perinatal Hepatitis B PHN serves a growing population of refugees and immigrants. The program provides case management, contact investigation of household members, monitoring of immunizations and titers (test for presence of antibodies) for exposed infants, and education to address cultural myths about Hepatitis B for pregnant women who are antigen-positive. The PHN collaborates with the medical provider, social worker, mental health worker, and family members at clinic visits and, through case management, makes any needed referrals. Program effectiveness is measured by improved outcomes in vaccine and serology completion for infants (from 92% to 100%), increases in the number of women referred to liver specialists for follow-up, and increases in the number of referrals of sexual partners and household members for follow-up (Przybilla, Johnson, & Hooker, 2009).

> *Sarah's first day of her public health nursing clinical experience with Jennifer begins right away on Monday morning. Sarah meets Jennifer at the Public Health Office at 7:30 a.m. She met Jennifer briefly a week earlier, but this is the first time that Sarah will have the opportunity to observe nursing through the eyes of a PHN.*
>
> *Sarah rides with Jennifer. Jennifer has three home visits scheduled for the morning, followed by two home visits in the afternoon. Jennifer briefly describes the three morning home visits, which are to families whom she knows from previous visits: (1) a 93-year-old woman with congestive heart failure who lives alone, (2) a toddler with an elevated lead level whose parents had emigrated from Mexico last year, and (3) a 17-year-old with a 3-month-old girl. After the morning visits, Jennifer plans to return to the office for a short time to make any follow-up phone calls and review plans for the afternoon home visits.*

See Table 6.3 on the next page for Jennifer's schedule.

## Expanded Description of Activities

**Asthma Coalition:** One of the school nurses in Aurora noticed that more and more children with asthma were coming to her office every year. She mentioned this concern to a local physician, who had also noticed an increase in pediatric patients needing asthma-related care. The school nurse contacted the public health department to find out whether it was aware of an increase in asthma rates in the county or state. The timing of that call was good—the public health nursing director had just learned of funds that were available for starting a coalition related to asthma in children. The state and county statistics were showing an increase in asthma cases over the past five years. Based on these conversations, a coalition was formed. Currently one of the PHNs is the chairperson of this coalition, which meets monthly to identify ways to increase public and provider awareness of methods to manage asthma. This coalition includes school nurses, nurse practitioners, physicians, PHNs, coaches, and parents of children with asthma.

**Diversity Coalition:** This is a group of community partners (educators, healthcare providers, local business owners) who are interested in supporting the various groups represented in Aurora. The overall goal of this group is to make Aurora a welcoming community for everyone. One of the elementary school teachers in town initiated this group, as he was observing segmentation of racial groups that led to tension not only in the elementary school but also in the community at large.

**Foot Care Clinic:** Twice a month, the PHNs hold a clinic to provide foot care for senior citizens at the community senior center. The PHNs worked with a podiatrist in the community and the public health medical director to develop a foot-clinic protocol and referral system. Because

**TABLE 6.3 Jennifer's Schedule**

| Time | Monday | Tuesday | Wednesday | Thursday | Friday |
|---|---|---|---|---|---|
| 8am–9am | Home visit: Hanson | Staff meeting | Prep for immunization clinic | Women, Infants, and Children Clinic | Intake, referrals, and nursing documentation |
| 9am–10am | Home visit: Garcia | Diversity Coalition meeting | Immunization clinic | Women, Infants, and Children Clinic | Weekly reflective supervision |
| 10am–11am | Home visit: Loften | Diversity Coalition: Collect county data for grant application | Immunization clinic | Women, Infants, and Children Clinic | Intake, referrals, and nursing documentation |
| 11am–12pm | Office: Follow up on calls, new referrals, nursing documentation | Intake, referrals, and nursing documentation | Meet with program manager to determine funding for Asthma Coalition | Women, Infants, and Children Clinic | Intake, referrals, and nursing documentation |
| 12pm–1pm | Lunch | Lunch | Lunch | Lunch | Lunch |
| 1pm–2pm | New Referral | Home visit: Ahmed | Prep for foot clinic at community center | Office: Follow up on phone calls and referrals, prep for afternoon home visits | Prep for immunization clinic |
| 2pm–3pm | New Referral | Home visit: Johnson | Foot care clinic | Home visit: Wallis | Immunization clinic |
| 3pm–4pm | Nursing documentation | Nursing documentation | Foot care clinic | Home visit: Froeland | Immunization clinic |

an identified need existed in the community to provide basic skin and nail care and assessment for elderly citizens, this has been a very popular clinic. Two PHNs staff the clinic.

**Immunization Clinic:** Each week, the public health office holds an immunization clinic where people can receive low-cost vaccinations for children or adults in their families. The clinic is held at the local health department, which is centrally located. It is a walk-in clinic, so no appointments are required. Each PHN takes a turn staffing the clinic. One PHN oversees the clinic by ordering vaccines, following current protocols for administration, and informing the PHNs of updated information.

**Phone Triage and Intake:** The PHNs all take turns providing intake services. During this time, the PHN works on documentation or projects at his or her desk and answers calls that come to the agency that require a PHN to assess and provide feedback. Examples of the types of calls include referrals for home visiting services, questions about where to get a car seat inspection, parents asking where to get vaccinations, or daycare providers worried about head lice.

**Reflective Supervision:** Each week PHNs in the agency meet with their supervisor for reflective supervision. This time is set aside for the nurse and supervisor to thoughtfully consider the families receiving home visiting services. The time allows the PHN to consider ethical or other challenges in providing services, and it allows the nurse to consider his or her own thoughts and reactions to each family.

**WIC Clinic:** Women, Infants, and Children (WIC) is a federally funded food program administered by states and counties that provides screening, nutrition counseling, and health referrals for pregnant and breastfeeding women and their children from birth to 5 years of age. In Aurora, PHNs and nutritionists from the Health and Human Services department staff this clinic twice a month at the public health nursing office. Jennifer's role is to provide height, weight, and hemoglobin checks for the children and pregnant women in the program.

Sarah's assignment for the day was to observe Jennifer's communication and actions. Sarah planned to take notes about her observations and communication between the PHN and her clients. See Sarah's notes.

## SARAH'S NOTEBOOK

| Activity | Sarah's Observations |
|---|---|
| **Visit 1:** Lily Hanson, a 93-year-old woman with congestive heart failure. Lives alone. | Arrived at a four-plex apartment building. The yard and building were maintained well, with big shade trees, grass, and flower beds surrounding the building. Lily's apartment was on the first floor (no steps). Jennifer knocked on the door and opened it slightly; Lily called to Jennifer to come in. Lily was sitting at the dining room table and using her portable oxygen, neatly dressed, with her pill bottles lined up. The apartment was well kept, with many photos on the walls. |
| | A fan was running quietly in the corner of the living room. Jennifer completed a heart and lung assessment and asked Lily about her activity level. Lily reported that even in the hot, humid weather, if she stayed indoors with the fans running, she felt comfortable. Jennifer filled Lily's pillbox for the week. Jennifer also asked Lily about alternate plans if her apartment became too hot for her to tolerate. Lily reported that she did have a window air conditioner, but it broke, and she did not have enough money to buy a new one. Jennifer suggested that Lily call the County Senior Support Network (SSN). The SSN has funds for elders in need of basic housing supplies. In this heat wave, Jennifer has learned that the SSN will provide air conditioners. |
| | Jennifer talked to Lily so naturally. Jennifer explained that she had known Lily for three years. The first year she came to visit, Lily was not friendly at all. She thought Jennifer was visiting to get information that would cause her to go to a long-term care facility. After that first year and many short conversations, Lily accepted that Jennifer was trying to help her maintain her independence so that she could continue to live in her apartment. Jennifer hypothesized that her persistence and nonjudgmental attitude helped Lily realize she was there to support her. |
| **Visit 2:** Toddler with an elevated lead level whose parents emigrated from Mexico last year | Drove to an older part of town with many single-family homes. Much of the paint had worn off or was peeling. In most of the yards, the grass was worn away, and there were many children's toys. Jennifer rang the doorbell, knocked, and called in the front window, but there was no response. There was no response to a phone call either. Jennifer explained that sometimes families might not be home even though an appointment had been made for the visit. Persons living in poverty experience more crises, and with fewer resources they might live from day to day, with less emphasis on future planning. I thought about how persons living with poverty might more often choose to meet survival needs and how these choices are consistent with Maslow's Hierarchy of Needs theory. |
| **Visit 3:** First-time 17-year-old mom, Jewel, who has a 3-month-old girl | Stopped at an old apartment building that had broken glass on the front steps. Entry security system was working. Jewel lives on the third floor. No elevator. Smelled musty. Jewel had the door open for us and responded cheerfully to Jennifer. It was 90 degrees out at 10 a.m. Jewel had the shades pulled to keep the sun out, but there were no air conditioners or fans in the efficiency apartment. Jennifer focused this visit on baby Kayla's development. She used the Ages and Stages Questionnaire that has questions specific to development expected for the age of the child. I noticed Jennifer also gave some suggestions to Jewel about what she could expect to happen in Kayla's development over the next few months. Jennifer gave information to Jewel about an organization that would help her get a fan and discussed how to prevent dehydration with the hot weather. During the visit, Jennifer coached Jewel in making a phone call to the apartment manager to report the glass on the front steps. |

*(continues)*

## SARAH'S NOTEBOOK (continued)

| Activity | Sarah's Observations |
| --- | --- |
| Office (and lunch) | Jennifer checked for messages and had one from the Garcia family—they will not be home today. Completed some charting. Checked for new referrals. Made calls to these families. |
| **New Referral:** Active case of tuberculosis (TB) | Met Mr. Adams at his house. Mr. Adams was diagnosed with pulmonary TB (tuberculosis) about 4 months ago. He likely acquired TB working overseas in a disaster relief effort. He recently moved to Aurora to be near his aging parents. Jennifer will be providing Direct Observed Therapy (DOT) for Mr. Adams. In DOT, Jennifer will observe Mr. Adams to make sure he takes his medication correctly. When TB medication is taken inconsistently, the TB bacteria can become resistant to medication. In comparison to Jennifer's interaction with Lily earlier today, this was a very formal meeting. Jennifer asked questions to get the intake information. She also inquired about Mr. Adams's preferences for DOT. After the discussion and a brief health history, Jennifer observed Mr. Adams taking the medication and left. |
| **New Referral:** Postpartum visit | We met Amy Chan. She is 2 weeks postpartum. Her baby boy is doing well. However, Amy is anxious and nervous about her son, as her first child died of Sudden Unexpected Infant Death (SUID) three years ago. Jennifer assessed the home environment for infant sleep practices, reviewed guidelines for safe infant sleep, and provided positive feedback regarding Amy's care for her son. Jennifer used the Edinburgh Postnatal Depression Scale (EPDS) to screen Amy for postpartum depression. Short messages and positive feedback seemed to help Amy. Jennifer suggested a support group for Amy. |

*Sarah speaks with Jennifer after the first day of her clinical experience. Jennifer explains that her planning for home visits needed to be flexible. Sometimes her plan needed to change because a client might have an unexpected health problem or family crisis. Sarah comments, "I don't know how I will ever become independent in my decision-making about what to do."*

*Jennifer suggests, "Let's review the day. Then we can analyze what we did today and which independent public health nursing interventions were accomplished. Also, I will have you look at my schedule for the rest of the week. You can begin to think about which interventions you would consider to be independent practice and how you might collaborate with others. We can discuss the skills and knowledge a PHN needs for these interventions."*

### Activity

Review Jennifer's schedule for the week (Table 6.3) and answer the following questions:

- Which public health interventions from the Public Health Intervention Wheel did Jennifer use?
- Which interventions were independent, and which were delegated functions?
- What skills and knowledge enabled Jennifer to practice independently?
- How did Jennifer collaborate with other individuals, groups, professionals, or organizations?

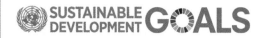

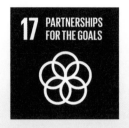 **SUSTAINABLE DEVELOPMENT GOALS**

**Scope of Nursing Practice in New Zealand**

**GOAL 17** New Zealand's new health strategy emphasizes prevention and early interventions aimed at ensuring that New Zealanders "live well, stay well, get well." Jane O'Malley, chief nursing officer, is leading the way toward using the health workforce to the maximum potential (full scope of practice for nurses). To improve health and access to care: 1) the Nursing Council of New Zealand can now determine the education, experience, competence, and supervision requirements to allow RNs to prescribe, and 2) a legislative change replaces the term *medical practitioner* with *health practitioner* in relevant laws. This increases the scope of practice for nurse practitioners in New Zealand (International Council of Nurses, 2017).

 **Healthy People**

**healthypeople.gov**

On the Healthy People 2020 website, go to "Topics & Objectives" and under "M" click "Maternal, Infant, and Child Health." Read about factors that affect pregnancy and childbirth. Go back to the Topics & Objectives page and under "S" click "Social Determinants of Health." Scroll to review examples of social and physical determinants of health. Refer to the 17-year-old mother described in Sarah's journal. Which determinants of health are important to consider and address for this young mother? Return to the "Maternal, Infant, and Child Health" page and click "Interventions and Resources" at the top of the page. Find one intervention among the suggestions that you could use to address the needs of this young family.

> *On Tuesday, Jennifer has a visit scheduled with a client being seen in the targeted home visit program, Mindy, who is 16 and lives with her mother. Mindy has a 6-month-old baby girl. Mindy's former boyfriend, the baby's father, had been physically abusive to Mindy during her pregnancy. Mindy has developmental delays and struggles with school and fitting in. Mindy was referred to public health nursing after her first prenatal clinic visit when she was six months pregnant. Mindy and Jennifer have developed a trusting relationship. Mindy has worked hard to follow through with good parenting practices and has been receptive to Jennifer. Jennifer checked her Facebook account last night and saw that Mindy had made a friend request to her. Jennifer feels torn between the professional, therapeutic, and supportive roles she provides for Mindy.*

## How to Establish Professional Boundaries in Public Health Nursing

Understanding professional boundaries is essential for all nurses. PHNs practice in environments that are sometimes more challenging for maintaining professional boundaries, such as in homes, schools, and other community settings that have different norms of behavior in contrast to the hospital setting. In the hospital setting, professional and client roles are more clearly defined. In community and home settings, relationships and the norms of interaction need to be differentiated from more casual social relationships. Sometimes students and PHNs find it difficult to keep from moving into a social friendship with the client as the relationship progresses over time. PHNs must clarify their role and the purpose of the relationship with clients to maintain professional boundaries. PHNs can also use dedicated reflective supervision time with their nursing supervisor to consider challenges around client relationships and boundaries.

*A Nurse's Guide to Professional Boundaries,* published by the National Council of State Boards of Nursing, provides guidelines for managing boundaries in nursing practice. See Table 6.4 for specific guidelines and their application to managing boundaries in public health nursing practice.

PHNs need to be aware of the potential for boundary violations in their interactions with individuals, families, and communities. Consider the following potential red flags that could lead to crossing boundaries (National Council of State Boards of Nursing, 2014, p. 5):

- Discussing intimate or personal issues with a patient
- Engaging in behaviors that could reasonably be interpreted as flirting
- Keeping secrets with a patient or for a patient
- Believing that you are the only one who truly understands or can help the patient

## TABLE 6.4 Boundaries and the Continuum of Professional Nursing Behavior

| Management of Boundaries | Examples of Nursing Actions |
| --- | --- |
| The nurse's responsibility is to delineate and maintain boundaries. | Sarah introduces herself as a nursing student working with Weaver County PH, shadowing Jennifer. |
| The nurse should work within the therapeutic relationship. | Jennifer has an open conversation with Mindy about why she cannot accept Facebook requests from clients. |
| The nurse should examine any boundary crossing, be aware of its potential implications, and avoid repeated crossings. | Sarah considers what it would mean for a nurse to have a non-work relationship on Facebook with a current or former client. |
| Variables such as the care setting, community influences, patient needs, and nature of therapy affect the delineation of boundaries. | Jennifer encourages Mindy to continue to share her personal experiences when Jennifer comes for visits and shows interest in Mindy's life as a parent. |
| The nurse should avoid situations where he or she has a personal, professional, or business relationship with the patient. | Jennifer declines Mindy's Facebook request and also discusses the agency policy with her supervisor. |
| Post-termination relationships are complex because the patient may need additional services. It may be difficult to determine when the nurse–patient relationship is completely terminated. | Jennifer works collaboratively with Mindy to ensure she feels competent as a parent. Jennifer helps Mindy understand when and why the home visiting services are no longer needed. |
| Be careful about personal relationships with patients who might continue to need nursing services. | Upon case closure, Jennifer takes time to celebrate Mindy's successes on a home visit and provides encouragement to Mindy to reach out to the agency with future needs. She does not use Facebook to stay in contact with former clients. |

*Source:* National Council of State Boards of Nursing, 2014, p. 3

- Spending more time than is necessary with a particular patient
- Speaking poorly about colleagues or your employment setting with the patient or family
- Showing favoritism
- Meeting a patient in settings besides those used to provide direct patient care or when you are not at work

Confusion about the nurse's role may occur when clients want to give gifts or offer money. Although PHNs do not wear uniforms, they need to choose professional-appearing attire that is comfortable. Individuals from some cultures might frown on clothing that they consider too revealing and might be reluctant to believe what the PHN is saying is important if the PHN is not professionally dressed. However, PHNs may also dress more casually in some settings, such as homeless shelters or schools, which may help clients feel more comfortable when talking to them. PHNs need to be alert for any situation or conversations that might result in self-disclosure. They need to ask themselves whether what they are doing is what a nurse would typically do. PHNs can use touch as a comfort measure but need to consider the meaning of any physical contact to the nurse and client. Touch and eye contact are not considered accepted practices in some cultures.

On some occasions, physical assessment is required, and although it is a norm for adults and children to remove clothes for physical exams in the hospital and clinic settings, removing clothes is not a norm in a community setting.

If infants and children require a physical examination, the PHN should ask the parent or the child, if old enough, to remove the child's clothes.

Maintaining professional boundaries does not mean being detached from clients. At the same time, the PHN does not fulfill the role of being a friend to a client. In interactions with clients, PHNs need to balance how they develop a trusting relationship with clients while maintaining their own separate professional identity.

### EVIDENCE EXAMPLE 6.4

#### Defining Boundaries in Public Health Nursing

Five PHNs who participated in a qualitative study described the challenge of defining boundaries as they worked with clients. They described situations of being persuaded to do something and then feeling regret that they had not said "no." The authors of the study suggested that one's professional ethical responsibility does not mean doing what others demand. Closer relationships that develop over a long-term time period with clients can lead to a sense of duty, which can result in over-involvement and possible development of a friendship, a potential professional boundary violation. "Each nurse has to make decisions that are not only based on quality standards, but also on their professional intuition and personal involvement" (Clancy & Svensson, 2007, p. 163).

## Activity

Discuss the following questions:

■ When is it helpful to share something personal about yourself with a client? When is it not helpful?

■ What are some red flags indicating that you might not be maintaining professional boundaries with clients?

■ Is it a boundary violation to attend a patient's baby shower? A funeral for a client? Why or why not?

■ How do you think Jennifer should handle Mindy's Facebook request?

## How Do Public Health Nurses Establish and Maintain Confidentiality?

Confidentiality in public health nursing often goes hand in hand with professional boundaries. Maintaining professional boundaries requires that PHNs keep health information private. PHNs must consider whom they speak to about clients and the confidentiality of their documentation processes. The Health Insurance Portability and Accountability Act (HIPAA), which specifies how health information may be communicated, is discussed in Chapter 7. Respecting patient confidentiality is a professional and legal duty. However, PHNs must also balance this duty against the need to disclose information to protect someone from harm, such as in situations of suicidal ideation. When children or vulnerable adults are involved, the duty to protect outweighs the duty to keep health information in confidence. Competing interests can exist, which means disclosure can be justified for the public good, such as child protection (Griffith, 2015).

❝ *Jennifer is well known at one of the apartment buildings in Aurora where many elderly adults live. Jennifer has made many visits to residents in this complex over the years. The residents, although not related, have become like family to each other and welcome Jennifer. They have an informal system of checking on each other daily and helping each other with trips to the grocery store or pharmacy. Often as Jennifer exits a client's apartment after a visit, several residents stop Jennifer to ask how her client is doing. The neighbors are genuinely concerned and want to be helpful in any way possible. Sarah notes that Jennifer does not offer any specific information, and after the visit she asks Jennifer how she usually responds to questions about the well-being of residents in the complex.* ❞

### EVIDENCE EXAMPLE 6.5
**Maintaining Boundaries and Confidentiality in Working With Families With Intimate Partner Violence**

Evanson (2006) investigated the role of PHNs who conducted home visits with families who had experienced intimate partner violence. The PHNs who worked in rural settings had more challenges in keeping confidentiality, helping women find resources, getting their own support, and keeping professional and personal boundaries. Although all the PHNs viewed setting boundaries as an essential part of their work with families who were experiencing intimate partner violence, Evanson concluded that the boundaries between personal and professional lives for rural PHNs are less clear than those for nonrural nurses. The rural PHNs had learned to be flexible with boundaries because they were highly visible in the community and often knew their clients personally through attending the same church, having children who were friends, or knowing mutual acquaintances. Personal ties were perceived as a barrier to disclosure of the interpersonal violence. Rural PHNs needed to be vigilant about maintaining confidentiality and at times needed to withhold the truth from others within a client's family or community. Evanson recommends that rural agencies provide support opportunities through staff meetings and case conferences to help nurses who work with families experiencing intimate partner violence cope with the emotional labor of their jobs.

## What Does Ethical, Legal, and Professional Accountability Mean in Public Health Nursing?

Ethical and professional standards and legal guidelines drive accountability in public health nursing practice. *Public Health Nursing: Scope and Standards of Practice* (ANA, 2013) specifies areas of accountability for PHNs (see Chapter 1). PHNs have more accountability to populations compared to nurses in other practice settings. The PHN is accountable for improving population health. Legal accountability is discussed in Chapter 7. See Chapter 1 for an explanation of ethical theory and a framework for analyzing ethical problems in public health nursing practice.

Public health ethics is driven by social justice. The aim is to create a flourishing community for all rather than satisfying individual self-interests. A bioethics perspective focuses more on autonomy and individual rights (Easley & Allen, 2007). Ethical challenges in public health nursing can result from the conflict between protecting the community and respecting individual autonomy. For example, individuals might be required to take medication to treat tuberculosis

## EVIDENCE EXAMPLE 6.6
### Ethics of Caring and Social Justice in Public Health Nursing Practice

Falk-Rafael and Betker (2012) interviewed ten expert public health nurses in Canada about how ethics guided their practice. Participants provided descriptions of situations that were consistent with caring, social justice, and social activism in their professional practice. The analysis revealed three themes: the moral imperative, the pursuit of social justice, and barriers to moral agency. Participants identified important values for interactions with clients (respect, autonomy, honesty, fairness, social justice, protection of human dignity) as imperative in their practice. They provided examples of addressing social determinants of health and advocating for health equity in social policy. Examples of barriers to moral agency identified by the PHNs included: 1) financial and administrative constraints, 2) feeling powerless to make changes, and 3) a shift to relying on electronic data for priority-setting that resulted in less involvement of the PHN with the community and a lack of priority-setting based on needs expressed by community members. Falk-Rafael and Betker proclaim that ethical practice for PHNs and their professional organizations requires caring through advocacy for social justice as vitally important to both the nursing profession and society (see Chapter 13).

## EVIDENCE EXAMPLE 6.7
### A School Nurse's Heroic Journey

Ellen Johnsen worked as a school nurse in Broken Arrow, Oklahoma, in the 1980s. Johnsen brought her concerns about a proposed unsafe and illegal medication administration policy to the school superintendent. A committee was formed to review the policy; however, school nurses were not included on the committee. They were invited to submit input by phone or mail. The committee proposed a revised policy that was consistent with the Oklahoma Nurse Practice Act. All medications, prescribed and over the counter (OTC), required physician orders. However, the superintendent rejected the committee's recommendation and proposed a policy draft that required parental permission but not a physician's order for OTC medications. The nurses were told if they did not agree with this policy, they would be replaced with school aides. Johnsen demonstrated a commitment to professionalism and standards of practice through her continued quest for a safe and legal policy. An analysis of her journey identified the following actions that demonstrate a commitment to professionalism and standards of practice in her leadership and change agent roles: She gathered information about professional standards; sought expert opinion on relevant laws, regulations, and policies; shared her knowledge with colleagues; collaborated on policy development; advocated for change in the face of barriers; and accepted the consequences of being a change agent. Although her contract was not renewed, Johnsen continued her quest for a safe and legal medication administration policy (Johnsen & Pohlman, 2017).

(even when they would prefer to choose otherwise) to protect others' health. Protecting individual rights to privacy might conflict with the need to share information to benefit the public's health, such as in the case of reporting cases of communicable diseases to the health department so that disease incidence can be monitored (Racher, 2007).

In the study by Clancy and Svensson (2007), PHNs expressed that they thought they had a greater sense of responsibility than hospital nurses, because the PHNs primarily worked on their own. They expressed that they felt alone with their worries and their uncertainties about what to do. Ethical decision-making does not occur in a vacuum. Resolutions are better with input from other experts in the field. PHNs need to seek out collegial and organizational support for their decision-making to ensure ethical, legal, and professional accountability.

### Activity

Consider the attributes of nursing professionalism found in Table 6.5. Which attributes did Ellen Johnsen demonstrate in her quest to achieve a safe and legal medication policy in her school district?

### TABLE 6.5  Attributes of Nursing Professionalism

| | |
|---|---|
| ■ Sense of nursing as a calling | ■ Critical thinking |
| ■ Self-regulating behaviors | ■ Intellectual and individual responsibility |
| ■ Presentation of self (image, attire, and expression) | ■ Respect for human dignity |
| ■ Personal integrity | ■ Protection of patients and the vulnerable |
| ■ Autonomy | ■ Well-developed group consciousness |
| ■ Knowledge and specialization | ■ Belief and participation in public service |
| | ■ Belonging to professional organization |

*Sources:* Akhtar-Danesh et al., 2013; Wynd, 2003

# What Should I Know About Delegation and Supervision in Public Health Nursing?

PHNs practice within their professional scope and standards of practice as well as within the guidelines of state Nurse Practice Acts, which define the legal parameters of nursing practice. Delegation is based on requirements addressed in each state's Nurse Practice Act. PHNs may be in the role of accepting delegated activities, such as carrying out provider orders for administering immunizations or monitoring respiratory status, and they also may be in the role of delegating specific functions to unlicensed assistive personnel (UAP) or licensed practical nurses (LPNs). UAPs include nurses' aides, certified nursing assistants, health aides, or other nonlicensed positions (ANA, 2012). Practice environments often include multiple services and interventions to promote the health of individuals, communities, and populations. The ability to work interprofessionally and to clearly identify the components of the delegation process is crucial to successful PHN practice. Weydt (2010) states:

> RNs are required to understand what patients and families need and then engage the appropriate care givers in the plan of care in order to achieve desired patient outcomes while maximizing the available resources on the patient's behalf. Delegation is an important skill that influences clinical and financial outcomes (para. 2).

Effective delegation is an essential nursing skill and is guided by three concepts the PHN must understand: *responsibility, accountability,* and *authority* (Weydt, 2010). The PHN has the *authority* to delegate specific tasks to individuals or groups, and these individuals or groups accept the *responsibility* for the tasks. However, at all times, the PHN retains *accountability* for the safety and quality of the outcome (Stanhope & Lancaster, 2012). Delegation is most effective when it is based on effective communication and mutual trust (Kaernested & Bragadottir, 2012).

The PHN must determine when and whether delegation is appropriate. The process for determination follows the steps of the nursing process (ANA, 2012). Some tasks should not be delegated because they fall in the realm of professional nursing—for example, counseling; health teaching; and activities that require nursing knowledge, skill, and judgment based on evidence or data (ANA, 2007). Tasks that can be delegated are more often repetitive and supportive in caregiving (Williams & Cooksey, 2004). It is important to note the emphasis on individuals or communities as partners in the plan of care and the importance of communication at all phases among healthcare consumers, UAPs, and PHNs. To determine whether delegation is appropriate, the American Nurses Association (2012) has identified six care provisions (see Table 6.6).

## TABLE 6.6 Care Provisions for Determining Effective Delegation

1. Perform an assessment of the healthcare consumer's:
   - Care needs and determine whether any cultural modifications are required.
   - Condition to determine whether it is stable and predictable.
   - Environment where the care will be provided.

2. Develop a plan of care with the healthcare consumer and his or her family, identifying the delegable task and intended outcome as part of the overall plan of care. Involving and educating healthcare consumers and their families about appropriate expectations of the roles of care providers promotes a safer environment and improved patient outcomes. The plan of care should include:
   - Baseline status of the healthcare consumer.
   - Specific unchanging task performance steps.
   - When and to whom the UAP needs to report if the baseline status changes.
   - Documentation of expectations as appropriate.

3. Analyze the following:
   - Is the task within the delegating registered nurse's (RN's) scope of practice?
   - Do federal or state laws, rules, or regulations support the delegation?
   - Does the employing organization/agency of the delegating RN and the UAP permit delegation?
   - Is the delegating RN competent to make the delegation decision?
   - Is the UAP competent to perform the delegated task?
   - Is RN supervision of the UAP available?

4. Monitor implementation of the delegated task as appropriate to the overall plan of care.

5. Evaluate the overall condition of the healthcare consumer and the consumer's response to the delegated task.

6. Evaluate the UAP's skills and performance of tasks and provide feedback for improvement, if needed.

*Source:* ANA, 2012

## Activity

Read the case study on the next page and analyze how a PHN could ensure that the Care Provisions of Delegation are followed when delegating to the family health aide. Then analyze how the Care Provisions of Delegation are represented in this case study.

## CASE STUDY
### Delegation

I received a referral on a 22-year-old and her 2-month-old baby. At my initial home visit, the baby appeared overweight and over-fed. The young mom had started him on rice cereal in a bottle at 2 weeks. Every time he cried, she gave him a bottle, even though he often struggled and tried to pull away from the nipple. I talked with her about feeding the baby and my concern about his weight, but she responded with, "Once he starts moving around, the weight will come off."

By 4 months of age, the baby was 27 pounds. By now I was very concerned and called both the nurse and the doctor at the clinic, but no action was taken. Next, I arranged a joint home visit with a nutritionist from WIC (Women, Infants, and Children Supplemental Food Program). We counseled the mom to feed the baby only when he was truly hungry.

Two weeks later, I returned to do an NCAST* feeding interaction and videotaped the mom feeding the baby. We watched the tape together and talked about hunger cues and how the baby did not appear hungry. The young mother listened but continued to feed the baby whenever he fussed or cried. It was as though she had no other way to comfort him other than to feed him. I was also becoming concerned about the baby's development, as he exhibited several delays in fine motor and language when I tested him.

At this point, I started visiting every 2 weeks and placed a family health aide in the home for 2 hours at a time 1 day a week. The aide's assignment was to role-model appropriate parenting and feeding. I also arranged to get a highchair for feeding the child through a nutrition program grant. Currently, I continue to coordinate services from the clinic, nutritionist, and family health aide. At the present time, the baby's weight has stabilized, and he has not gained any more weight.

*NCAST (Nursing Child Assessment Satellite Training) is an objective and systematic assessment of interactions between parent and child (30 hours of continuing education). It can alert the nurse to areas of concern and the need for teaching. It has been used as legal documentation in court cases of child abuse.

*Source:* Minnesota Department of Health [MDH], Office of Public Health Practice, 2006

Discuss how these Care Provisions of Delegation do or could take place in this case study:

- Perform an assessment of the healthcare consumer.
- Develop a plan of care with the healthcare consumer and his or her family.
- Analyze delegation factors.
- Monitor implementation of the delegated task as appropriate to the overall plan of care.
- Evaluate the overall condition of the healthcare consumer and the consumer's response to the delegated task.
- Evaluate the UAP's skills and performance of tasks and provide feedback for improvement, if needed.

## Do I Need to Become Registered to Become a Public Health Nurse?

*Public Health Nursing: Scope and Standards of Practice* identifies the baccalaureate degree in nursing as the credential for public health nursing practice (ANA, 2013). In addition, the Association of Community Health Nurse Educators (ACHNE) assumes the minimum requirement for entry-level public health or community nursing practice is a baccalaureate nursing degree (ACHNE, 2009). There are several routes to achieving this entry-level education preference. Nurses with associate degrees may choose to enter RN-to-BSN programs, or graduates with a baccalaureate degree or higher in another major may choose an "accelerated" nursing program. Accelerated programs may offer a master's degree (check individual institutions) for this select group of students. For students interested in advanced studies in the area of public health nursing, the doctor of nursing practice (DNP) or the PhD are degrees that support practice and research in the field.

You can look at your state's Nurse Practice Act to determine whether a baccalaureate degree is required for the practice of public health nursing in your state. Some states require certification or registration for the title of PHN. The baccalaureate is the preferred entry into practice degree.

> *Sarah is very excited about public health nursing and asks Jennifer how she could obtain public health nursing certification. Jennifer recommends that Sarah read the Nurse Practice Act in whichever state she practices nursing after she graduates with her baccalaureate degree in nursing. Sarah can also contact the board of nursing in that state to learn more about nursing practice guidelines specific to that area.*

### Examples of Legal Requirements in Nurse Practice Acts

- California, Hawaii, Iowa, Minnesota, New York, North Carolina, South Carolina, and Wisconsin require a baccalaureate degree for PHN practice.
- In California, Minnesota, New York, and South Carolina, licensure acts or rules have language that defines the scope of public health nursing practice and reserves the use of the title "public health nurse" for those professional nurses who meet specific criteria.
- In California, PHN certification requires training in child abuse and neglect, and a PHN certificate is needed to use the title of "public health nurse" (California Board of Registered Nursing, 2006).

## Public Health Nursing Practice in a Variety of Public and Private Healthcare Settings

PHNs provide care for individuals, families, and communities in many settings as well as in local and state health departments. This section provides a description of how nurses in home care, school, corrections, and faith community settings use public health nursing knowledge and skills in their practice.

- **Home Care:** Home visiting nurses in New York, West Virginia, and Ohio provided a specific intervention to facilitate chronic disease management for elderly clients enrolled in Medicare. The nurses made monthly visits to clients, using behavior change approaches and empowerment strategies to work with clients on managing chronic disease. They used handbooks to encourage physical activity. Public health interventions implemented by the home visiting nurses included case finding, health teaching, counseling, and case management. Following the intervention, the group receiving the home visits had less difficulty bathing and experienced less dependence in walking (Friedman, Li, Liebel, & Powers, 2014).

- **Schools:** Five nursing students from a local college of nursing partnered with a school district in Dakota County, Minnesota, to carry out an aggregate assessment of children with seizure disorders in five elementary schools. They identified health determinants at the individual and systems levels of practice and identified risk factors at the systems level of practice. They found that lunch room, playground, and transportation staff did not know how to respond to a student having a seizure. In response, the students: 1) developed a handout and PowerPoint presentation for school teachers and staff with input from the Minnesota Epilepsy Society, and 2) created a laminated business-card-size "Seizure Action Steps" that could be attached to staff name tag lanyards. These Seizure Action Step cards were distributed to all teachers and staff district-wide. The cards have increased staff comfort levels in having access to quick guidelines about actions needed if a child has a seizure. This systems-level health teaching intervention—implemented in partnership with the district Health Services Coordinator, who is a licensed school nurse—was an independent nursing action (contributed by Stacie O'Leary, health service coordinator, and Patricia Schoon, assistant professor, Metropolitan State University).

- **Correctional Facilities:** The Washington County, Minnesota, Sheriff's Office contracts with the local Department of Public Health & Environment to provide nursing services to inmates in the Washington County jail. The Correctional Health Nursing supervisor in the jail medical unit attends weekly Re-entry Assistance Program (RAP) team meetings that are facilitated by Community Corrections staff. The goal of the RAP is to provide multidisciplinary support to inmates who are preparing to be released from jail into the community. The collaboration between Corrections, Jail Medical, the Workforce Center, Community Financial Services, and other providers allows inmates to ask questions and get concrete assistance and guidance around barriers to successful re-entry. The Correctional Health Nursing supervisor provides referrals for physical and dental healthcare and assists with facilitating overall medical care needed upon release (contributed by Jill Timm, senior program manager, Washington County Department of Public Health & Environment).

- **Faith Communities:** Pappas-Rogich and King (2014) conducted a survey of 247 faith community nurses (FCNs) to identify their use of faith community nursing functions and practice standards and how often they implement Healthy People 2020 leading indicators in their practice. More than 50% of FCNs in the study used the following indicators in their practice weekly or monthly: 1) promote daily physical activity, 2) promote good nutrition and healthier weight, and 3) promote emotional health and well-being. FCNs partnered with many organizations in the community, including hospitals, local public health departments (LHDs), senior service agencies, faith-sponsored agencies, and hospices. Also, 30% of FCNs reported participating in partnerships with health system–sponsored FCN programs.

## Ethical Application

When working with individuals and families, PHNs often must balance acting in the professional role with building a trusting relationship. In the attempt to find this balance in working with at-risk families, a PHN might encounter tension between different ethical perspectives. If a PHN emphasizes the expert role, the client might feel inadequate or judged.

The client might need a "friend" and want to view the PHN as a friend. However, framing the relationship as a friendship implies expectations of sharing and obligation that might fall outside the professional role. Professional caring does not mean being a friend but carries the responsibility of ethical action based on promoting good for the client, contributing to a flourishing community, and strategizing to reduce oppression for clients and families who receive public health services.

See Table 6.7 for an application of ethical perspectives to maintaining professional boundaries. Think about the related scenarios in this chapter: 1) the adolescent mother asked Jennifer to be her friend on Facebook; and 2) residents in the apartment building where Jennifer visited several elderly clients asked her how her clients were doing.

## TABLE 6.7  Ethical Action in Maintaining Professional Boundaries

| Ethical Perspective | Application |
| --- | --- |
| Rule ethics (principles) | ■ Use expert public health nursing knowledge to promote good and prevent harm to clients and families.<br>■ Keep health information confidential to protect the client. |
| Virtue ethics (character) | ■ Be compassionate in recognizing the hardships and health challenges encountered by clients and families.<br>■ Use caring interactions to communicate confidence in the client's ability to make positive health decisions.<br>■ Focus on building trusting relationships as a basis for mutual goal setting. |
| Feminist ethics (reducing oppression) | ■ Connect families to resources that reduce some of the inequities they experience because of poverty.<br>■ Establish a relationship with the client that communicates valuing others as equal individuals. |

## Activity

For either of the two scenarios discussed earlier in the chapter (the Facebook incident and the apartment residents asking about the well-being of clients), analyze the resolution to the ethical problem by answering the following questions:

■ Which values related to the situation do you see as important to you as a professional and as a person?

■ Who do you think you should be as a PHN (important virtues)?

■ Based on your values and who you should be, what would you do in this situation?

■ Which ethical perspectives (rule ethics, virtue ethics, and feminist ethics) support your chosen action?

## ! KEY POINTS

■ Nurse Practice Acts in each state and the scope and standards of public health nursing provide expectations for PHNs' professional accountability.

■ The Public Health Intervention Wheel defines the independent interventions that PHNs implement in their practice.

■ Professional boundaries can be more challenging to maintain in public health nursing, given the community setting and long-term relationships with clients.

■ Protection of patient confidentiality can be more challenging for PHNs to ensure in rural communities, where many residents know the PHNs.

■ HIPAA provides legal standards for handling protected health information.

■ PHNs can use the six Care Provisions of Delegation identified by the ANA to guide their delegation responsibilities.

■ Nurses in a variety of settings use expert public health knowledge and skills in interventions with individuals, families, communities, and systems.

## REFLECTIVE PRACTICE

Nurses who practice in healthcare organizations, such as hospitals, are constantly reminded about rules and regulations that guide their nursing practice. They are surrounded by other nursing staff and supervisors whom they can quickly ask for guidance in any situation that might seem confusing. In many situations, PHNs do not have the security of having other nurses and nursing administrators immediately available to them. School nurses are often the only nursing professionals in the building. PHNs who make home visits might feel isolated and unsure of which response conforms to ethical and legal actions. PHNs must be knowledgeable about the scope of professional practice and guidelines for ethical and legal practice. They need to provide rationales that are based on ethical, legal, and professional guidelines to support their choice of nursing actions.

Read the case study and write your answers to the following questions. Then discuss them with your classmates.

1. How does the scope of public health nursing practice (see Chapter 1) guide the responsibilities of the PHN in this case study?

2. What do you think are the most relevant interventions for the PHN to implement from the Public Health Intervention Wheel?

3. What is the PHN's ethical and legal accountability for the boyfriend's domestic violence?

4. What concerns do you have about maintaining confidentiality and professional boundaries in this case study?

5. Which Cornerstones of Public Health Nursing do you think are consistent with supporting the PHN's interventions in working with this family?

6. How would you ensure ethical practice on your part in working with this family?

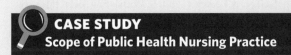

## CASE STUDY
### Scope of Public Health Nursing Practice

You are a PHN with approximately 40 high-risk families in your caseload. One of your clients is a 17-year-old adolescent, Mariana, who has an 11-month-old baby boy, Adan, whom she delivered at 34 weeks gestation with a birth weight of 4 pounds 1 ounce. Mariana lives in a trailer court off and on with an unemployed boyfriend who has hit her twice in the past month. She will not report the assaults because he is on probation for selling drugs and would immediately go to prison. She states, "He has promised it will never happen again."

Mariana's boyfriend not only isolates her from family and friends; he has pressured her to drop out of an alternative school, where she had successfully secured onsite licensed childcare and school bus transportation. She was on track to achieve her high school diploma this year. Mariana is unable to acquire her WIC vouchers for purchase of healthy foods because she has no transportation to the WIC office. In addition, Mariana has missed several healthcare appointments for Adan and herself. Her healthcare provider has requested PHN assistance in helping this family keep medical appointments.

Your initial referral to the family was for the premature birth of Adan, who had respiratory complications and spent 3 weeks in the hospital before he came home. Mariana is estranged from her mother, reporting, "She kicked me out when she found out I was pregnant." She appears to have minimal parenting skills but is receptive to your visits and is working on developing parenting skills. She has declined your referral to Early Childhood and Family Education (ECFE) activities.

Adan was within normal developmental limits for the first six months of his life but is now starting to exhibit some delays. You suspect that his frequent illnesses are contributing to the developmental delays. He suffers from chronic upper respiratory illnesses and otitis media. Mariana smokes a half pack of cigarettes per day and has not been receptive to discussing smoking cessation.

Mariana's lack of a routine lifestyle, increased levels of stress, lack of sleep, and poor nutrition has negatively affected both her and Adan. Mariana revealed she took a pregnancy test last week and is pregnant again. Her smoking is putting both Adan and the unborn child at risk.

*Source:* Adapted from a case study developed by the Minnesota Department of Health, n.d.

## APPLICATION OF EVIDENCE

Jennifer, the PHN from Weaver County Health Department, has received a referral from the county's Child Protection Services. The referral was originally made by an RN who worked at the local hospital and suspected possible child abuse of a 2-year-old named Marcie who had a minor injury that required a visit to the emergency department. The child protection worker did not find any evidence of child abuse or neglect but asked to have a PHN follow up to promote positive parenting practices with the child's parents.

▪ Which independent nursing interventions could Jennifer use in working with the child's parents? How are these interventions consistent with the Nurse Practice Act in your state?

▪ What should Jennifer remember about maintaining professional boundaries as she meets with Marcie's parents?

▪ During the visit, Jennifer discovers that Marcie attends the same community daycare as one of Jennifer's children, although the two children are not in the same group. What will Jennifer need to do to maintain confidentiality in the small community setting?

## References

Akhtar-Danesh, N., Baumann, A., Kolotylo, C., Lawlor, Y., Tompkins, C., & Lee, R. (2013). Perceptions of professionalism among nursing faculty and nursing students. *Western Journal of Nursing Research, 35*(2), 248–271. doi:10.1177/0193945911408623

American Holistic Nurses Association. (2016). Nurse Practice Act (NPA) analysis summary December 2016. Retrieved from http://www.ahna.org/Home/Resources/State-Practice-Acts

American Nurses Association. (2007). *Registered nurses utilization of nursing assistive personnel in all settings* [Position statement]. Retrieved from http://ana.nursingworld.org/MainMenuCategories/HealthcareandPolicyIssues/ANAPositionStatements/uap.aspx

American Nurses Association. (2012). *Principles for delegation by registered nurses to unlicensed assistive personnel (UAP).* Silver Spring, MD: Author.

American Nurses Association. (2013). *Public health nursing: Scope and standards of practice.* Silver Spring, MD: Author.

American Nurses Association. (2015). *Code of ethics for nurses with interpretive statements.* Silver Spring, MD: Author.

Association of Community Health Nurse Educators. (2009). *Essentials of baccalaureate nursing education for entry level community/public health nursing.* Wheat Ridge, CO: Author.

Beck, A. J., & Boulton, M. L. (2015). Trends and characteristics of the state and local public health workforce, 2010–2013. *American Journal of Public Health, 105*(S2), S303–S310.

California Board of Registered Nursing. (2006). *California Nursing Practice Act with regulations and related statutes.* Charlottesville, VA: Matthew Bender & Company, Inc.

Clancy, A., & Svensson, T. (2007). "Faced" with responsibility: Levinasian ethics and the challenges of responsibility in Norwegian public health nursing. *Nursing Philosophy, 8*(3), 158–166.

Easley, C. E., & Allen, C. E. (2007). A critical intersection: Human rights, public health nursing, and nursing ethics. *Advances in Nursing Science, 30*(4), 367–382.

Evanson, T. A. (2006). Intimate partner violence and rural public health nursing practice: Challenges and opportunities. *Online Journal of Rural Nursing and Health Care, 6*(1), 7–20.

Falk-Rafael, A., & Betker, C. (2012). Witnessing social injustice downstream and advocating for health equity upstream: "The trombone slide" of nursing. *Advances in Nursing Science, 35*(2), 98–112.

Friedman, B., Li, Y., Liebel, D. V., & Powers, B. A. (2014). Effects of a home visiting nurse intervention versus care as usual on individual activities of daily living: A secondary analysis of a randomized controlled trial. *BMC Geriatrics, 14*(1), 24.

Griffith, R. (2015). Understanding the code: Exceptions to the duty of patient confidentiality. *British Journal of Community Nursing, 20*(7), 356–359.

Henry Street Consortium. (2017). *Entry-level population-based public health nursing competencies.* St. Paul, MN: Author. Retrieved from www.henrystreetconsortium.org

Institute of Medicine. (2015). Assessing progress on the Institute of Medicine report *The Future of Nursing.* Retrieved from https://www.nurse.com/blog/2015/12/10/iom-releases-progress-report-on-future-of-nursing-2020-goals/

International Council of Nurses. (2017). Patient centred care, New Zealand. Retrieved from https://www.icnvoicetolead.com/case-study/patient-centred-care-new-zealand/

Jarrin, O. G. (2010). Core elements of U.S. Nurse Practice Acts and incorporation of nursing diagnosis language. *International Journal of Nursing Terminologies and Classifications, 21*(4), 166–176. doi:10.1111/j.1744-618x.2010.01162.x

Johnsen, E. F., & Pohlman, K. J. (2017). Historic leadership: One courageous school nurse's heroic journey—Part 2. *NASN School Nurse, 32*(2), 94–99. doi:10.1177/1942602X16688322

Kaernested, B., & Bragadottir, H. (2012). Delegation of registered nurses revisited: Attitudes towards delegation and preparedness to delegate effectively. *Nordic Journal of Nursing Research & Clinical Studies, 32*(1), 10–15.

Minnesota Department of Health. (n.d.). *Case study: Scope of public health nursing practice.*

Minnesota Department of Health, Office of Public Health Practice. (2006). *Wheel of public health interventions: A collection of "getting behind the wheel" stories, 2000–2006.* Retrieved from http://www.health.state.mn.us/divs/opi/cd/phn/docs/0606wheel_stories.pdf

Minnesota Nurses Association. (2013). Scope of practice issues addressed with changes to Nurse Practice Act. *Minnesota Nursing Accent, 85*(1), 10.

National Council of State Boards of Nursing. (2014). *A nurse's guide to professional boundaries.* Retrieved from https://www.ncsbn.org/3757.htm

Pappas-Rogich, M., & King, M. (2014). Faith community nursing: Supporting Healthy People 2020 initiatives. *Journal of Christian Nursing, 31*(4), 228–234. doi:10.1097/CNJ.0000000000000104

Przybilla, J., Johnson, A., & Hooker, C. (2009). Perinatal hepatitis B prevention: Adapting public health services to meet the changing needs of a diverse community. *Public Health Reports, 124,* 454–457.

Racher, F. E. (2007). The evolution of ethics for community practice. *Journal of Community Health Nursing, 24*(1), 65–76.

Russell, K. A. (2012). Nurse Practice Acts guide and govern nursing practice. *Journal of Nursing Regulation, 3*(3), 36–42. Retrieved from http://www.journalofnursingregulation.com/article/S2155-8256(15)30197-6/fulltext

Schaffer, M. A., Anderson, L. J. W., & Rising, S. (2016). Public health interventions for school nursing practice. *Journal of School Nursing, 32*(3), 195–208. doi:10.1177/1059840515605361

Schaffer, M. A., Keller, L. O., & Reckinger, D. (2015). Public health nursing activities: Visible or invisible? *Public Health Nursing, 32*(6), 711–720. doi:10.1111/phn.1291

Stanhope, M., & Lancaster, J. (2012). *Public health nursing: Population-centered health care in the community.* Maryland Heights, MO: Elsevier.

Weydt, A. (2010). Developing delegation skills. *OJIN: The Online Journal of Issues in Nursing, 15*(2). Manuscript 1. (May 31). Retrieved from http://www.nursingworld.org/MainMenuCategories/ANAMarketplace/ANAPeriodicals/OJIN/TableofContents/Vol152010/No2May2010/Delegation-Skills.html

Williams, J. K., & Cooksey, M. M. (2004). Navigating the difficulties of delegation: Learn to improve teamwork in the unit by delegating duties appropriately. *Nursing, 34*(9), 32.

Wynd, C. A. (2003). Current factors contributing to professionalism in nursing. *Journal of Professional Nursing, 19*(5), 251–261. doi:10.1016/S8755-7223(03)00104-2

Zero to Three. (2017). Reflective supervision. Retrieved from https://www.zerotothree.org/resources/407-reflective-supervision

Zupancic-Albin, A. (2017). The Nurse Practice Act: Learn it, know it, live it. *Johns Hopkins Nursing.* Retrieved from http://magazine.nursing.jhu.edu/category/spring-2017/

# COMPETENCY #5

## Works Within the Responsibility and Authority of the Governmental Public Health System

■ **Marjorie A. Schaffer**
with Bonnie Brueshoff and Raney Linck

*Dan was recently employed as a public health nurse (PHN) by a county health department. After two months on the job, he is asked to assist other PHNs in responding to a recent outbreak of measles. All confirmed cases to date are in the Somali population. Unfortunately, the Somali communities have been targeted with misinformation about vaccine risks and have subsequently struggled with low rates of MMR immunization.*

*Dan has never worked for the government. Through the orientation process, he begins to wonder whether he will ever understand how the different levels of government work together. He refers to his orientation materials for Population-Based Public Health Nursing Competency #5, which focuses on working with governmental systems. He comments to his supervisor, Carol, "This competency has so many parts. How will I ever understand what all these terms mean for the work I am doing?"*

---

### DAN'S NOTEBOOK

**COMPETENCY #5** Works Within the Responsibility and Authority of the Governmental Public Health System

A. Describes the relationship among the federal, state, and local levels of public health system

B. Identifies the individual's and organization's responsibilities within the context of the Essential Public Health Services and Core Functions

C. Understands practice implications for laws, regulations, and rules relevant to public health

D. Adheres to legal mandates such as data privacy and mandated reporting

E. Differentiates the public health model from the medical model

F. Understands the independent public health nursing role as described in the Scope and Standards of Public Health Nursing

G. Describes the role of government in the delivery of community health services

H. Identifies components of the healthcare system:

    1) Funding streams such as Medicare, Medicaid, Prepaid Medical Assistance Plan (PMAP), categorical grants

    2) Programs utilized by state and local health departments, such as Women, Infants, and Children (WIC) program, home visiting, and school health

    3) Community resources

*Source:* Henry Street Consortium, 2017

*(continues)*

**DAN'S NOTEBOOK** *(continued)*

**USEFUL DEFINITIONS**

**Funding Stream:** Source of revenue for public health programs and services.

**Local Public Health Department:** An "administrative or service unit of local or state government concerned with health, and carrying some responsibility for the health of a jurisdiction smaller than the state" (National Association of County and City Health Officials [NACCHO], 2016, p. 12).

**Medical Model:** Focuses on the individual; concerned with restoring health for individuals who seek care.

**Public Health Infrastructure:** The underlying framework for the public health system, which includes: 1) a qualified workforce, 2) up-to-date data and information systems, and 3) capable agencies for assessing and responding to public health needs (Healthy People 2020, 2017b).

**Public Health Model:** Focuses on the health of populations; concerned with promoting, protecting, and maintaining the health of every citizen.

**Statutory Authority:** A set of rules or a statute that gives an agency authority to determine rules to carry out assigned duties (Minnesota Department of Health [MDH], 2016).

## Taking Responsibility for Improving Population Health

PHNs work in all levels of government; in urban, suburban, and rural settings; and in a variety of community agencies and organizations. Federal, state, and local governments all provide essential resources for contributing to the public's health. This chapter discusses how levels of government work together to promote public health and how PHNs deliver population-based public health services in these settings, agencies, and organizations.

## How Are the Federal, State, and Local Levels of Public Health Connected?

At the *federal* level, the U.S. Department of Health and Human Services (DHHS) oversees many other agencies that focus on the health and well-being of U.S. citizens. One of these agencies is the Centers for Disease Control and Prevention (CDC). The CDC keeps track of disease outbreaks and health statistics and protects the health and quality of life for U.S. populations. The CDC website is a good source for statistics and other information you need for public health interventions. For example, a PHN could use the CDC website to find updated statistics on state and national obesity trends and evidence-based strategies for obesity prevention.

Other agencies that come under the DHHS umbrella oversee Medicare and Medicaid Services; research and healthcare quality; substance abuse and mental health services; and the safety of food, cosmetics, medications, biological products, and medical devices. For example, a PHN could access information on food-safety alerts, such as the

contamination of ground beef (salmonella, typhimurium) and salad bars (norovirus).

*State* health departments often work with both federal and local levels of government. State health departments regulate facilities and organizations that influence health and health services. Examples of healthcare facilities regulated by the state include hospitals, clinics, and nursing homes. State functions include financing and administering programs (Stanhope & Lancaster, 2016) and offering technical assistance to local health departments for program development and services. The organization and functions of state healthcare departments can differ greatly among the states. Regardless of the organizational structure, a strong partnership between state and local health departments is essential to promote and protect the health of populations.

*Local* public health departments (LHDs) include both city and county health departments. They get directives from the state and federal levels and report to their local elected board members. Local agencies display considerable variability in the populations they serve and how they accomplish their work. Table 7.1 identifies characteristics of LHDs found in the 2016 National Profile of Local Health Departments report (NACCHO, 2016).

LHDs often take actions to comply with state health department regulations and federal guidelines. In Dakota County in Minnesota, when a PHN received a report on a suspected case of measles, the PHN (local level) documented information from the Minnesota Department of Health (state level) and followed up on the measles contacts. The PHN reached all contacts and recommended contacts be in quarantine for the incubation period for showing symptoms of measles. In addition, relevant surveillance activities were

## ...aracteristics of Local Health Departments

| ...teristic | Data |
|---|---|
| ...erved | ▪ Fewer than 50,000 persons: 61% of LHDs<br>▪ 500,000 or more: 6% of LHDs |
| ...expenditures | ▪ 2008: $63 per person<br>▪ 2016: $48 per person |
| ...s of partners | ▪ Emergency responders (98% of LHDs)<br>▪ K–12 schools (98% of LHDs)<br>▪ Hospitals (95% of LHDs)<br>▪ Media (95% of LHDs) |
| ...istered nurses | ▪ 94% of LHDs employ registered nurses<br>▪ Median number of nurses ranged from 1 in LHDs serving populations under 10,000 to 542 for LHDs serving populations greater than 1 million<br>▪ Registered nurses comprise 18% of the LHD workforce (not all are PHNs)<br>▪ Overall percentage of nurses decreased by 28% between 2008 and 2016, related to health department budget cuts for programs and staffing |
| Other public health staff in LHDs | ▪ 91% of LHDs employ office and administrative support staff<br>▪ Larger LHDs also often employ epidemiologists, statisticians, information systems specialists, public information professionals, health educators, and public health physicians |

*Source:* NACCHO, 2016

conducted by the PHN per MDH (state) and CDC (federal) guidelines.

 **Healthy People** On the Healthy People 2020 website, go to "Topics and Objectives," and under "P" click **healthypeople.gov** "Preparedness." Government agencies, nongovernmental organizations, the private sector, communities, and individuals work together to "strengthen and sustain communities' abilities to prevent, protect against, mitigate the effects of, respond to, and recover from incidents with negative health effects" (Healthy People 2020, 2017a, para. 1). What are some ways that PHNs can use the information in this section to contribute to accomplishing this goal? Think about actions that will address the needs of individuals, families, and communities during a major health incident. Which levels of government will be involved in PHN responses? See Table 7.2 in this chapter.

## How Do the Essential Public Health Services and Core Functions Guide the Public Health Department and Your Work as a Public Health Nurse?

In the United States, PHNs and other public health professionals who work for governmental public health agencies have a scope of practice based on *core public health functions* and the *essential services of public health* (Institute of Medicine [IOM], 1988).

### EVIDENCE EXAMPLE 7.1
#### Three Levels of Government Working Together in Emergency Preparedness

LHDs work with the state and federal levels of government to provide emergency preparedness services. At the local level, 45% of LHDs reported they responded to an all-hazards event in the past year and 90% participated in an emergency preparedness exercise (NACCHO, 2016). PHNs have specific skills for preparing for and responding to disasters. In addition to acting as first responders in disaster events, PHNs use a population approach to collaborate on policy development, disaster response plans, and disaster drills and training (Jakeway, LaRosa, Cary, & Schoenfisch (2008). PHNs contribute to the following four disaster phases (Jakeway et al., 2008, p. 355):

▪ **Mitigation:** Prevent a disaster or emergency; minimize vulnerability to effects of an event

▪ **Preparedness:** Ensure capacity to effectively respond to disasters and emergencies

▪ **Response:** Provide support to people and communities affected by disasters and emergencies

▪ **Recovery:** Restore systems to functional level

See Table 7.2 for an example of how the three levels of government work together in emergency preparedness.

**TABLE 7.2 Emergency Preparedness Example**

| | Local | State | Federal |
|---|---|---|---|
| Planning | LHDs write all-hazards plans to direct local emergency responses, including staffing of Open Points of Dispensing (PODs), communications with the public and other partners, and Department Operations Center (DOC) on setup and procedures.<br><br>LHDs conduct exercises to test plans in order to practice skills and identify areas for improvement. | The state health department consults with LHD on plans and writes grant requests regarding required plan elements and required exercises that need to be completed in order to receive grant funding. | The Centers for Disease Control and Prevention (CDC) is the funding source for both state and local health departments. The CDC creates and conducts a biannual assessment, the Operational Readiness Review, to measure the overall status of both state and local preparedness around the 15 Public Health Preparedness Capabilities. |
| Prevention and Risk Mitigation | LHDs complete a Hazard and Vulnerability Assessment with Emergency Management to evaluate greatest risks in the jurisdiction (geographical area). Based on those risks, the LHD can do community outreach and provide trainings to mitigate some of the adverse effects of different emergencies. | The state health department regularly communicates and meets with LHD staff to provide training and consultation and interpret CDC guidance. The state employs regional consultants to individually work with the LHDs and coordinate risk and prevention activities across the region. | The CDC stockpiles medications and supplies based on assessed public health risks such as a future influenza pandemic, bioterrorism, or emerging infectious agents. These are called Strategic National Stockpiles (SNS). The CDC also funds development of vaccines and other prophylactic pharmaceuticals to prepare for future needs. |
| Response | The LHD sets up a Department Operations Center from which the Incident Command will run the response to a Public Health Emergency. This response could be staffing a hotline, communicating with the public, setting up a shelter, or dispensing prophylactic medication or vaccine through a Point of Dispensing (POD). | The state public health agency provides situational updates, subject matter experts, and emergency messaging to the public. The state can request emergency medications, vaccines, equipment, and supplies from the Strategic National Stockpile and push that out to the LHD to dispense to the public. | The CDC interacts with international partners to coordinate international public health emergency responses, such as the 2015 Ebola outbreak. The CDC also can help deploy staff to state and local partners for assistance. This is called the Epidemic Intelligence Service (EIS). They have medical response teams available to assist state and local partners when local resources are depleted. |
| PHN Role | PHNs working in LHDs hold leadership roles in incident command and can provide subject matter expertise regarding the health implications of an emergency. At a Point of Dispensing, nurses staff the roles of screening (assessing for contraindications, allergies, or drug interactions), dispensing, and education. | PHNs working at the state help provide subject matter expertise around infectious pathogens, mass dispensing guidelines, and public health interventions. The majority of emergency preparedness work at the state level falls under the population-based section of the Public Health Intervention Wheel. Many emergency preparedness interventions are consistent with the PHN role. | PHNs at the CDC are involved in many preparedness roles, including serving as experts in vaccine guideline development. PHNs are part of the disease response teams at the national level that are deployed to local responses as needed. Nurses serve in leadership roles in emergency preparedness and planning as well. |

Contributed by Christine Lees, MPH, BSN, PHN, Dakota County Public Health and Amalia Roberts DNP, RN, PHN, Dakota County Public Health

Figure 7.1 demonstrates the relationship between the core functions and the essential services that government agencies and their staff must carry out (*Source:* CDC, 2014).

The three core functions are:

- **Assessment:** Community assessment of population health needs by monitoring and investigating levels of population health and illness
- **Policy Development:** Development of health policies, goals, plans, and interventions to meet priority community health needs
- **Assurance:** Measurement of outcomes of health policies, goals, plans, and interventions and the competency and adequacy of public health professionals to determine whether a community's priority health needs have been met in an efficient, effective, and timely manner

The Ten Essential Services of Public Health (CDC, 2014) in Figure 7.1 need to be carried out by PHNs and other public health professionals to maintain the health of a community and its diverse populations. Table 7.3 outlines these essential services and provides examples of each.

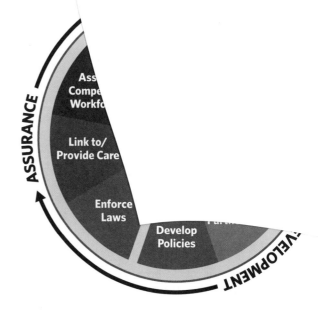

**FIGURE 7.1** Essential Public Health Services and Core Functions
*Source:* CDC, 2014

## TABLE 7.3  Ten Essential Services of Public Health, With Examples

| Essential Service | Example |
| --- | --- |
| 1. Monitor Health | ■ Carry out community assessment to determine levels of health and illness in community and populations. |
| 2. Diagnose and Investigate | ■ Check lead levels of preschool children, infants, and toddlers at risk for lead poisoning. <br> ■ Offer diabetes screening in the Native American community. |
| 3. Inform, Educate, and Empower | ■ Teach first-time parents how to care for their new baby. <br> ■ Provide car seat education to new parents. |
| 4. Mobilize Community Partnerships | ■ Develop a network of community services for elderly people within the community. |
| 5. Develop Policies | ■ Work with county board members to develop a policy for playground safety in local communities. |
| 6. Enforce Laws | ■ Report suspected child abuse or neglect. <br> ■ Monitor compliance with immunization laws for school children. |
| 7. Link to/Provide Care | ■ PHNs and emergency department staff develop a referral and follow-up system for homebound elderly who visit the emergency department and then return home. |
| 8. Assure Competent Workforce | ■ Update public health nursing staff on the influenza virus. <br> ■ Teach rural PHNs how to do well-water testing. <br> ■ Precept nursing students. |
| 9. Evaluate | ■ Carry out evaluation studies to determine the effectiveness of public health nursing programs, such as home visiting to new families. <br> ■ Evaluate programs that LHDs contract with for service provision. |
| 10. System Management and Research | ■ Determine needs for public health services and service gaps in the community. <br> ■ Provide data to justify claims that tax dollars improve the public's health and demonstrate a return on investment. |

*Source:* CDC, 2014

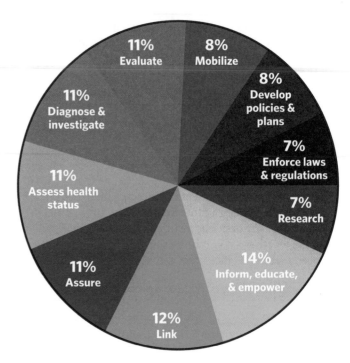

**FIGURE 7.2** Percentage of PHNs' Time Dedicated to Essential Services (*n* = 57)

The following section shows how PHNs accomplish the work that is outlined in the essential services and core functions and contribute to the well-being of populations. In a survey of 57 PHNs working in local and state governments and representing 28 states, they identified the amount of time spent providing each of the essential services. The percentage of time spent on each essential service ranged from 7% to 14% (Keller & Litt, 2008). See Figure 7.2.

> *Dan remembers seeing the Public Health Core Functions in his orientation manual—assessment, policy development, and assurance. He says to Carol, "Let's see if I understand how this works."*
>
> *"For the measles outbreak, I can see assessment happening when we are identifying how many children in the targeted age group live in our county. For policy development, we are following the directives given by the CDC and the state department of health for vaccine administration. I can see how we are working with and through others to ensure that as many children as possible have access to the vaccine. Assurance occurs when we make sure the vaccine is accessible to the population groups that need to be vaccinated and that the vaccine has been administered to them."*
>
> *Carol affirms Dan's analysis of how the core functions were represented in the response efforts to the measles outbreak. Dan then says, "I am not sure about all those essential services. Do PHNs conduct all ten in response to the measles outbreak?"*
>
> *Carol answers, "Let's analyze how each of the essential services occurs when our health department responds to the measles outbreak. Let's develop a handout to put into the orientation manual to help everyone understand how we are providing the essential services."*

See Table 7.4 for the handout that Dan and Carol developed.

## Application of Ten Essential Services to Measles Outbreak Response

A measles outbreak occurred in Minnesota in late March of 2017. This was the worst measles outbreak in Minnesota since 1990. A total of 79 cases were reported, which primarily affected the Minnesota Somali community. All local health departments in Minnesota had a role in preventing the spread of this infectious disease, involving activities such as active awareness and risk communication with medical providers.

## How Do Public Health Nurses Use Statutory Authority?

*Statutory authority* refers to the statutes (laws) and rules through which the government gives authority to agencies to carry out specific duties. In the public health arena, PHNs are responsible for adhering to public health laws that have been enacted to protect and promote the health of communities. Public health laws may be federal, state, or local, but many are implemented at the local level.

Public health law is often established in response to critical public health problems that affect populations. Mello and colleagues (2013) identified three criteria for determining opportunities for establishing public health law: 1) the

**TABLE 7.4  Ten Essential Services: Measles Outbreak Response by Local Public Health**

| Essential Service | Application Example |
| --- | --- |
| 1. Monitor health | Monitored data on those at risk due to being unvaccinated, and monitored clinic and hospital data of reported cases provided by Minnesota Department of Health |
| 2. Diagnose and Investigate | Communicated with summer camps and daycares on symptoms to watch for and resources available |
| 3. Inform, Educate, and Empower | Worked with local media outlets and sent a Health Advisory to medical providers on the outbreak, including what to watch for and report |
| 4. Mobilize Community Partnerships | Worked with Somali community leaders and organizations to reach the at-risk population |
| 5. Develop Policies | Adopted policies from CDC and state department of health on vaccine recommendations |
| 6. Enforce Laws | Activated response by utilizing the Health Department Emergency Response Plan |
| 7. Link to/Provide Care | Coordinated with the Department of Human Services regarding childcare licensing regulations and potential changes needed due to outbreak |
| 8. Ensure Competent Workforce | Provided training for staff to assist with contact investigation and follow-up to ensure competence for roles and responsibilities |
| 9. Evaluate | Once outbreak was over, a "hot wash" was conducted to document the response work and lessons learned |
| 10. System Management and Research | CDC vaccine information posted on website, which included basic information and vaccination guidance |

law targets a significant public health problem, 2) factors contributing to the public health problem are understood well enough to change behavior through law, and 3) a feasible intervention can be implemented.

Public health law is potentially an effective tool for improving population health outcomes. However, competing interests and values about laws may affect individual choice. This adds complexity to enacting laws that address threats to individual and population health. It is important to provide objective and timely evidence to support legal policy that contributes to improving population health. Major trends in public health law and practice include the following focus areas (Hodge et al., 2013):

- The Affordable Care Act
- Emergency legal preparedness
- Health information privacy and data sharing
- Tobacco control
- Drug overdose protection
- Food policy
- Vaccination requirements and exemptions
- Sports injury law and policy
- Public health accreditation
- Maternal and child health

Public health laws influence funding for public health programs. For example, emergency preparedness programs received major funding following bioterrorism events and threats. Funding increases the number of public health practitioners employed in emergency preparedness programs.

Public health laws also protect the health of the public. PHNs need to understand public health law and how it protects individual, family, and community safety. Laws concerned with public health include public health nuisance; quarantine; mandated reporting of communicable disease; mandated reporting of suspected abuse and neglect of children, the disabled, and the elderly; and commitment. See examples of local public health laws in Table 7.5.

For PHNs who practice in school settings, a federal law titled the Family Educational Rights and Privacy Act (FERPA) protects the privacy of student educational records (U.S. Department of Education, 2015; U.S. DHHS and the U.S. DoE, 2008). When the school contracts for school nursing services from a community agency, the school nurse is obligated to follow the school data privacy policy for educational records (Association of State and Territorial Health Officers [ASTHO], 2015).

The Network for Public Health Law (https://www.networkforphl.org/) compiles information and resources about public health law at all levels of government. It identifies primary legal issues and offers technical assistance for a variety of topics.

## TABLE 7.5  Public Health Law Examples

| Type of Law | Key Features | Example |
|---|---|---|
| Civil commitment | Protects mentally ill individuals from danger to themselves or others; addresses process of obtaining a court order to obtain treatment for mental illness when individuals are unable or unwilling to seek treatment voluntarily and need protection from harming themselves or others due to illness. Civil commitment laws vary across states. | PHNs collaborate with family members, other health professionals, community agencies, and the government in the civil commitment process by providing information about the process and referring to resources. |
| Data privacy | The federal government administers the Health Insurance Portability and Accountability Act (HIPAA) of 1996. PHNs are accountable for ensuring the data-privacy aspect of HIPAA. In some states, laws specify that information important for ensuring public health can be disclosed. | Minnesota's Data Sharing Law allows the sharing of immunization data with schools and childcare providers without parental permission. Healthcare providers can share information about communicable diseases with the state health department without patients' permission. Otherwise, the sharing of individual and family healthcare information requires that clients sign a release of information form authorizing sharing of information. |
| Mandated reporting of suspected child abuse or neglect | Professionals in relevant disciplines who have a reason to believe a child is being neglected or abused are obligated to report the information to the local welfare agency. Many states also offer civil immunity for people who make reports, and penalties if suspected child abuse is not reported (Pozgar, 2005). | PHNs are mandated reporters for suspected child abuse and neglect. |
| Mandated reporting of communicable disease | Mandates reporting of communicable diseases so that occurrence of the disease can be monitored. | During the H1N1 epidemic in 2009, surveillance of incidence of H1N1 cases helped determine the number of flu clinics to be offered and whether schools needed to close. |
| Public health nuisances | Include conditions that threaten the health of the public and require response or action from the local health department. Examples are: garbage accumulation, sewage, noise, junked cars, abandoned swimming pools, rodent infestation, and faulty electrical wiring or plumbing. | Top three complaints were mold, garbage houses, and accumulation of rubbish or junk (MDH, 2017c). |
| Quarantine | Provides for isolating individuals or groups to prevent the spread of communicable disease; restricts activities or travel of an otherwise healthy person with possible exposure to a communicable disease to prevent disease transmission. | Can be used to reduce the effects of bioterrorism or pandemic events, such as the spread of avian influenza or Ebola. |
| School-entry laws | Mandate evidence of vaccination for specific communicable diseases or a legal exemption signed by a parent. | School-entry laws, in place since the 1960s, have led to increased vaccination rates and decreased rates of childhood communicable diseases (Horlich, Shaw, Gorji, & Fishbein, 2008). Some parents might object to compulsory vaccinations for their children because of medical reasons or religious/cultural beliefs. |

*Sources:* Minnesota Department of Health, 2003, 2005, 2015, 2016, 2017a, 2017b; Minnesota Department of Health State Community Health Services Advisory Committee, 1992; National Alliance on Mental Illness, 2016; Office of the Reviser of Statutes, 2016

## THEORY APPLICATION

### Comparison of the Public Health and Medical Models

As you think about how government organizations guide and deliver public health services, and the responsibilities of the government and PHNs for improving the health status of individuals and populations, consider how PHNs use a public health model in contrast to a medical model. One difference is that the public health model focuses on populations, whereas the medical model focuses on individuals. Another difference is the public health focus on prevention of disease as opposed to the medical model focus on treatment of disease. In the public health model, healthcare is viewed as a right, whereas in the medical model, healthcare is a service. PHNs can use the public health model to help frame their practice as prevention-oriented and population-based. See Table 7.6. Consider how the public health model differs from the traditional medical model when planning interventions to improve health status among populations to ensure that interventions are consistent with the mission of public health.

Some services are provided in both public health and medical settings, but their approaches to healthcare differ. For example, childhood screening is provided in public health programs to improve the well-being of the population of children in the community. From the perspective of the medical model, an individual child is screened on routine visits in a clinic to evaluate that child's health status.

In 2008, the Minnesota state legislature signed into law the Statewide Health Improvement Program, changed to Statewide Health Improvement Partnership in 2017 (SHIP). SHIP is designed to reduce risk factors for chronic disease; reducing these risk factors ultimately decreases healthcare costs. Partnership strategies engage communities in implementing evidence-based interventions to reduce obesity and tobacco use. SHIP awards community-level grants to support public health solutions in Minnesota counties. Since SHIP strategies have been implemented, the adult obesity rate in Minnesota has decreased in comparison to obesity rates in surrounding states from 27.6% in 2014 to 26.1% in 2015 (Minnesota Department of Health, 2017d). Many partners work together to improve health, including schools, businesses, apartment owners and managers, farmers, hospital, clinics, faith communities, and local government.

### TABLE 7.6 Differences Between the Public Health and Medical Models

| Public Health Model | Medical Model |
| --- | --- |
| Mission is to promote, protect, and maintain the health of every citizen. | Mission is to restore health to those who seek care (i.e., treatment and cure). |
| Focus is on the primary health needs of communities and populations. | Focus is on the primary health needs of individuals. |
| Health seen as a birthright of every citizen. | Healthcare seen as a service to be sought. |
| Goal is client/family and population self-sufficiency. | Goal is providing quality service to meet immediate medical care needs. |
| Focus is on prevention. | Focus is on treatment. |
| Seeks to protect the public's health before problems arise. | Seeks to meet the needs of patients who present for care of an existing problem. |
| Reaches out to identify individuals, families, and populations with service needs (case-finding). | Addresses the needs of patients who present for care. |
| Focus is on populations, the community, and the family. | Focus is on the individual. |
| Provides services that others cannot or will not provide. | Generally provides services that are reimbursable. |
| Seeks social change to improve the health status of populations. | Seeks change to improve health status of an individual. |
| Provides services primarily in community settings. | Provides services primarily in healthcare facilities. |
| Provides health-promotion services in the home and might provide services to meet medical needs or refer those individuals with medical needs to a home care agency. | Provides home care services for medical needs related to disease and disability. |

" *After the flurry of responses to the measles outbreak had subsided, Dan reflects on how his work differs from that of his previous position as a nurse for a pediatric clinic. Dan comments to his supervisor, Carol, "I never realized how the government is responsible for public health. I now think about people who need the MMR vaccine not as individuals, but as populations. We prioritized which populations were at risk. We also made sure that the vaccine was available to everyone, regardless of whether they could pay for the vaccine. In the clinic, we followed a medical model that approached clients as individuals."*

*Carol adds, "Yes, the public health model is oriented to finding people who need health services rather than always waiting for people to identify their needs. In addition, public health is oriented toward changing health and social systems to create environments that encourage improvement in health status. By reaching out to those populations most in need of the vaccination, we have actually created an environment that will help keep people healthy in the communities served by our agency."* "

## How Do the Scope and Standards of Public Health Nursing Guide the Public Health Nurse in Independent Practice?

The great majority of interventions implemented by PHNs represent independent nursing practice and are consistent with interventions delineated by the Public Health Intervention Wheel. *Public Health Nursing: Scope and Standards of Practice*, published in 2013 by the American Nurses Association, is also important for guiding the professional role expectations and actions of PHNs (see Chapter 1). The document has two sections—standards of practice and standards of professional performance. The standards of practice detail how the nursing process is applied in public health nursing. Table 7.7 analyzes how each of these role expectations occurred in the response to the measles outbreak.

## How Is the Government Involved in the Delivery of Community Health Services?

Often, governmental organizations collaborate with private and nonprofit organizations to deliver community health services. Governmental organizations may provide funding, oversight, consultation, and other resources to support the public health work of private and nonprofit organizations. How do the core functions of assessment, policy development, and assurance take place in the following evidence examples?

---

### EVIDENCE EXAMPLE 7.3
#### Childhood Obesity Prevention

A program in School District 197 in Dakota County, Minnesota, is consistent with the public health model approach. SHIP funding was awarded to the school district to encourage students to eat a variety of fruits and vegetables. The program is based on the following premises: 1) obesity contributes to diseases that affect a population (heart disease, diabetes, and other chronic diseases); 2) disease and health problems result from individual vulnerability and environmental factors, and 3 of 5 Minnesotans are overweight or obese due to insufficient physical activity and unhealthy eating (Minnesota Department of Health, 2017d); and 3) interventions should be targeted toward changing environmental factors. Interventions include:

▪ During lunch each week, students have an opportunity to taste a less common fruit or vegetable.

▪ After tasting, students fill out a survey on their interest in having the new food on the lunch menu.

▪ Foods with favorable ratings among the students are included in school lunch menus, when feasible.

▪ Parents are encouraged to send lunches or snacks that include vegetables and fruits instead of less healthy alternatives such as chips and candy.

▪ In addition, sugary drinks were banned from school vending machines, which was a policy developed by the state Department of Education in collaboration with the Department of Agriculture.

School nurses and parents reported children were willing to try new foods. Stacie O'Leary, the health service coordinator for the school district, observed the project goal led to making an environmental change in the school district.

**TABLE 7.7  Standards of Professional Performance—Application to Measles Outbreak in Minnesota**

| Standard | Example |
|---|---|
| Ethics | Recognized that the outbreak is about unvaccinated children versus specific communities or ethnic groups |
| Education | Provided education materials to childcare centers and summer camps on signs and symptoms of measles and where to refer to for any concerns |
| Evidence-Based Practice and Research | Accessed information from the CDC for vaccine safety and adverse reactions |
| Quality of Practice | Adhered to CDC vaccination recommendations, including the exceptions to be made for providing earlier vaccinations per CDC |
| Communication | Held meetings in communities with populations at risk to dispel the misinformation about vaccine risks, including the Somali community where key Somali leaders were involved |
| Leadership | Activated Incident Command Structure to coordinate the response and work with local organizations |
| Collaboration | Worked with MDH and other LHDs to provide outreach and surveillance to the population at risk |
| Professional Practice Evaluation | Completed After Action/Improvement Plan that follows guidelines from the Homeland Security Exercise and Evaluation Program |
| Resource Utilization | Worked with the Minnesota Vaccines for Children Program that provides free or low-cost vaccines for eligible children through age 18 |
| Environmental Health | Promoted practices that reduced exposure to those most at risk within the community |
| Advocacy | Provided outreach throughout the county to promote and encourage measles vaccination and communicate clinic schedules |

## EVIDENCE EXAMPLE 7.4
### Government Collaboration With Communities

- The Minnesota Health Department adopted a statewide Breastfeeding-Friendly Health Department (BFHD) program to support initiating and maintaining breastfeeding for 12 months and beyond. One of the ten steps for being a BFHD is collaborating with community partners. For example, the BFHD initiative recommends collaborating with community partners to ensure access to breastfeeding classes, educating the community on breastfeeding support, encouraging local public places to provide a breastfeeding-friendly environment, and providing workplace lactation support training to local businesses. The initiative aims to establish breastfeeding as a community norm (MDH, 2017e).

- The Orange County Health Department California created a coalition called Waste Not Orange County. The coalition advocates for food security screening in primary healthcare settings and food donation sites. They educate the community about food donations, identify individuals and families experiencing food insecurity, and connect them to sources of food. They partner with Food Finders, which is a nonprofit organization that picks up excess food from hospitals, restaurants, and supermarkets and distributes it to food shelves. The coalition implemented a health inspection protocol, using volunteers to educate businesses about food donations and market the coalition's activities to the business community. To incentivize food donations, the coalition awarded window seals to participating businesses and featured a photo of the business on their coalition website (Garcia-Silva, Handler, & Wolfe, 2017).

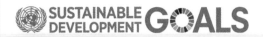

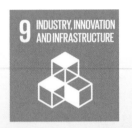

**Mobile Outreach Nurse-Led Clinic USA**

**GOAL 9** Nurses are firsthand witnesses to client needs and healthcare system challenges, which positions them to create innovative solutions. Elisabeth Knight, a nurse practitioner, brings health services to rural and low-income areas of southern Arizona, where many lack access to healthcare and insurance. Along with a medical assistant and a driver, Elisabeth provides health clinics in a truck equipped with exam rooms and a lab. Services include preventative care, basic wellness advice, management of chronic conditions, and prenatal and birth care to expectant mothers. The Arizona legislature provided funding for the mobile clinic. The College of Medicine at the University of Arizona, Tucson, oversees the program. The mobile clinic serves 2,400 people yearly; everyone is accepted, regardless of their income and ability to pay. Elisabeth observed, "Part of what we're able to do is teach people to manage their chronic conditions by providing the tools, information and knowledge they need to take care of themselves, which helps us keep them out of the emergency room" (International Council of Nurses, 2017).

## What Should the Public Health Nurse Know About the Healthcare System?

The United States healthcare system is financed by a combination of public and private entities that provide services to insured, underinsured, and uninsured populations. Private healthcare organizations may be for-profit or non-profit. Many government programs provide services using a combination of federal, state, and local funds. Local health departments often provide services to low-income residents. PHNs can assist community residents with referrals to clinics that are free or have sliding fee scales and connect them with insurance navigators for accessing healthcare coverage.

Table 7.8 identifies major programs and funding sources in the U.S. Healthcare System.

The ACA included provisions for health promotion initiatives to contribute to better health outcomes and reduce costs. As part of the ACA, the National Prevention Strategy: America's Plan for Better Health and Wellness (National Prevention Council, 2011) has four major strategies:

1. Building healthy and safe community environments
2. Expanding quality preventive services in clinical and community settings
3. Empowering people to make healthy choices
4. Eliminating health disparities

The seven priority areas are: (1) tobacco-free living, (2) preventing drug abuse and excessive alcohol use, (3) healthy eating, (4), active living, (5) injury and violence-free living, (6) reproductive and sexual health, and (7) mental health and emotional well-being. The National Prevention Strategy identifies evidence-based recommendations for reducing the incidence of preventable death and major illness.

Several other federal agencies are responsible for overseeing health research, dissemination of health information, and health regulations to protect public health and safety. These include (Mossialos, Djordjevic, Osborn, & Sarnak, 2017):

- **Centers for Disease Control and Prevention:** Conducts research and programs to protect public health and safety
- **National Institutes of Health:** Oversees biomedical and health-related research
- **Health Resources and Services Administration:** Supports strategies to improve healthcare access
- **Agency for Healthcare Research and Quality:** Conducts evidence-based research
- **Food and Drug Administration:** Regulates food, tobacco products, pharmaceutical drugs, medical devices, and vaccines

Because of the high cost of healthcare, service delivery is changing. New ways of structuring healthcare aim to improve health outcomes and reduce costs. Recent initiatives include (Mossialos et al., 2017):

- **Healthcare or Medical Home:** A patient-centered model that emphasizes care coordination and continuity of care.
- **Accountable Care Organization (ACO):** Provider networks that take on contractual responsibility for providing quality care for a defined population.
- **Bundled payments:** Organizations providing care are reimbursed with a single payment for all services delivered by multiple providers for a single episode of care, such as surgical or chronic illness care.

In addition, the U.S. healthcare system has implemented special Information Technology infrastructures to maintain public health in four areas. See Table 7.9. A program called Electronic Health Record (EHR) Meaningful Use is creating a secure electronic reporting infrastructure for real-time

## TABLE 7.8  Major U.S. Healthcare System Programs and Funding

| Component | Description |
| --- | --- |
| Centers for Medicare and Medicaid Services (CMS)<br><br>Established by Congress in 1965 followed by many incremental legislative changes | Federal agency administers Medicare, a federal program for adults 65 and older and some people with disabilities.<br><br>Works in partnership with state governments to administer Medicaid. |
| The Affordable Care Act (ACA)<br><br>Established by Congress in 2010 | "…established 'shared responsibility' between the government, employers, and individuals for ensuring that all Americans have access to affordable and good-quality health insurance. However, health coverage remains fragmented, with numerous private and public sources, as well as wide gaps in insured rates across the U.S. population" (p. 173).<br><br>The ACA gives states the option of expanding Medicaid through subsidies from the federal government. |
| Private insurance—individual or employer | Regulated at state level.<br><br>"In 2014, state and federally administered health insurance marketplaces were established to provide additional access to private insurance coverage, with income-based premium subsidies for low- and middle-income people" (p. 173).<br><br>Medicare beneficiaries have the option of purchasing private supplemental insurance to cover additional health services and cost-sharing. |

*Source:* Mossialos et al., 2017

## TABLE 7.9  Public Health IT Structures

| Public Health Reporting System | Description |
| --- | --- |
| Syndromic Surveillance (SS) | SS examples include monitoring for injury trends, such as bicycle accident–related injuries; tracking the burden of disaster-related conditions in hospitals following a natural disaster, such as a tornado; and tracking the severity of asthma and upper respiratory tract infections during allergy season.<br><br>79% of local health departments (LHDs) have implemented in 2016, with 3% in process. |
| Immunization Information Systems (IIS) | Creates a centralized repository of all immunization data with two-way electronic record exchanges that include sending and receiving immunization histories for individuals and related demographic information, as well as observations about an immunization event, such as reactions or eligibility for a funding program.<br><br>85% of local health departments (LHDs) have implemented in 2016, with 3% in process. |
| Electronic Laboratory Reporting (ELR) | State and local laws require the reporting of particular lab results to public health agencies regarding communicable diseases such as anthrax, botulism, smallpox, and more. Through reporting, these agencies can act quickly to control the spread of the disease (e.g., vaccinating or treating close contacts of a patient, identifying contaminated foods, or uncovering industrial practices that cause toxic exposures).<br><br>49% of local health departments (LHD) have implemented in 2016, with 8% in process. |
| Cancer Registry | Population-based cancer surveillance is essential for coordination of care, activities, and resource allocation to decrease the mortality and morbidity of this disease, which is the second-leading cause of death in the United States.<br><br>Cancer registries exist in all 50 states, Washington D.C., Puerto Rico, and the U.S. Pacific islands. |

*Sources:* CDC, 2013, 2017a; Georgia Department of Health, 2017; International Society for Disease Surveillance, 2012; NACCHO, 2016; Savage, 2011

analysis. The goal is that whenever a provider charts healthcare data in a hospital or clinic EHR, the data is automatically submitted to public health agencies. This provides an early warning system for bioterrorism, communicable disease outbreaks, as well as insights in how to prepare for and provide better care during extreme weather events and mass gatherings like major sporting events (Yoon, Ising, & Gunn, 2017).

The Institute for Healthcare Improvement (IHI) developed the Triple Aim Initiative as a framework for improving health system performance. The three dimensions that healthcare policymakers need to pursue are: 1) improving the patient experience, 2) improving the health of populations, and 3) reducing the per capita cost of healthcare (IHI, 2017). See Figure 7.3.

IHI emphasizes that all three dimensions need to be addressed simultaneously:

IHI believes that to do this work effectively, it's important to harness a range of community determinants of health, empower individuals and families, substantially broaden the role and impact of primary care and other community based services, and assure a seamless journey through the whole system of care throughout a person's life (IHI, 2017, para. 5).

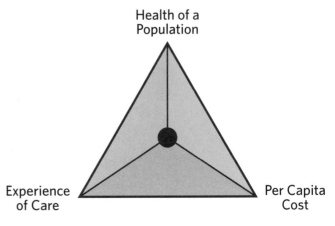

**FIGURE 7.3** Triple Aim Initiative

## EVIDENCE EXAMPLE 7.5

### ACA Outcomes

Since implementation of the ACA, access to healthcare has increased in the United States. The groups with the greatest gains in access include young adult, Hispanic, black, and low-income populations, which demonstrates some progress in reducing health disparities. In addition, cost control measures have reduced some expenses. Incentives to reduce avoidable hospital readmissions for Medicare patients have decreased the 30-day readmission rate nationally. Since Medicare payments to the lowest-performing hospitals were reduced in 2012, hospital-acquired conditions decreased by 17% over a 3-year period. Although healthcare spending following ACA implementation has slowed, data through July 2016 showed that national healthcare spending had increased 4.9% in the previous year (Mossialos et al., 2017).

## EVIDENCE EXAMPLE 7.6

### Impact of ACA on PHN Daily Work

Edmonds, Campbell, and Guilder (2016) surveyed 1,143 PHNs across the United States on their knowledge, perceptions, and practices under the ACA. Forty-five percent of PHNs reported their work changed due to the ACA. PHN activities related to ACA provisions included: integration of primary care and public health, provision of clinical preventive services, care coordination, client navigation, establishing private-public partnerships, implementation of population health strategies and population health data assessment and analysis, community health assessment, involvement with medical homes and Accountable Care Organizations, and maternal and child health home visiting services.

## EVIDENCE EXAMPLE 7.7

### Comparison of U.S. Healthcare System With Other High-Income Countries

The United States has worse health outcomes and higher care costs in comparison with ten other high-income countries (Australia, Canada, France, Germany, Netherlands, New Zealand, Norway, Sweden, Switzerland, and the United Kingdom). The U.S.:

- Ranks last in overall healthcare system performance
- Ranks last in access, equity, and healthcare outcomes
- Ranks next to last in administrative efficiency
- Ranks fifth in care process (prevention, safe care, coordination, patient engagement)
- Has worse population health outcomes in infant mortality and life expectancy at age 60

Out of the 11 countries in the study, the U.S. was the only country that did not have universal access to healthcare. Access to primary care in the U.S. is poor, which means there is "inadequate prevention and management of chronic diseases, delayed diagnoses, incomplete adherence to treatments, wasteful overuse of drugs and technologies, and coordination and safety problems" (Schneider, Sarnak, Squires, Shah, & Doty, 2017).

Some health policy experts recommend adding a fourth aim (Quadruple Aim), which addresses the goal of improving the work environments for healthcare providers, clinicians, and staff (Bodenheimer & Sinksy, 2014).

The ACA does address Triple Aim dimensions to some degree. However, given the U.S. political climate, the future of the ACA is uncertain. Differing values and beliefs about the right to healthcare and partisan politics have contributed to the inability of the 2017 Congress to move forward with a clear healthcare agenda.

## Understanding Funding Streams in Local Public Health Departments

In your PHN role, you might be called on to contribute to planning and writing grant applications for funds for specific public health programs. Funding for local public health comes from a mix of local, state, and federal funds, fees, and reimbursements. Because there are multiple sources of funding for public health, budgets are complex and vary each fiscal year. Sources of funding include local taxes, Medicaid, Medicare, client fees, Local Public Health Act state funds, federal Temporary Assistance for Needy Families (TANF), and private insurance (Riley, Gearin, Parrotta, Briggs, & Gyllstrom, 2013).

Public health programs and funding sources vary across states. For example, in Minnesota, for clients receiving Medicaid (low-income adults, children, pregnant women, and individuals with disabilities), state law authorizes the Prepaid Medical Assistance Program (PMAP). This program provides managed care, which includes regular preventive services and illness care, and may include dental care, free car seats, disease management programs for members with chronic conditions, and smoking cessation programs.

Categorical grants are a potential source of funding for local public health programs. Categorical grants, awarded by federal and state governments, are competitive, may have specific eligibility criteria, and are often project-oriented. An example is the Maternal and Child Health Block Grant Program (Title V), the nation's oldest federal-state partnership, which aims to improve the health and well-being of women and children. Funds are distributed to states (who distribute to local health departments) based on a formula and require a match; every 4 dollars of federal Title V money received must be matched by at least 3 dollars of state or local money.

Funding sources often respond to current crises, such as bioterrorism and opioid overdosing. Public health funding is dependent on a flourishing economy; a downturn in the economy means that public health resources might be more limited. Research studies show that there is strong relationship between local public health spending and performance of public health departments (MDH, 2012). PHNs have an important role to play in advocating for population health through presenting data about public health needs and collaborating with other public health professionals and organizations to make a case for funds needed to implement effective public health programs.

## Programs of Local Public Health Departments

In larger health departments, you might become more specialized with skills and knowledge for a specific public health program, such as follow-up for clients with tuberculosis or family-planning clinics. In rural health departments, your skill set and knowledge may have to be broader, because you might work in a variety of programs and settings. Although variation exists among programs that LHDs provide, some public health services are provided more frequently, such as immunizations and surveillance and epidemiology for communicable/infectious diseases. In addition, population-focused home visiting programs can be offered that target specific vulnerable or high-risk populations, such as parenting adolescents.

LHDs have numerous responsibilities and activities; percentages of the occurrence of specific activities in local health departments are the following (NACCHO, 2016):

- Communicable disease surveillance (93%)
- Adult immunization provision (90%)
- Child immunization provision (88%)
- Environmental health (85%)
- Tuberculosis screening (84%)
- Tuberculosis treatment (79%)
- Food service establishment inspection (78%)
- Food-safety education (77%)
- Schools/daycare centers (74%)
- Population-based nutrition services (74%)
- Maternal and child health (69%)
- Women, Infants, and Children (WIC) (66%)
- Home visits (60%)
- Family planning (53%)

The NACCHO 2016 report showed that emergency preparedness has become an important responsibility of public health, with 81% of health departments providing emergency preparedness training to staff. Data from this report noted that LHDs provided screening for a number of diseases and conditions in addition to tuberculosis, including high blood pressure, blood lead, diabetes, cancer, and cardiovascular conditions. Additional health services that may be provided by LHDs are prenatal care, well child clinics, oral health, home healthcare, primary care, and mental health and substance abuse services.

Increasingly, LHDs are employing informatics specialists, given the growth in the use of information technology (IT). Information technology use by LHDs has increased in all categories since the 2008 NACCHO report, particularly for the use of electronic records. The NACCHO 2016 report identified the following uses of IT in local health departments:

- Have electronic immunization registries (85%)
- Electronic disease reporting systems (79%)
- LHD website 78%
- Use Facebook (65%)
- Have electronic health records (EHRs) or plan to implement EHRs (37%)
- Use Twitter (25%)

## Community Resources

PHNs are expected to have knowledge about the many resources that are available to individuals, families, and communities and the referral process needed to receive services from those resources. LHDs cannot carry out their mission without community partnerships and resources. PHNs build cooperative partnerships with community agencies, organizations, other professionals, and community groups to respond to community health concerns. (See Chapter 8.) Many nonprofit organizations are vital partners

that assist in working on and achieving public health goals. Nonprofit organizations provide services that contribute to the well-being of persons, communities, or society and do not aim to make a profit. They might be funded by grants or donations and sometimes receive funds from governmental organizations.

> *Dan notes that nurses from the Medical Reserve Corps are volunteering to help staff some of the immunization clinics. He asks one of the nurses, Grace, how she became involved in the Medical Reserve Corps. Grace comments, "I have a regular job at the hospital in my community, but when I heard about the Medical Reserve Corps, I decided I wanted to help my community if a disaster occurred. I am a volunteer. I found out about this organization when some of my friends went to New Orleans to help with health needs after Hurricane Katrina."*
>
> *Dan later speaks with his supervisor, Carol, about the Medical Reserve Corps.* Carol says, "Since Hurricane Katrina, many healthcare workers in our state have signed up to be in the program, and now it includes more than 7,000 volunteers. This program strengthens the public health response, which we call public health infrastructure, when a disaster occurs. Local coordinators oversee the program and provide training and support so that volunteers are ready to respond to the disaster. Our health commissioner can mobilize volunteers when they are needed."*
>
> *Dan responds, "The Medical Reserve Corps is a great community resource. I am going to tell my friends from my last job at the hospital about this wonderful volunteer opportunity."*
>
> *NACCHO, 2017

### EVIDENCE EXAMPLE 7.8

**Community Resources**

- The Minnesota Visiting Nurse Agency (MVNA) is a nonprofit organization that provides family-centered and community-based public health nursing services to clients from diverse racial, ethnic, and socioeconomic backgrounds. PHNs coordinate care with healthcare providers and local community agencies. In their family health program, PHNs support family self-sufficiency and use of community resources, such as WIC, Minnesota Family Investment Program (MFIP), schools, Early Childhood Family Education, Follow Along, Child and Teen Checkups, Help Us Grow, and Way to Grow (MVNA, 2017).

- In a qualitative study that explored public health interventions used in school nursing practice, the school nurses (SNs) in the study referred students and families to many community resources, including vision and hearing assessment and care, insurance, free or low-cost medical care, teen pregnancy, clothing, shelter, dental, mental health, and child protection. SNs who practiced in rural schools described barriers to finding needed community resources due to fewer resources, lack of transportation, parents' work schedules, and a lack of healthcare organizations willing to provide care for children receiving Medicaid (Anderson et al., 2017).

## Ethical Application

PHNs might encounter an ethical problem regarding immunizations for children if parents are concerned that immunizations can cause their children harm (for example, the worry about the measles vaccination causing autism). An important role for PHNs is to know about evidence on the effects of immunizations to communicate to parents. (See Table 7.10 for the application of ethical perspectives to immunization.)

**TABLE 7.10  Ethical Action in Providing Immunizations to Children**

| Ethical Perspective | Application |
|---|---|
| Rule ethics (principles) | ■ Promote justice by providing access to immunizations for families with children, which is consistent with school-entry laws.<br>■ Prevent harm to the children by promoting immunization for this population.<br>■ Use evidence about the effectiveness of immunizations and debunk misinformation to provide education about benefits. |
| Virtue ethics (character) | ■ Respect individual parental rights to refuse immunization for their children per the law, which allows parental exemption based on religious or other values. |
| Feminist ethics (reducing oppression) | ■ Be aware of using authority in a manner that oppresses parents.<br>■ Encourage parents' voices and perspectives in making decisions about what to do. |

## KEY POINTS

■ All levels of government (local, state, and federal) have responsibility for promoting public health and often work together.

■ Three core functions of public health and ten essential services determine the goals of public health departments.

■ PHNs who are employed by governmental agencies are responsible for upholding specific laws that protect the public health.

■ The public health model focuses on populations and prevention, in contrast to the medical model, which focuses on individuals and provides healthcare services in response to illness and injury.

■ The U.S. healthcare system has poorer healthcare outcomes in comparison to other high-income countries.

■ The Triple Aim Framework—which focuses on improving the patient care experience, improving population health, and reducing healthcare costs—is an innovative approach for guiding strategies to improve health system performance.

■ Funding for public health comes from public and private sources and determines the programs and services that local public health departments can provide.

■ Local public health departments work with nonprofit organizations to improve the health status of populations.

 REFLECTIVE PRACTICE

Governmental organizations develop and enforce laws and regulations to prevent disease and promote the health of populations. They also provide the resources needed to improve public health. These resources include staff members with expert knowledge and funds to support public health programs and services. As a PHN working for a governmental organization, it is both a responsibility and an honor to contribute to improved population health through one's expert knowledge and skills. Consider how PHNs use their expert knowledge and skills in governmental responses to natural disasters and severe weather.

Locate your state health department web page on emergency preparedness for natural disasters. Select a natural disaster that may potentially impact the health of the population. Consider how PHNs are involved in helping communities respond to a natural disaster.

■ What are the responsibilities of the local, state, and federal levels of government in responding to the disaster?

■ How could community resources be involved in responding to the consequences of the disaster (disease prevention and health promotion)?

■ How would PHN actions in response to the disaster be consistent with the Cornerstones of Public Health Nursing? (See Chapter 1.)

## APPLICATION OF EVIDENCE

1. Which essential services would be most relevant in responding to the natural disaster of flooding in a community?

2. Give a practice example that illustrates each of the three core functions for responding to a flood in a community.

3. Refer to Table 7.7, which identifies the ANA Standards of Professional Performance for Public Health Nursing. How do the following standards apply to the example of a flooding disaster: education, collaboration, resource utilization, leadership, and advocacy?

4. Which public health laws and legal issues do PHNs need to keep in mind when responding to a flood disaster?

## References

American Nurses Association. (2013). *Public health nursing: Scope and standards of practice.* Silver Spring, MD: Author.

Anderson, L. J. W., Schaffer, M. A., Hiltz, C., O'Leary, S. A., Luehr, R. E., & Yoney, E. L. (2017). Public health interventions: School nurse practice stories. *The Journal of School Nursing, 34*(3), 192–202. doi:10.1177/1059840517721951

Association of State and Territorial Health Officers. (2015). *Public health and schools toolkit: Comparison of FERPA and HIPAA Privacy Rule for accessing student health data.* Retrieved from http://www.astho.org/programs/preparedness/public-health-emergency-law/public-health-and-schools-toolkit/comparison-of-ferpa-and-hipaa-privacy-rule/

Bodenheimer, T., & Sinksy, C. (2014). From triple to quadruple aim: Care of the patient requires care of the provider. *Annals of Family Medicine, 12*(6), 573–576.

Centers for Disease Control and Prevention. (2013). Electronic laboratory reporting (ELR). Retrieved from http://www.cdc.gov/EHRmeaningfuluse/elr.html

Centers for Disease Control and Prevention. (2014). The public health system and the 10 essential public health services. Retrieved from https://www.cdc.gov/stltpublichealth/publichealthservices/essentialhealthservices.html

Centers for Disease Control and Prevention. (2017a). National Program of Cancer Registries (NPCR). Retrieved from https://www.cdc.gov/cancer/npcr/index.htm

Centers for Disease Control and Prevention. (2017b). *National voluntary accreditation for public health departments* [Fact sheet]. Retrieved from https://www.cdc.gov/stltpublichealth/hop/pdfs/nvaph_factsheet.pdf

Edmonds, J. K., Campbell, L. A., & Guilder, R. E. (2016). Public health nursing practice in the Affordable Care Act era: A national survey. *Public Health Nursing, 34*(1), 50–58. doi:10.1111/phn.12286

Garcia-Silva, B., Handler, E., & Wolfe, J. (2017). A public–private partnership to mitigate food insecurity and food waste in Orange County, California. *American Journal of Public Health, 107*(1), 105–107.

Georgia Department of Public Health. (2017). Meaningful use. Retrieved from https://dph.georgia.gov/meaningful-use

Healthy People 2020. (2017a). Preparedness. Retrieved from https://www.healthypeople.gov/2020/topics-objectives/topic/preparedness

Healthy People 2020. (2017b). Public health infrastructure. Retrieved from https://www.healthypeople.gov/2020/topics-objectives/topic/public-health-infrastructure

Henry Street Consortium. (2017). *Entry-level population-based public health nursing competencies.* St. Paul, MN: Author. Retrieved from www.henrystreetconsortium.org

Hodge, J. G., Jr., Barraza, L., Bernstein, J., Chu, C., Collmer, V., Davis, C., … Orenstein, D. G. (2013). Major trends in public health law and practice: A network national report. *The Journal of Law, Medicine & Ethics, 41*(3), 737–745. doi:10.1111/jlme.12084

Horlich, G., Shaw, F. E., Gorji, M., & Fishbein, D. B. (2008). Delivering new vaccines to adolescents: The role of school-entry laws. *Pediatrics, 121,* S79–S84. doi:10.1542/peds.2007-1115i

Institute for Healthcare Improvement. (2017). The IHI Triple Aim initiative. Retrieved from http://www.ihi.org/Engage/Initiatives/TripleAim/Pages/default.aspx

Institute of Medicine. (1988). *The future of public health.* Washington, DC: National Academies Press.

International Council of Nurses. (2017). Mobile outreach nurse led clinic, USA. Retrieved from https://www.icnvoicetolead.com/case-study/mobile-outreach-nurse-led-clinic-usa/

International Society for Disease Surveillance. (2012, November). *Electronic syndromic surveillance using hospital inpatient and ambulatory clinical care electronic health record data: Recommendations from the ISDS Meaningful Use Workgroup.* Retrieved from https://knowledge-repository.s3.amazonaws.com/recommendations/Recommendations_2012_11_MU_Recommendations.pdf

Jakeway, C. C., LaRosa, G., Cary, A., & Schoenfisch, S. (2008). The role of public health nurses in emergency preparedness and response: A position paper of the Association of State and Territorial Directors of Nursing. *Public Health Nursing, 25*(4), 353–361. doi:10.1111/j.1525-1446.2008.00716.x

Keller, L. O., & Litt, E. A. (2008). *Report on public health nurse to population ratio.* Association of State and Territorial Directors of Nursing (ASTDN). Retrieved from http://dph.georgia.gov/sites/dph.georgia.gov/files/ASTHOReportPublicHealthNursetoPopRatio2008.pdf

Mello, M. M., Wood, J., Burris, S., Wagenaar, A. C., Ibrahim, J. K., & Swanson, J. W. (2013). Critical opportunities for public health law: A call for action. *American Journal of Public Health, 103*(11), 1979–1988. doi:10.2105/ajph.2013.301281

Minnesota Department of Health. (2003). *Communicable disease reporting and HIPAA*. Retrieved from http://www.health.state. mn.us/divs/idepc/dtopics/reportable/rule/hipaacomm.html

Minnesota Department of Health. (2005). *2005 updates to the law on isolation and quarantine*. Retrieved from http://www.health. state.mn.us/divs/idepc/dtopics/infectioncontrol/ps/iqlaw.html

Minnesota Department of Health. (2012). *Financing local public health services in Minnesota: Trends in local tax levy expenditures*. Retrieved from http://www.health.state.mn.us/ divs/opi/pm/ran/docs/1210ran_lhdfinancing.pdf

Minnesota Department of Health. (2015). *Building a solid founda-tion for health: 2015 report to the Minnesota Legislature on public health system development*. Retrieved from http://www. health.state.mn.us/divs/opi/resources/docs/1501legreport.pdf

Minnesota Department of Health. (2016). Child protection. Retrieved from http://www.dhs.state.mn.us/main/ idcplg?IdcService=GET_DYNAMIC_ CONVERSION&RevisionSelectionMethod= LatestReleased&dDocName=id_000152

Minnesota Department of Health. (2017a). Communicable disease rule, Chapter 4605. Retrieved from http://www.health.state. mn.us/divs/idepc/dtopics/reportable/rule/rule.html

Minnesota Department of Health. (2017b). *Immunization data sharing, HIPAA, and MIIC*. Retrieved from http://www. health.state.mn.us/divs/idepc/immunize/registry/hipaa.html

Minnesota Department of Health. (2017c). *Local public health act performance measures, data book 2016*. Retrieved from http://www.health.state.mn.us/divs/opi/annualreporting/ docs/library/2016_databook.pdf

Minnesota Department of Health. (2017d). The Statewide Health Improvement Partnership. Retrieved from  http://www. health.state.mn.us/ship/

Minnesota Department of Health. (2017e). Breastfeeding friendly health departments. Retrieved from http://www.health.state. mn.us/divs/oshii/bf/healthdeptBFF.html

Minnesota Department of Health State Community Health Services Advisory Committee. (1992). *Controlling public health nuisances: A guide for community health boards*. Retrieved from http://www.health.state.mn.us/divs/eh/local/chsboardguide.pdf

Minnesota Visiting Nurse Agency. (2017). Family health. Retrieved from https://www.mvna.org/family-health/

Mossialos, E., Djordjevic, A., Osborn, R., & Sarnak, D. (Eds.). (2017). *International profiles of health care systems*. The Commonwealth Fund. Retrieved from http://www. commonwealthfund.org/publications/fund-reports/2017/may/ international-profiles

National Alliance on Mental Illness. (2016). *Understanding the Minnesota civil commitment process*. Retrieved from http:// www.namihelps.org/civilcommitmentbookletfinal-2016.pdf

National Association of County and City Health Officials. (2016). *2016 national profile of local health departments*. Retrieved from http://nacchoprofilestudy.org/wp-content/uploads/2017/10/ ProfileReport_Aug2017_final.pdf

National Association of County and City Health Officials. (2017). Medical Reserve Corps. Retrieved from http://www.naccho.org/ programs/public-health-preparedness/medical-reserve-corps

National Prevention Council. (2011). National prevention strategy. U.S. Department of Health and Human Services, Office of the Surgeon General. Retrieved from https://www.surgeongeneral. gov/priorities/prevention/strategy/index.html

Office of the Reviser of Statutes. (2016). *Minnesota Statutes. 626.556 Reporting of maltreatment of minors*. Retrieved from https://www.revisor.mn.gov/statutes/?id=626.556

Pozgar, G. D. (2005). *Legal and ethical issues for health profession-als*. Sudbury, MA: Jones and Bartlett.

Riley, W. J., Gearin, K. J., Parrotta, C. D., Briggs, J., & Gyllstrom, M. E. (2013). Tax levy financing for local public health fiscal allocation, effort, and capacity. *American Journal of Preventive Medicine, 45*(6), 776–781. doi:10.1016/j.amepre.2013.08.012

Savage, R. (2011, August 15). *HL7 Version 2.5.1: Implementation guide for immunization messaging, release 1.3*. Centers for Disease Control and Prevention and American Immunization Registry Association. Retrieved from http://www.cdc.gov/ vaccines/programs/iis/technical-guidance/downloads/ hl7guide-2011-08.pdf

Schneider, E. C., Sarnak, D. O., Squires, D., Shah, A., & Doty, M. M. (2017). *Mirror, mirror 2017: International comparison reflects flaws and opportunities for better U.S. health care*. Commonwealth Fund. Retrieved from http://www. commonwealthfund.org/interactives/2017/july/mirror-mirror/

Stanhope, M., & Lancaster, J. (2016). *Public health nursing: Population-centered health care in the community*. St. Louis, MO: Elsevier, Inc.

U.S. Department of Education. (2015). Family Educational Rights and Privacy Act (FERPA). Retrieved from https://www2.ed.gov/ policy/gen/guid/fpco/ferpa/index.html

U.S. Department of Health and Human Services and the U.S. Department of Education. (2008). *Joint guidance on the applica-tion of the Family Educational Rights and Privacy Act (FERPA) and the Health Insurance Portability and Accountability Act of 1996 (HIPAA) to student health records*. Retrieved from https://www2.ed.gov/policy/gen/guid/fpco/doc/ ferpa-hipaa-guidance.pdf

Yoon, P. W., Ising, A. I., & Gunn, J. E. (2017, July 10). Using syn-dromic surveillance for all-hazards public health surveillance: Successes, challenges, and the future. *Public Health Reports, 132*(Suppl. 1), 3S–6S.

# COMPETENCY #6
## Utilizes Collaboration to Achieve Public Health Goals

■ **Marjorie A. Schaffer**
*with Melissa L. Horning and Carol J. Roth*

> *Jake is a public health nursing student who has 10 years of experience in the acute care setting as an associate degree nurse. His expertise has been in the area of cardiac care, working in the Coronary Care Unit at a local hospital. Jake has returned to school to complete a baccalaureate degree in nursing. The community surrounding the university that Jake attends has identified a need to address healthcare access for the homeless population. A local church approached the university to work with it to develop a clinic for the homeless by using resources in the community and students for the delivery of care for this underserved population. Jake's preceptor, Linda, a public health nurse (PHN), is representing the local public health department at planning meetings. Jake will have the opportunity to learn how professionals, community members, and organizations collaborate to contribute to the development of a community clinic that serves a vulnerable population. Jake has many questions, such as: Whom would he collaborate with to contribute to this goal? Whom should be invited to be partners in the collaboration? How does such a diverse group work together? What is the PHN's responsibility in collaborative work?*
>
> *Before Jake attends the first planning meeting with Linda, he picks up his notebook to review the population-based public health nursing competency list and concentrates on Competency #6, which focuses on collaborative practice.*

## JAKE'S NOTEBOOK

**COMPETENCY #6** Utilizes Collaboration to Achieve Public Health Goals

A. Demonstrates effective participation on interprofessional teams

B. Develops relationships and builds partnership with communities, systems, individuals, and families

C. Utilizes community assets and community engagement to empower communities, systems, individuals, and families

*Source:* Henry Street Consortium, 2017

### USEFUL DEFINITIONS

**Collaboration:** Working together "to achieve a common goal through enhancing the capacity of one or more of the members to promote and protect health" (Keller, Strohschein, Lia-Hoagberg, & Schaffer, 2004, p. 456).

**Community Asset:** "Anything that can be used to improve the quality of community life," including people, physical structures, community services, and businesses (KU Center for Community Health and Development, 2017).

**Community Engagement:** Collaborating with community members or community organizations to mutually participate in problem-solving to address issues that affect their well-being (National Institutes of Health, 2011).

**Interprofessional Collaboration:** Creating collective action to address the complexity of client needs and creating a team culture that integrates the perspectives of each professional and facilitates mutual team member respect and trust (D'Amour, Ferrada-Videla, Rodriguez, & Beaulieu, 2005).

**Partnership:** Individuals or organizations sharing ideas, experiences, skills, and resources to address problems through mutual decision-making and action (Wilson & Mabhala, 2009).

## Accomplishing More by Working Together

PHNs work with many individuals and community organizations. Collaboration can be between two or more individuals or between organizations. PHNs collaborate with representatives of the population, other professionals, and organizations to contribute to healthcare planning and promote health (American Nurses Association [ANA], 2013).

A study about public health nursing practice analyzed how PHNs collaborated with individuals, communities, and systems. At the *individual level,* PHNs said their goal was to make a difference in the lives of their clients by focusing on "doing with" rather than on "doing for" (Aston, Meagher-Stewart, Edwards, & Young, 2009). They wanted to empower their clients to take responsibility and ownership for health decisions. The PHNs identified several strategies for empowering their clients: begin with the client's perspective, tune into the readiness of the client, assess holistically (refer to Public Health Nursing Competency #9 in Chapter 11), and build rapport with the client.

At the *community level,* Aston et al. (2009) suggested strategies to encourage community member participation in health programs and initiatives. The PHNs involved community members in decision-making groups, focused on community assets, and gave positive feedback and encouragement by affirming what was working well. The PHNs involved people who normally might not have the opportunity to participate in decision-making groups, such as youth living in poverty and mothers who were isolated. At every group meeting, the PHNs asked, "So who is missing and who needs to be here?" PHNs often initiate the process of uniting people around a problem they all care about. PHNs encourage group ownership and often look for community members to take the lead in problem solving. PHNs can assist with the group process, but ideally community members should control the flow and process toward finding and implementing solutions. Collaboration works best when everyone has the opportunity to share thoughts and ideas. One PHN in the study used the word *catalyst* to describe an approach that draws the voices and participation of community members. This means that someone needs to initiate the collaborative process, which then continues to develop with the input of the people who contribute their perspectives and skills to the collaboration.

At the *systems level,* the PHNs in the study connected community members and groups to existing social networks, including neighborhood groups; community organizations, such as churches; or programs that provide food. These connections helped to create a participatory infrastructure. The PHNs linked people and community organizations that were working on similar goals but had not yet worked together. As a result, partnerships were built that advocated for clients and linked agencies, contributing to

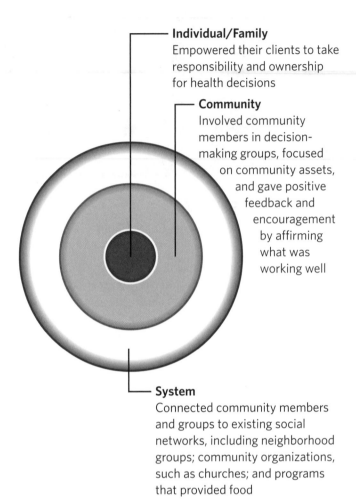

**Individual/Family**
Empowered their clients to take responsibility and ownership for health decisions

**Community**
Involved community members in decision-making groups, focused on community assets, and gave positive feedback and encouragement by affirming what was working well

**System**
Connected community members and groups to existing social networks, including neighborhood groups; community organizations, such as churches; and programs that provided food

**FIGURE 8.1** How PHNs Work With Individuals, Communities, and Systems

better services for clients. One PHN talked about finding "the movers and shakers" in the community through reaching out to community groups, such as men's or women's groups, church groups, and community health boards. These strategies encourage the collective voice of community members and foster citizen participation. PHNs can also bring their expertise in health promotion to existing collaborative groups that are already established in communities (Aston et al., 2009).

Consider how PHNs collaborate with individuals and families, community groups, and systems in the collaboration example in Table 8.1. A local church hosts a Wellness Center to serve the needs of people living in the community who have health needs and difficulty accessing healthcare. Many clients need dental care, so PHNs collaborate at all levels of practice and across professions to respond to this need. Figure 8.1 also elaborates on how PHNs collaborate with individuals and families, communities, and systems.

## TABLE 8.1 Collaboration Example

| Level of Practice | Example |
| --- | --- |
| Individual | When clients at the Wellness Center complain of toothaches, PHNs refer them to low-cost dental care and arrange transportation to the community site where dental care is provided. |
| Community | PHNs collect information on agencies and organizations that provide low-cost dental care and create a pamphlet to communicate that information to potential clients and other community locations where people in need can learn about resources. In addition, PHNs could provide social marketing to local schools about resources for dental care. |
| Systems | PHNs advocate for policy change to include dental care in health programs that serve individuals and families without employer-provided insurance. |

## TABLE 8.2 Best Practices for Collaboration

- Effective leadership
- Commitment of the participants
- Shared values and a sense of purpose
- Mutual respect for team members
- Linkages between groups and individuals
- Identification of strategies and resources to achieve the goals, and a structure to support the collaborative work
- Internal systems to support the structure (e.g., communication mechanisms, a place to meet, time available in assigned workload)

# Best Practices for Collaboration

With the input of several stakeholders (individuals and organizations), the pooling of expertise and resources (e.g., knowledge, expertise, lived experience, money) can lead to expanded ideas and strategies for improving population health outcomes. Together with community partners and other professionals, PHNs strive to identify mutual goals and expected outcomes for the collaboration. See Table 8.2 for a summary of best practices for effective collaborative action.

# Collaboration With Other Professionals and Communities

Depending on their practice setting, PHNs work with a variety of other professionals, groups, and organizations. For example, a PHN working in a school collaborates with teachers, families, students, school administration, primary care providers, other health and special education professionals, social workers, and groups that address such health needs as chronic illness and mental health services. The following are possible partners in public health nursing networks:

**Education collaborators:**
- Childcare programs and providers
- Colleges and universities
- Early childhood development programs
- Head Start
- Literacy programs/English as a second language learner programs
- Schools
- Special education

**Holistic healthcare team members:**
- Alcoholics Anonymous
- Audiologists
- Chemical dependency programs
- Clinical nurse specialists
- Complementary/alternative therapy programs
- Dental care providers (dentists, dental hygienists, dental assistants)
- Home care agencies
- Mental health centers and providers
- Nutritionists
- Occupational therapists
- Physical therapists
- Planned Parenthood
- Primary care providers (physicians, nurse practitioners, physician assistants)
- Psychologists
- Services for children with special needs
- Services for vision and hearing impaired
- Speech therapists
- Traditional/Native healers

**Housing and food collaborators:**
- Battered women's shelters
- Congregate dining
- Food shelves
- Free and reduced-price school meal programs
- Homeless shelters
- Housing programs
- Meals on Wheels
- Supplemental Nutrition Assistance Programs (SNAP)
- Women, Infants, and Children (WIC)

**Legal collaborators:**
- Law enforcement
- Legal aid
- Ombudsmen

**Social Service collaborators:**
- Child protection and welfare programs
- Energy assistance
- Financial assistance
- Jobs and training services
- Social services
- Transportation services
- Vulnerable adult programs

**Community collaborators:**
- Artists
- Businesses
- City councils/county boards
- Clergy and religious/faith leaders
- Community action programs
- Community residents
- Community service organizations (Rotary, Lions)
- Environmental health programs
- Extension agents
- Musicians
- Volunteers

*Interprofessional collaboration* is essential for developing effective partnerships that improve health outcomes in public health nursing practice. Interprofessional collaborative practice engages communities and populations. Teamwork and team-based care involve engaging other health professionals, specific to the care environment, to participate in client-centered problem solving. The Interprofessional Education Collaborative Expert Panel (2011) identified four domains or competencies of interprofessional practice (see Table 8.3).

The values/ethics competency means that collaborators take on a "community/population orientation, grounded in a sense of shared purpose to support the common good in healthcare, and reflect a shared commitment to creating safer, more efficient, and more effective systems of care" (Interprofessional Education Collaborative Expert Panel, 2011, p. 170). For roles and responsibilities, PHNs need to understand their own professional role and responsibilities as well as those of other professions. To communicate effectively on interprofessional teams, PHNs need to avoid professional jargon and demonstrate a readiness to work together by being available, showing interest, and actively listening. A consideration for effective teamwork is having respect for the professional expertise among diverse members of the team while staying focused on the goal of the collaboration (Interprofessional Education Collaborative Expert Panel, 2011).

The "professional" part of interprofessional collaboration refers to individuals who have specific knowledge and skills that they can use to contribute to community well-being.

**TABLE 8.3 Domains and Actions Consistent With Interprofessional Collaboration**

| Domain | Action Example |
|---|---|
| Values/ethics for interprofessional practice | Acting with honesty and integrity in all relationships and modeling respect, confidentiality, and dignity for clients and team members |
| Roles and responsibilities for collaborative practice | Communicating one's role and responsibilities to clients/families, community groups, and other professionals |
| Interprofessional communication practices | Actively participating in timely, sensitive, and instructive sharing/feedback |
| Teamwork and team-based practice | Engaging other professionals in shared problem solving and decision-making |

Interprofessional education occurs when the various professions "learn about, from, and with each other to enable effective collaboration and improve health outcomes" (WHO, 2010, p. 7). However, because professionals from different professions have different perspectives, practices, and terminology, they may encounter barriers to effective teamwork. How can you anticipate and reduce potential barriers to effective teamwork in interprofessional collaboration?

- Work to understand differences among team members' culture, language, lifestyles, and beliefs
- Listen, be fully attentive, and truly hear
- Acknowledge and express appreciation
- Exhibit empathy and understanding
- Display courtesy and consideration
- Be accountable and professional
- Abide by the organizational professional code of conduct

*Source:* Brewer, 2012, p. 33

PHNs work with many people who have different educational backgrounds, different experiences, and different philosophies of life from their own and from each other. They encounter different perspectives about which issues are most important and what should be done to address specific health concerns. It is important to become familiar with common differences to avoid making assumptions about the viewpoints of community partners and members of the community. Sometimes tension and conflict occur as collaborators work through different perspectives and ideas about how to respond to a problem. Constructive conflict may help move the group toward change. In most cases, the accomplishments of the collaboration are far more than what one individual or one professional group could accomplish alone. Conflict that can be worked through has the potential to lead to effective collaboration and positive change.

As you begin your practice, ask questions of people with different educational preparation and roles about what they think about a situation. Many will be pleased that you ask about their perspectives. Differences can be as basic as using different terminology for similar work, practices, or interventions. What you call an assessment might be called something different in another profession. Also, take enough time to communicate and make sure that all collaborators are on the same page. Time limitations and a sense

## EVIDENCE EXAMPLE 8.1
### Interprofessional Collaboration

As you read through these examples of interprofessional collaboration, think about your community and how you could collaborate with other professionals to improve the health of the population.

■ Eckstrom and colleagues (2016) described a fall risk reduction project that involved an interprofessional collaboration approach. An interprofessional teaching team provided education to an interprofessional clinical team about how to implement the American Geriatrics Society and British Geriatrics Society guidelines to reduce the fall risk for older adults in Oregon. The clinical teams included representatives from medicine, nursing, pharmacy, and social work in ambulatory, long-term care, hospital, and home health settings. The project increased fall risk reduction activities of professionals in these settings.

■ A study by Clancy, Gressnes, and Svensson (2012) found that interpersonal and relationship skills were viewed as most important for interprofessional collaboration in a survey of PHNs, physicians, midwives, and child protection workers from Norwegian municipalities and social services. All participants ranked trust, respect, and collaborative competence as most important in interprofessional collaboration. Thirty percent of participants reported that conflict among professionals was common. The authors suggested that structural changes—such as co-locating professionals, which could increase the potential for face-to-face communication—would likely decrease territorial thinking based on professional expertise.

## THEORY APPLICATION
### Normative Group Development

To collaborate effectively with people representing different organizations, an understanding of group dynamics is useful. Tuckman developed a theory that explains the norms for group development (1965). PHNs can apply this theory to new situations of working with interprofessional teams. See Table 8.4. The stages of normative group development predict how a collaborative group develops its relationships and interaction patterns for working on a common public health goal. There are four stages: forming, storming, norming, and performing. After the forming phase, most groups will move through a storming phase. Conflict-management skills can be helpful in the storming phase to identify participant interests and positions, create new options through brainstorming, and negotiate a plan for moving forward (Bazarman, 2005). In the norming phase, group members begin to unify as a group. After moving through the norming phase into the performing phase, the group aims to work together collaboratively to achieve an agreed-upon goal. A healthy, functioning group creates energy that moves the group toward goal accomplishment.

### TABLE 8.4 Normative Group Development

| Forming | Storming | Norming | Performing |
|---|---|---|---|
| ■ Members work to understand one another.<br>■ The group determines its boundaries and focus.<br>■ Group leaders emerge. | ■ Conflict emerges.<br>■ Some members may be resistant to following group direction.<br>■ People express concern about the right way to do things. | ■ Trust develops.<br>■ Members identify as a group.<br>■ The group experiences cohesion in choosing a goal. | ■ The group focuses on accomplishing tasks.<br>■ Members establish rules for working together. |

*Source:* Tuckman, 1965

of urgency in responding to a public health problem can sometimes create barriers to collaboration. However, time spent getting to know one another can help to establish trust among the collaborators and prevent tension and conflict, which would likely take more time to resolve at a later point or even result in the collaboration's failure.

> *The first planning meeting Jake attends includes 31 other people (the pastor, the assistant pastor, a police liaison, two social workers, four nurses from various clinical backgrounds, two alternative healers, two chiropractors, two community members, two people from the church's board of directors, a director from a local clinic, a block nurse coordinator, three homeless persons, two faculty from the university Jake is attending, two staff members from the surrounding homeless shelters, an insurance representative, a local physician, a musician, and two other nursing students). The group meets early in the evening to accommodate the participants' different schedules. It takes most of the first meeting to introduce everyone and to allow each person to share an opinion of what the wellness clinic's vision would be.*
>
> *Jake is shocked to realize that for such a large group to come to a consensus about a vision, at least six meetings would be needed. He realizes the group members needed time to talk so that they could determine their goals and how they were going to work together. During the initial meeting, the police liaison, who is also a social worker and a member of the church, emerges as the natural leader of the project. His skills and experiences have prepared him for a leadership role. He also has experience working with the homeless population in the neighborhood. After the meeting, Jake asks his preceptor, Linda, several questions. He wonders how a group of people with such a variety of backgrounds and experiences could create one plan. What will the group do if everyone has different ideas about how to develop the clinic? Which services does the clinic need to provide to meet the needs of the homeless population?*
>
> *As the meetings progress, some community members drop out of the group, feeling frustrated as they perceive that their ideas are not being considered. As Jake continues to work on the planning team, he realizes that conflict-management skills and leadership skills are essential to work with such a large group. Jake marvels at the ability of the police liaison to create calm in a tense situation and focus on the group's vision to serve the homeless population through this community outreach project. Decision-making involves negotiation and compromise among the group members.*
>
> *New members will sometimes come to one meeting and then be gone at the next. This spotty attendance means that at each meeting, time is needed to introduce new members and explain the vision and review the group's planning phase. After about 10 meetings, a core group of community members have been identified through their commitment and attendance at meetings. Jake observes that this smaller group more easily comes to a consensus about the project's vision and purpose and that the members begin to trust each other and understand their roles in the group.*
>
> *Each group member is focused on the delivery of services to assist the homeless. Each member brings unique gifts and contributions to the table. Jake is excited to be a part of this collaborative endeavor. He is asked to develop a flyer to promote and advertise the wellness clinic, which will be open on Wednesday evenings.*

---

### Activity

- Identify the forming, storming, norming, and performing stages in the preceding scenario.
- Discuss actions members of the group might take to reduce potential barriers to effective interprofessional collaboration.

---

## Building Partnerships With Communities, Systems, Individuals, and Families

Partnerships are needed to implement many public health strategies to improve population health. In organizational and systems-level partnerships, many factors need to be addressed, including use of resources, personnel, and power-related factors that influence decision-making. There are often challenges when creating and maintaining partnerships; however, the benefits of working together are often very rewarding (Wilson & Mabhala, 2009).

Effectively collaborating and developing partnerships requires equality among the partners (Casey, 2008; Drahota et al., 2016). Equality in collaborative relationships is promoted through listening, being respectful, shared decision-making, appreciating differences and mutual goals, and developing trust. To encourage effective collaborative relationships with communities, professionals need to give up control and recognize that all members bring diverse and valuable expertise, lived experiences, and skillsets to the partnership (Campbell, Whitcomb, Culver, & McClanahan, 2015; Casey, 2008). Collaborative relationships work best if they are nonhierarchical in nature. Partnership roles are determined based on knowledge or expertise rather than on professional role, function, or education level (Casey, 2008). Ineffective relationships result from power or control inequities (Casey, 2008; Drahota et al., 2016). To reduce power and control inequities, you need to pay attention to how the partnership is structured, who directs resources, and how much time participants are expected to commit to partnership work.

Factors found to facilitate effective partnerships include the following (Campbell et al., 2015; Casey, 2008; Drahota et al., 2016):

- Establishing trust, commitment, and respectful relationships among partners

- Having mutually shared values, goals, and outcomes

- Sharing resources and balancing power and control

- Having effective, clear, and open communication and decision-making

- Establishing clearly defined roles and a conflict-resolution plan together

- Recognizing and building on strengths and assets of the partners and individuals and communities

**Healthy People**
**2020**
**healthypeople.gov**

The Healthy People 2020 website offers suggestions useful for collaboration and building partnerships. On the website: 1) click "Healthy People in Action," 2) click "Stories from the Field," 3) click two or three map points to read the featured story, and 4) identify the role of partnership in the success story. Then consider how PHNs could use Healthy People 2020 goals, tools, and resources as they collaborate with professionals and communities.

The Culture of Health action areas consist of the following:

- ***Making health a shared value*** is critical for government, business, communities, and all individuals to thrive, as we all are interdependent upon one another. As Paul Wellstone once said, "We all do better, when we all do better" (Wellstone.org, 1999, para. 7). Taking steps to make health a shared value requires working within the social environment and shifting mindsets to focus on health as a collective, fostering a sense of community and promoting civic engagement through activities like voting and volunteering (RWJF, 2015; Trujillo & Plough, 2016).

- ***Fostering cross-sector collaborations*** is necessary to create a Culture of Health. If PHNs work alone or even with others within public health or healthcare sectors, they will not have the resources or power to create the necessary changes to foster a culture where all people can be healthy. Thus, cross-sector collaborations are critical to bringing diverse groups and interests together, like government, businesses/industry, education, healthcare and public health, and community organizations. By incorporating each group's knowledge, resources, and strengths, cross-sector collaborations can have greater influence and impact on the policies and environments that influence population health, well-being, and equity to build a Culture of Health (RWJF, 2015).

## Building a Culture of Health: Partnership and Collaboration

An important skill for PHNs is learning how to develop collaborative community partnerships to bring about community and systems change for improving health (Fawcett, Schultz, Watson-Thompson, Fox, & Bremby, 2010; Towne & Valedes, 2017). Collaborating to establish effective partnerships is essential for building a "Culture of Health."

What is a Culture of Health? The Culture of Health is a systems-level initiative that brings together all stakeholders who aim to improve health outcomes. As coined by Robert Wood Johnson Foundation (RWJF, 2015), a Culture of Health is where all individuals, communities, and societies can enjoy good health to grow, live, work, and play. Through an extensive research process, RWJF developed the Culture of Health Action Framework, shown in Figure 8.2, as a guide for how governments, organizations, and health professionals can work together to build a culture that increases population health, well-being, and equity. The four action areas overlap and are interconnected; one action area in particular focuses on collaboration and partnership (RWJF, 2015; Trujillo & Plough, 2016). As you read about each of the four RWJF action areas, consider how important collaboration and partnership is for each action area.

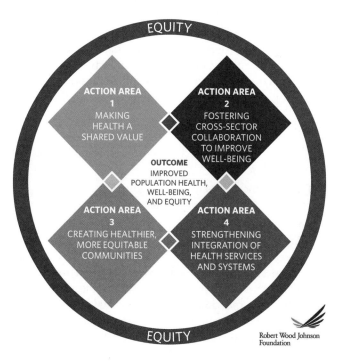

**FIGURE 8.2** Culture of Health Action Framework
*Source:* © 2015, Robert Wood Johnson Foundation.
Used with permission.

▪ *Creating healthier more equitable communities* focuses on ensuring all people and communities have equitable opportunities and resources in their neighborhoods to achieve health and well-being. To create healthier, more equitable communities, a PHN must work through policies and systems to impact the built, social, and economic environments by decreasing residential segregation and increasing access to affordable housing, healthy foods, safe communities, and quality education at all levels (RWJF, 2015).

▪ *Strengthening the integration of health services and systems* emphasizes that to improve health outcomes for all and reduce healthcare costs, all individuals need to both be able to access affordable, holistic healthcare services across the spectrum of medical, dental, and mental healthcare services and receive needed social and public health services. When working together, integrated healthcare, public health, and social services can best facilitate health promotion, disease prevention, and chronic disease management through effective primary, secondary, and tertiary prevention (RWJF, 2015).

Cross-sector collaboration requires the support of quality partnerships, investments, and policies (RWJF, 2015). While each of these four action areas is critical for working toward building a Culture of Health and increasing health equity, well-being, and population health, cross-sector collaboration is critical to moving much of the work forward. Factors that can facilitate success of cross-sector collaboration and partnerships include (Libbey & Miyahara, 2011; Mattessich & Rausch, 2014):

▪ Clear, shared vision with common goals that are considerate of the culture, backgrounds, and environments of each partner in the cross-sector collaboration

▪ Skilled, devoted leadership with defined roles of responsibility

▪ An understanding of each of the partner organizations and mutual respect for what each brings to the partnership

▪ Financial incentives from both government and corporate businesses to support the partnership

You likely have already noticed that there are many similarities between these factors that facilitate success of cross-sector collaborations to build a Culture of Health and those that facilitate successful partnerships at individual, community and systems levels. Just like successful partnerships at the individual, community, and systems levels, developing and sustaining quality cross-sector partnerships for collective action is not easy. Yet, the outcomes of successful cross-sector collaborations propel PHNs toward creating a Culture of Health. Successful cross-sector collaboration outcomes include improvements to services provided, policy change, and improvements to and awareness of how social, built, and economic environments (e.g., transportation availability, safety of neighborhoods, availability of affordable housing) influence health (Mattessich & Rausch, 2014).

## Activity

Consider who the cross-sector collaborators are with whom PHNs work to build a Culture of Health.

## EVIDENCE EXAMPLE 8.2
### Cross-Sector Collaboration in Action

▪ The Twin Cities Mobile Market is a "grocery store on wheels" that works to increase access to affordable healthy foods by bringing them to the doorsteps of under-resourced communities. Led by a skilled, devoted leader, Ms. Porter, the Twin Cities Mobile Market is possible because of the successfully developed cross-sector collaboration and partnerships with wholesalers, grocery stores, local farmers, local government (including public health departments and nurses), public and private housing agencies, healthcare systems and insurance companies, community organizations and partners, philanthropic and government funders, SNAP-Ed programs, legislation, and researchers. This cross-sector collaboration makes it possible for the Twin Cities Mobile Market to serve under-resourced community sites each month, and currently, 50% of all Twin Cities Mobile Market sales are for fruits and vegetables (Twin Cities Mobile Market, 2017).

▪ An exemplar of cross-sector collaboration is Community of Care in rural Cass County, North Dakota, which started as a pilot project of the Good Samaritan Society to help older residents remain in their homes as long as safely possible. Today, Community of Care is supported by human service funds, grants, and other community financial sources. Staffing includes an executive director, a faith community nurse, a care coordinator, a part-time bookkeeper, a volunteer coordinator, and a cadre of community volunteers. Cross-sector collaboration has resulted in expansion of services to community members, including transportation to healthcare appointments, referrals to state health insurance counseling, yard work, minor home repairs, low-impact exercise classes, blood pressure screening, music and memory programs, a health newsletter, and health education activities. Community wellness fairs are offered in partnership with local university nursing students. The outreach activities include home visits to residents who are living in the rural parts of the county, as well as providing referral assistance to the family members of the residents. A goal of one of the grants that helps support Community of Care is to reduce hospital readmission rates through the efforts of collaboration (Community of Care, 2017).

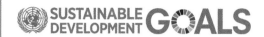

**Rural Nursing in South Africa**

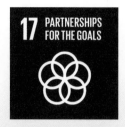

**GOAL 17** In South Africa, there is a shortage of doctors and nurses in rural areas and a greater need for access to healthcare. Healthcare needs include contraception and antenatal care, immunizations, and reducing the spread of tuberculosis and HIV. Guin Lourens, along with eight fellow nurses, established an organization called Rural Nursing of South Africa to increase nursing leadership in responding to identified healthcare needs. This organization partners with the Rural Health Advocacy Project, the Rural Doctors Association of South Africa, and Rural Rehab South Africa to respond to gaps in rural healthcare (International Council of Nurses, 2017).

In the following activity, find an example of how PHNs could actively participate in cross-cultural collaboration with other stakeholders to promote health in a population.

### 🌐 Online Activity

Visit the Community Tool Box website (http://ctb.ku.edu/en) compiled by the KU Center for Community Health and Development at the University of Kansas, a designated World Health Organization Collaborating Centre for Community Health and Development. Check out the tool box resources that can be used to support and guide collaborative public health nursing actions and work with partners at individual, community, and systems levels. Which resources would be useful to you and the PHNs you work with during your public health clinical experience? Which resources on this website do you think are helpful for PHNs to stay up-to-date on the best practices of collaboration and partnership?

## Collaborating Through Community Engagement

Community engagement involves collaborating with a community agency, a community safety-net organization, or community members to meet mutual needs that empower the community and the target population. It is important to acknowledge that community engagement work can involve the community at different levels, from very little community involvement to full community involvement (National Institutes of Health, 2011; Potter & Willis, 2013). For example, community engagement activities with less community involvement include outreach and consultation, in which information is often provided to the community. These activities may be the start of long-term and lasting community partnerships and collaborations; however, at these lower levels of community involvement, there is often less trust, flow of information, and communication, and thus there is less potential for impact.

In comparison, community engagement activities with the greatest levels of community involvement are those rooted in collaboration with shared leadership between partners and the highest levels of trust, information sharing, communication, and impact (Bagnall, White, & South, 2017; National Institutes of Health, 2011). Community engagement is best developed locally by drawing on the knowledge and experience of community and volunteer organizations to find and locate people from the community to take on peer and lay roles in health initiatives (Bagnall et al., 2017).

There is not a "one size fits all" approach to engaging communities. Public Health England and National Health Service England identified four different options to choose from to fit with the community context and type of health initiative for doing community engagement work (Bagnall et al. 2017). These options include:

1. Strengthening communities by building on community capacities to act together on health and the social determinants of health

2. Developing volunteer and peer roles that focus on enhancing individuals' capabilities to provide advice, information, and support or organize health activities in their own or other communities

3. Building collaborations and partnerships to involve communities and local services working together at any stage of the planning cycle, from identifying needs through to implementation and evaluation

4. Increasing access to community resources by connecting people to community resources, practical help, group activities, and volunteer opportunities to meet health needs and increase social participation

PHNs strive for strong collaborations and partnerships with community agencies and members. Therefore, you should always aim to increase the level at which the community is involved in community engagement work, which is an advocacy intervention. Within your public health nursing clinical experience, you may become involved in community engagement activities. Ultimately, the services and interventions you provide should empower and engage those you are working with, enrich the healthcare abilities of the agency/community partner, and build organizational capacity. By acknowledging and building on the strengths that already exist, you are adding to the community's assets and strengthening its ability to manage its own healthcare needs. Public health nursing advocacy through community engagement involves empowering vulnerable populations and their communities through capacity-building, collaborations, and partnerships. Table 8.5 provides a checklist of key steps to take to ensure community engagement work will be successful.

> *Jake realizes that the tone of the meetings has changed to a collaborative relationship of listening to each other, respecting differences, and valuing each other's input in the process—traits representative of an effective partnership. The members who are homeless are key partners and helpful in identifying needs and offering suggestions for delivery of services. Jake feels the strength of the bond of the collaborative partnership team in a shared vision. Jake observes that the team members are sharing resources and ideas with the group and striving for positive outcomes for the wellness clinic.*
>
> *When Jake's preceptor, Linda, asks him which characteristics and skills he thinks are needed for partnerships to be effective in planning such a challenging project, he answers that being committed, tactful, and persistent are important. He comments that it was really hard when people dropped out of the planning group in the early stage. However, the people who stayed with the project demonstrated they are committed and persistent. Jake also says that he thinks it is very important to have people in the group who have some influence in the community.*

## Using Community Assets to Empower Communities, Systems, Individuals, and Families

To be effective collaborators, PHNs must recognize and emphasize community assets in planning interventions to promote public health. PHNs along with community groups and organizations, such as churches, social service agencies, and neighborhoods, can identify assets within the community that provide building blocks for public health initiatives. An intervention that builds on a foundation of community assets is sometimes referred to as a *strength-based intervention*, which means that an intervention is selected and/or enhanced because it is already a resource or strength that exists within the community.

### TABLE 8.5 Checklist for Successful Community Engagement

❏ Learn about the community, the community safety-net organization, and at-risk populations.

❏ Develop trusting relationships with the community and diverse at-risk populations.

❏ Identify public health nursing activities beneficial to the organization, at-risk populations, and students.

❏ Collaborate with and engage the community agency in the planning, implementation, and evaluation of public health nursing activities.

❏ Develop culturally sensitive public health nursing services that are respectful of diverse populations.

❏ Create public health nursing services that are asset based, building on the strengths of the community agency, community resources, and at-risk populations.

❏ Be flexible in developing and implementing public health nursing services.

❏ Provide public health nursing services that strengthen an ongoing relationship with the community agency.

*Sources:* Builds on work of Broussard, 2011; Schoon, Champlin, & Hunt, 2012

## Asset Mapping: A Tool for Strengthening Communities

Karen Goldman and Kathleen Schmalz (2005) contrast a needs-based assessment approach with an asset-based assessment approach. Looking for the community's needs results in assessing what is wrong with the community and determining how "to fix" the problems, while looking for assets results in building on community strengths and mobilizing resources within the community to promote community health (see Table 8.6).

Assessing community assets means listening carefully to the voices of community members through interviews, meetings, focus groups, and asset-based inventories. Asset-based inventories identify strengths of individuals, community groups, and community organizations. Strategies to conduct an inventory may also include conducting a walking or windshield survey in which community strengths are noted, and using maps to document assets with a Geographic Information System (GIS). Additionally, other sources of information might include community websites; town directories; bulletin boards; and listings of business, organizations, and institutions (KU Center for Community Health and Development, 2017).

Asset mapping can benefit the community in several ways. This approach empowers people to think more positively and encourages them to discover their abilities and resources to contribute to their own health and meeting

## TABLE 8.6  Needs Assessment vs. Asset Mapping

| Needs Assessment | Asset Mapping |
|---|---|
| ▪ Community need is based on deficiency or problem.<br>▪ Looks at what is wrong with the community and how to fix it.<br>▪ Leads community to seek assistance rather than using in-house skills and change agents.<br>▪ Discourages community members. | ▪ Community assets include people, places, businesses, and organizations that can be mobilized for improvement.<br>▪ Focuses on positive aspects (strengths).<br>▪ Leads community to look within for solutions and resources to solve problems. |

*Source:* Goldman & Schmalz, 2005

## TABLE 8.7  Questions for Community Groups to Promote Thinking About Assets

| Asset Category | Questions |
|---|---|
| Physical | What are two or three physical assets in your community (neighborhood, buildings, parks, space, land, natural resources)? |
| Individual | What are your talents, experience, perspectives, and skills?<br><br>What do you care about?<br><br>What do you know about?<br><br>Whom do you know? |
| Associations | What is your participation in formal or informal voluntary groups, networks, and organizations of individuals who gather to do or enjoy something they cannot do alone?<br><br>Which groups are you part of?<br><br>Which groups do you know about? |
| Institutions | Which institutions (such organizations as businesses, nonprofit agencies, government, and schools) are located in your community?<br><br>What do these organizations contribute to your community? |
| Economic | What is something you spend money on?<br><br>What is something you make or do that people would pay you for?<br><br>Where do you invest your money?<br><br>What are unique economic assets in your community? |

*Sources:* Hamerlinck, 2013; Snow, 2004

their goals for the future. They also learn to listen and value the contributions of others. Asset mapping is an inclusive process, which results in highlighting information and resources that can be used to mobilize individual and community assets (Kretzmann & McKnight, 1993; Morgan & Ziglio, 2010).

John Kretzmann and John McKnight (1993) have identified five categories of community assets: physical, individual, associations, institutions, and economic. Luther Snow (2004) and John Hamerlinck (2013) propose asset-mapping questions, which can be adapted to help community groups explore their assets (see Table 8.7).

Once the community group has identified its assets, the next step is to review and consider how these assets can be tapped. In a group exercise, group members can list assets on pieces of paper or sticky notes and talk about how they are connected and can be used to improve the health and well-being of the community (Snow, 2004).

An asset-based approach to working with communities brings both strengths and challenges. Whiting, Kendall, and Wills (2012) discuss assets from a health promotion perspective. They identify categories of health assets and development assets (individual level) and public health asset frameworks (generally focus on community assets). Table 8.8 describes both strengths and challenges of the asset-based approach for individuals and communities.

> *Jake realizes the importance of knowing community assets and working with other professionals. The pastor knows the neighborhood and community well and has space and people resources for serving the meal on Wednesday evenings to the homeless. The social worker has experience with chemical dependency patients and the skills needed to address drug-abuse issues or concerns among the homeless. Another nurse is a mental health specialist who knows about useful referrals for homeless people. The police liaison knows many people who are homeless and is very well respected in the community. The insurance representative can help find resources to increase people's access to healthcare by identifying funding options and programs. The PHN knows about social service resources and possible sources of healthcare funding. Jake, as a nursing student, brings his gifts of delivery of care by doing blood pressure screenings, health teaching, and foot care at the wellness clinic. The programs planned at the wellness clinic are services the collaborative community members can offer or find others to come in and provide.*
>
> *Jake is present the first night the wellness clinic opens. As he sits down to share a meal with some of the individuals who visited the wellness clinic, he realizes the value in this statement: "It takes a community to take care of its own." The strengths of each collaborative partner are needed to develop the wellness clinic.*

**TABLE 8.8  Strengths and Challenges of an Asset-Based Approach**

| Strengths | Challenges |
|---|---|
| ▪ Helps people think positively about their circumstances | ▪ Requires financial investment |
| ▪ Helps to obtain a common view of what is important | ▪ Is initially time-consuming |
| ▪ Can be fun for the clients/participants involved | ▪ May be challenging emotionally and physically |
| ▪ Is realistic because it identifies what is already available | ▪ May be resisted if current practice is viewed as effective |
| ▪ Is inclusive | ▪ May identify assets that are not useable |
| ▪ Is a form of discovery | ▪ May highlight assets identified by various stakeholders, rather than by communities or individuals |
| ▪ Facilitates interdependencies | ▪ Proves difficult to sustain, particularly within the current political and socioeconomic climate |
| ▪ Centers on effectiveness | |
| ▪ Facilitates hearing and valuing others | |
| ▪ Provides the information necessary for the mobilization of assets | |
| ▪ Promotes the population as a producer of health, rather than as a service user | |
| ▪ Encourages people to realize their ability to contribute to the development of health | |
| ▪ Facilitates the identification of a range of health-promotion factors | |
| ▪ Helps to develop more sustainable initiatives | |
| ▪ Seeks to empower people | |
| ▪ Helps to identify ways for individuals to use their talents | |

*Source:* Whiting, Kendall, & Wills, 2012, pp. 27–28

## EVIDENCE EXAMPLE 8.3
### Asset Mapping

▪ The University of Chicago launched an initiative that employed local youth to conduct a block-by-block census of community assets on the South Side of Chicago. The population of the geographic area was primarily African American and Hispanic, with 32% living at poverty level and a 22% unemployment rate. Partnerships included three community-development organizations. College-age adults mentored and supervised 54 high school youth participants. Over 8,000 assets in 28 sectors or categories were identified in the census. The largest sectors were food, trade services, and religious worship. The project provided data about local assets that can be tapped to help build a Culture of Health by sharing language and principles (Lindau et al., 2016).

▪ An initiative to address childhood obesity used asset mapping to identify individual and community strengths in the targeted population, a public school district in upstate New York. The goal was to reduce television viewing time.

Partners in the initiative included childcare staff, school and college staff and faculty, primary healthcare staff, local businesses, social and faith-based organizations, the local library, and students from all educational levels. Partners networked to involve others in the community; community groups offered 40 different after-school and weekend activities in 11 public locations for preschool children and their families in a sponsored "TV turn off week." Community groups collaborated on a variety of family activities, such as sports, lessons, music, dancing, and arts and crafts. Outcomes based on feedback from questionnaires and partner debriefing sessions indicated that: 1) more parents enrolled their children in programs, which promoted physical activity (*individual/family level*); 2) the library decided to continue to offer storytelling hours (*community level*); and 3) childcare providers changed their policies for viewing media (*systems level*) (Baker et al., 2007).

## Ethical Application

When PHNs collaborate with other professionals, community members, and community organizations, ethical concerns often center on selecting interventions that promote social justice for vulnerable populations that have fewer resources for improving their health. However, as PHNs work to promote a healthier life for community members, they must also consider how community members are going to view and experience the interventions they develop. In addition, collaboration often requires courage to work with others who have different views and persistence to keep working together even amid disagreements and tension about the right way to proceed. All voices need to be heard in the decision-making process. In collaboration, an emphasis on community assets leads to inclusion, diversity, empowerment, and advocacy. See Table 8.9 for the application of ethical perspectives to collaboration.

### TABLE 8.9 Ethical Action in Collaboration

| Ethical Perspective | Application |
| --- | --- |
| Rule Ethics (principles) | ▪ The goal is beneficence or promoting good (improvement in health status) for the community and community members.<br>▪ Encourage autonomy of community members by ensuring that their perspectives contribute to determining interventions to improve health. |
| Virtue Ethics (character) | ▪ Be courageous in working with those with different views and perspectives.<br>▪ Be persistent in working through disagreements and tension in collaboration with others. |
| Feminist Ethics (reducing oppression) | ▪ Encourage including the voices of all stakeholders in the collaboration.<br>▪ Respect everyone.<br>▪ Strive for equality in the provision of programs and services.<br>▪ Emphasize community strengths.<br>▪ Advocate for individuals and community groups who have less power. |

"When Jake first started the community health course, he believed that, although important, the delivery of services to persons who were homeless was someone else's concern, not his. He also wondered why individuals who were homeless were included in the planning group. In the early meetings, he observed that the participants who represented the homeless population were very quiet, so many other members of the group were talking about what they thought homeless people wanted. In the third meeting, the police liaison who had emerged as the group's leader asked the members who represented the homeless population to offer their opinions on some of the ideas that had been expressed. He explained that they were "experts" on what it meant to be homeless and would therefore have good ideas about which services and resources would best help meet their health needs. The police liaison also did not back away from conflict but continued to emphasize the common goal of the group. In later meetings, participants who represented the homeless population began to share more about their experiences.

After being a part of the project and actually spending time with individuals who were homeless, Jake now understands why it is important to include people who have experienced homelessness in planning the clinic. The planning group empowers the group members who are homeless to participate as equal partners and take a leadership role in creating solutions.

As Jake provides foot care for a middle-age man one evening, the man shares his story of how he worked for a big company, lost his job as the company downsized, coped by drinking, lost his house and his family, and finally lost his sense of self-respect. As Jake reflects on this story, he concludes that each of us could find ourselves in a similar situation. Through collaboration, Jake realizes that a community can use its strengths and resources to make a difference."

Acknowledgment: Chapter narrative development by Joyce Bredesen, DNP, RN, PHN

## KEY POINTS

- PHNs collaborate with many partners, including other nurses, health professionals, lay workers, community members, healthcare and community organizations, businesses, and government organizations.
- When building interprofessional collaboration relationships, pay attention to the following: teamwork, communication practices, roles and responsibilities, and values.
- Effective partnerships share a common goal and require respect for and equality among partners.

- Partnership development requires trust between partners and a commitment to spend the time needed to develop that trust.
- Collaborative partnerships for promoting the Culture of Health and health of the public should work to have high levels of community engagement
- Collaborative partnerships should integrate community assets that contribute to the identification and design of intervention strategies in collaboration with community members.
- Tools for identifying community assets include community engagement and asset mapping.

## REFLECTIVE PRACTICE

Developing a clinic for the homeless is a complex project that involves many stakeholders and community organizations. Before partners begin to collaborate, reflecting on the goals of the collaborative project is essential. When partners are gathered together, they need to reach consensus on a shared goal. Now that you have learned about collaboration and the knowledge and skills needed to collaborate effectively, consider the following questions:

1. What does Jake need to consider about effective partnerships before collaborating to develop a clinic for the homeless?

2. Consider strategies for overcoming barriers to interprofessional collaboration. For the scenario about the clinic for the homeless, what do you see as possible barriers the team might encounter? What can they do to effectively manage those barriers?

3. What information about the population and community organizations will be needed for planning? What is an effective way to gather the information?

4. What would be important to include on the agenda for the first planning meeting?

5. What actions will support cross-sector collaboration?

6. How can the group explore individual and community assets that can be mobilized?

7. Which additional questions will you need to ask to partner effectively in developing a clinic for the homeless population? How will the group meaningfully engage all partners?

8. Refer to the Cornerstones of Public Health Nursing in Chapter 1. Which of the Cornerstones are consistent with and support the development of a clinic for individuals and families who are homeless?

After you have worked through these questions, develop an outline of possible partners and collaborative strategies. Propose relevant Public Health Intervention Wheel interventions and the level of each intervention that may be part of the expected outcome and action plan.

## APPLICATION OF EVIDENCE

1. Which responses would you expect from the planning group based on Tuckman's Theory of Normative Group Development (Tuckman, 1965)?

2. Which partnership guidelines would you apply to increase the likelihood of partnership success?

3. How could you use asset mapping or community engagement to achieve partnership goals?

# References

American Nurses Association. (2013). *Public health nursing: Scope and standards of practice.* Silver Spring, MD: Author.

Aston, M., Meagher-Stewart, D., Edwards, N., & Young, L. M. (2009). Public health nurses' primary health care practice: Strategies for fostering citizen participation. *Journal of Community Health Nursing, 26,* 24–34.

Bagnall, A. M., White, J., & South, J. (2017). Community engagement: What the NICE guidance means for community practitioners. *Primary Health Care, 27*(6), 29–33. doi:10.7748/phc.2017.e1192

Baker, I. R., Dennison, B. A., Boyer, P. S., Sellers, K. F., Russo, T. J., & Sherwood, N. A. (2007). An asset-based community initiative to reduce television viewing in New York state. *Preventive Medicine, 44*(5), 437–441. doi:10.1016/j.ypmed.2006.11.013

Bazarman, M. H. (Ed.). (2005). *Negotiating, decision making and conflict management.* Cheltenham, UK: Edward Elgar Publishing United.

Brewer, K. (2012). Making interprofessional teams work for nurses, patients. *American Nurse Today, 7*(3), 32–33.

Broussard, B. B. (2011). The bucket list: A service-learning approach to community engagement to enhance community health nursing clinical learning. *Journal of Nursing Education, 50*(1), 40–43. doi:10.3928/01484834-20100930-07

Campbell, L. A., Whitcomb, K., Culver, M., & McClanahan, C. (2015). Community engagement: Leveraging resources to improve health outcomes. *Nursing Administration Quarterly, 39,* E26–E30. doi:10.1097/NAQ

Casey, M. (2008). Partnership—Success factors of interorganizational relationships. *Journal of Nursing Management, 16,* 72–83. doi:10.1111/j.1365-2934.2007.00771.x

Clancy, A., Gressnes, T., & Svensson, T. (2012). Public health nursing and interprofessional collaboration in Norwegian municipalities: A questionnaire study. *Scandinavian Journal of Caring Sciences, 27*(3), 659–668. doi:10.1111/j.1471-6712.2012.01079.x

Community of Care. (2017). Community of care, Cass County, North Dakota. Retrieved from http://communityofcarend.com/

D'Amour, D., Ferrada-Videla, M., Rodriguez, L., & Beaulieu, M. (2005). The conceptual basis for interprofessional collaboration: Core concepts and theoretical frameworks. *Journal of Interprofessional Care, 19*(Suppl. 1), 116–131. doi:10.1080/13561820500082529

Drahota, A., Meza, R. D., Brikho, B., Naaf, M., Estabillo, J. A., Gomez, E. D., … Aarons, G. A. (2016). Community-academic partnerships: A systematic review of the state of the literature and recommendations for future research. *The Milbank Quarterly, 94*(1), 163–214. doi:10.1111/1468-0009.12184

Eckstrom, E., Neal, M. B., Cotrell, V., Casey, C. M., McKenzie, G., Morgove, M. W., . . . Lasater, K. (2016). An interprofessional approach to reducing the risk of falls through enhanced collaborative practice. *Journal of American Geriatrics Society, 64*(8), 1701–1707. doi:10.1111/jgs.14178

Fawcett, S., Schultz, J., Watson-Thompson, J., Fox, M., & Bremby, M. (2010). Building multisectoral partnerships for population health and health equity. *Preventing Chronic Disease, 7*(6), A118. Retrieved from http://www.cdc.gov/pcd/issues/2010/nov/10_0079.htm

Goldman, K. D., & Schmalz, K. J. (2005). "Accentuate the positive!" Using an asset-mapping tool as part of a community-health needs assessment. *Health Promotion Practice, 6*(2), 125–128. doi:10.1177/1524839904273344

Hamerlinck, J. (2013, March 18). *Map your assets.* Presentation given at Minnesota Campus Compact conference.

Henry Street Consortium. (2017). *Entry-level population-based public health nursing competencies.* St. Paul, MN: Author. Retrieved from www.henrystreetconsortium.org

International Council of Nurses. (2017). *Rural nursing, South Africa* [Case study]. Retrieved from https://www.icnvoicetolead.com/case-study/rural-nursing-south-africa/

Interprofessional Education Collaborative Expert Panel. (2011). *Core competencies for interprofessional collaborative practice: Report of an expert panel.* Washington, DC: Education Collaborative.

Keller, L. O., Strohschein, S., Lia-Hoagberg, B., & Schaffer, M. A. (2004). Population-based public health interventions: Practice-based and evidence-supported. Part 1. *Public Health Nursing, 21*(5), 453–468. doi:10.1111/j.0737-1209.2004.21509.x

Kretzmann, J. P., & McKnight, J. (1993). *Building communities from the inside out: A path toward finding and mobilizing a community's assets.* Chicago, IL: ACTA Publications.

KU Center for Community Health and Development. (2017). *Identifying community assets and resources.* Retrieved from http://ctb.ku.edu/en/table-of-contents/assessment/assessing-community-needs-and-resources/identify-community-assets/main

Libbey, P., & Miyahara, B. (2011). *Cross-jurisdictional relationships in local public health.* Retrieved from http://www.rwjf.org/content/dam/farm/reports/reports/2011/rwjf69317

Lindau, S. T., Vickery, K. D., Choi, H., Makelarski, J., Matthews, A., & Davis, M. (2016). A community-powered, asset-based approach to intersectoral urban health system planning in Chicago. *American Journal of Public Health, 106*(10), 1872–1878. doi:10.2105/AJPH.2016.303302

Mattessich, P. W., & Rausch, E. J. (2014). Cross-sector collaboration to improve community health: A view of the current landscape. *Health Affairs, 33*(11), 1968–1974. doi:10.1377/hlthaff.2014.0645

Morgan, A., & Ziglio, E. (2010). Revitalising the public health evidence base: An asset model. In A. Morgan, E. Ziglio, & M. Davies (Eds.), *Health Assets in a Global Context* (pp. 3–16). doi:10.1007/978-1-4419-5921-8_1

National Institutes of Health. (2011). *Principles of community engagement* (2nd ed.). NIH Publication No. 11-7782. Retrieved from https://www.atsdr.cdc.gov/communityengagement/index.html

Potter, K., & Willis, J. (2013). Community development and building capacity. In D. Sines, S. Aldridge-Bent, A. Fanning, P. Farrelly, K. Potter, & J. Wright (Eds.), *Community and public health nursing* (5th ed., pp. 22–35). Hoboken, NJ: Wiley-Blackwell.

Robert Wood Johnson Foundation. (2015). Measuring what matters: Introducing a new action framework. Retrieved from https://www.rwjf.org/en/blog/2015/11/measuring_what_matte.html

Schoon, P. M., Champlin, B., & Hunt, R. (2012). Developing a sustainable foot care clinic in a homeless shelter within an academic-community partnership through curricular integration and faculty engagement. *Journal of Nursing Education, 51*(12), 714–718. doi:10.3928/01484834-20121112-02

Snow, L. K. (2004). *The power of asset mapping.* Herndon, VA: Alban Institute.

Towne, K. M., & Valedes, R. (2017). Nurse partnerships across the public health system. *Nursing Management, 48*(1), 15–17. doi:10.1097/01.numa.0000511186.41289.5a

Trujillo, M. D., & Plough, A. (2016). Building a culture of health: A new framework and measures for health and health care in America. *Social Science & Medicine, 165,* 206–213. doi:10.1016/j.socscimed.2016.06.043

Tuckman, B. W. (1965). Development sequences in small groups. *Psychology Bulletin, 63*(6), 384–399.

Twin Cities Mobile Market. (2017). About the Twin Cities Mobile Market. Retrieved from https://www.wilder.org/Programs-Services/tcmm/Pages/default.aspx

Wellstone.org. (1999). *Sheet metal workers speech.* Speech by Paul Wellstone. Retrieved from http://www.wellstone.org/legacy/speeches/sheet-metal-workers-speech

Whiting, L., Kendall, S., & Wills, W. (2012). An asset-based approach: An alternative health promotion strategy? *Community Practitioner, 85*(1), 25–28.

Wilson, F., & Mabhala, M. (Eds.). (2009). *Key concepts in public health.* London, UK: Sage Publications.

World Health Organization. (2010). *Framework for action on interprofessional education and collaborative practice.* Retrieved from http://whqlibdoc.who.int/hq/2010/WHO_HRH_HPN_10.3_eng.pdf

# COMPETENCY #7

## Effectively Communicates With Communities, Systems, Individuals, Families, and Colleagues

■ **Marjorie A. Schaffer**

*with Raney Linck, Linda J. W. Anderson, Carol J. Roth, and Desiree Holmquist*

> *On the first day of public health clinical, the PHN preceptor, Gail, has three nursing students pull up the latest report on sexually transmitted diseases (STDs) from the Centers for Disease Control (CDC, 2016). The facts are startling. The U.S. now has the highest total number of cases of chlamydia, gonorrhea, and syphilis in its history. However, in recent years, more than half of state and local STD programs have had budget cuts. "Since our STD clinic has closed due to funding cuts, I really need your help in creating a prevention and treatment campaign."*
>
> *Gail is clear about the urgency. "Chlamydia is the most commonly reported communicable disease in our region. The incidence has quadrupled since 1996. In addition, our region has seen a recent spike in babies born with congenital syphilis." She explains that the ideal campaign would include a poster for people waiting in the public health clinic and some sort of social media outreach to promote awareness of STDs and sexual health.*
>
> *The three students assess their own strengths. Emily gives great presentations in class, Hannah is a skilled writer of academic papers, and Darius is the "techie" of their group. They review their materials for population-based health nursing competency #7, which focuses on communication. They realize that clearly defining their target audiences is key, including learning about their values, needs, and health literacy. Unique aspects of writing and creating a poster and pamphlet need to be considered. Emily wants to create a short online presentation and needs to explore digital tools (such as PowerPoint, VoiceThread, YouTube, podcasts, and Prezi). Darius quickly finds many online resources but needs to evaluate them carefully for accuracy, functionality, and relevance to the specific audience.*

---

### STUDENT NOTEBOOK

**COMPETENCY #7  Effectively Communicates With Communities, Systems, Individuals, Families, and Colleagues**

A. Interacts respectfully, sensitively, and effectively with everyone

B. Utilizes sound teaching/learning strategies that tailor communication to target individual, family, community, organizational, or system audiences

C. Selects appropriate communication methods to reach target audience(s)

D. Presents accurate demographic, statistical, programmatic, and scientific information

*Source:* Henry Street Consortium, 2017

*(continues)*

## STUDENT NOTEBOOK (continued)

### USEFUL DEFINITIONS

**Health Literacy:** "The degree to which individuals have the capacity to obtain, process, and understand basic health information and services needed to make appropriate health decisions" (Ratzan & Parker, 2000, p. 36).

**Motivational Interviewing:** A counseling technique that focuses on behavioral change through emphasizing a side-by-side companionable approach that supports the client's own values and reasons for change, in contrast to a traditional approach of expert provider and passive recipient (Miller, 2004).

**Social Marketing:** The use of "commercial marketing principles and technologies, for programs developed to influence the knowledge, attitudes, values, beliefs, behaviors, and practices of the population of interest" (Keller, Strohschein, Lia-Hoagberg, & Schaffer, 2004, p. 456).

**Tailoring:** Using information about client characteristics to design communication of content that is more relevant to the client (Hawkins, Kreuter, Resnicow, Fishbein, & Dijkstra, 2008).

**Targeting:** Messages are designed to reach a specific population sub-group (Schmid, Rivers, Latimer, & Salovey, 2008).

---

Learning communication strategies for working with individuals and families is an essential component of your nursing education. You often learn about communicating with colleagues as you focus on leadership strategies, teamwork, and delegation in a leadership course. However, strategies for communicating with communities and systems involve additional skills, including applying teaching/learning principles that integrate knowledge about the learner (individual or community), learning how to clearly organize and present data and health information, and using technology in communication.

## How Do Public Health Nurses Interact Respectfully, Sensitively, and Effectively With Everyone?

PHNs use a repertoire of basic communication skills in all their work. Effective interpersonal communication, involving the use of self, is especially essential for counseling and health teaching interventions. The intention of this type of communication is to empower clients to participate in decisions about their health. Keep in mind that the client might be an individual, a family, or a community group. The following list contains tips for effective communication with individuals and families:

- Use active listening.
- Model "I" messages (I think…, I feel…).
- Paraphrase and summarize the client's statement to confirm its meaning.
- Pay attention to silence and nonverbal communication.

- Consider the client's comfort with degree of physical space between persons.
- Ask open-ended questions.
- Consider how cultural traditions, values, beliefs, and practices of both client and PHN influence health communication.
- Provide language assistance to individuals and families with limited English proficiency.
- Consider the context of the communication environment—protect privacy and confidentiality.
- Use touch if it enhances the communication and is acceptable to the client.

*Sources:* Green, 2006; Kreuter, Lukwago, Bucholtz, Clark, & Sanders-Thompson, 2003; Minnesota Department of Health, 2001

PHNs also may need to communicate with clients through the assistance of a trained interpreter. Table 9.1 suggests strategies for working with interpreters.

Developing relationships can be challenging for PHNs in situations where clients and families may not see a need for involvement with public health nursing services. When individuals and families do perceive a need for assistance, PHNs still need to negotiate a relationship that empowers clients to make decisions for improving their health.

The development of a trusting, purposeful, and goal-directed relationship that protects client dignity, autonomy, and privacy is an important foundation for effective communication of health information (National Council of State Boards of Nursing, 2014; Registered Nurses' Association of Ontario [RNAO], 2002/2006). Expert knowledge in the following areas contributes to PHNs' capacity to develop

**TABLE 9.1  Tips for Working With Interpreters**

| Situation | Tips |
|---|---|
| Prior to Face-to-Face Meetings | ■ If possible, meet with the interpreter before the meeting to clarify technical terms, provide any written materials, and discuss seating arrangements. |
| | ■ Brief the interpreter about the client's data privacy rights. |
| During the Meeting | ■ Identify the role of the interpreter with the client(s). |
| | ■ Place the interpreter in the client's sight line. |
| | ■ Provide good lighting so the interpreter can be seen. |
| | ■ Speak at your normal pace. Interpreters will ask you to slow down or repeat if necessary. |
| | ■ Speak in first person—speak to the interviewee, not the interpreter. |
| | ■ Enunciate your words, but do not use a loud voice. |
| | ■ Use short sentences and group your thoughts—ask only one question at a time. |
| | ■ Use words, not gestures, to convey the meaning of words/phrases. |
| | ■ Avoid acronyms, jargon, and technical terms—explain terms. |
| | ■ Remember to pause and ask if there is understanding or a need for clarification, and be prepared to restate the questions in a different way if you are misunderstood. |
| | ■ Watch for nonverbal signs—excessive head nodding, smiling, or nervous laughter can be cues that the message was not understood. |
| | ■ Avoid private conversations—everything will be interpreted. |
| | ■ One person should speak at a time. If you are facilitating a group discussion, be aware that the interpreter will be several seconds behind. |
| | ■ Avoid asking the interpreter for opinions or comments regarding the content of the meeting. |
| | ■ Provide a short break every hour. |
| | ■ Say "thank you" to both the client(s) and the interpreter. |
| After the Meeting | ■ Have a brief post-meeting interview with the interpreter to assess the meeting. |
| | ■ Document outcomes of the meeting. |

*Sources:* D. Holmquist (personal communication, September 2017); Minnesota Department of Human Services, 2005

effective relationships: interpersonal caring and development theory; culture, diversity influences, and determinants of health; health/illness; the broad influences on healthcare and healthcare policy; and systems (RNAO, 2002/2006).

Consider what it means to have a "therapeutic alliance," which focuses on collaboration in communication. A *therapeutic alliance* happens when the client and the PHN interact collaboratively to determine goals for improved health through a respectful and trusting relationship. This sets the stage for client readiness to receive health information and, consequently, take action in response to the health information (Spiers & Wood, 2010; Zugai, Stein, & Roche, 2015).

For the examples in Evidence Example 9.1, consider how attention to relationship development contributes to client responses.

## Motivational Interviewing: A Strategy for Health Behavior Change

PHNs use motivational interviewing (MI) to encourage positive health behaviors (VanBuskirk & Wetherell, 2014). *Motivational interviewing* is a specific kind of counseling strategy in which the professional helps clients become aware of their values and the reasons they might have for changing their behaviors. The purpose of MI is to encourage clients to move away from behaviors that hurt their health toward behaviors that improve their health. The collaborative approach of MI is a dialogue, in contrast to giving advice or instruction (Harvard Medical School, 2011). The Stages of Change Model is useful for guiding communication to motivate clients to adopt healthy behaviors.

## EVIDENCE EXAMPLE 9.1
### Developing Relationships

■ Harden (2010) summarized evidence on relationship-building in programs that provide home visiting to psychologically vulnerable families characterized by child maltreatment, mental health challenges, or other psychological risks. Relationships between families and home visitors are critical for engaging families in the home visiting program and contributing to positive outcomes. These relationships are based on trust, empathy, responsiveness, and nonjudgmental and optimistic attitudes from the home visitor. Evidence shows that building relationships with high-risk families who have had negative experiences with past service providers requires patience, creativity, and persistence in relationship-building. In addition, matching home visitors and families who have similar backgrounds, culture, and language may improve family engagement.

■ In a qualitative study in Norway, Glavin and Saeteren (2016) explored the experiences of ten new Somali mothers with their perinatal care. PHNs provided home visits and saw new mothers and their infants in the well child clinics. Somali mothers reported PHNs were available for questions, explained everything, and were "kind" and "good." Through interviews, the researchers discovered that the new mothers had poor language skills and were not well integrated into Norwegian society. They recommended that PHNs should use an interpreter and encourage new mothers to learn the Norwegian language. The researchers recommended that integration into Norwegian society could be facilitated by offering immigrant mothers the opportunity to participate in maternity groups at the well child clinics, which could strengthen social relationships.

■ In a community level example, PHNs effectively used relationships in risk communication when they provided counseling sessions for mothers of children at health check-ups in Fukushima City, Japan, following the 2011 nuclear disaster. PHNs provided information on radiation risks and addressed mothers' concerns for child safety. They supported residents in making informed decisions and empowered them to take an active role in understanding the risks in their environment (Goto et al., 2014).

## THEORY APPLICATION
### Stages of Change (Transtheoretical Model)

The Stages of Change Model is applicable to both individual behavior change and organizational change. Although there are five stages—see Table 9.2—clients may cycle back to earlier stages.

PHNs can determine the relevant step of behavior change the client is experiencing and then use MI to encourage the client to change health behaviors. Some clients might move through these steps quickly, whereas others might remain at one step for a longer period of time. The PHN follows the clients' cues in MI, because the emphasis is on empowering clients to make decisions that benefit their health. "Empowerment is a process of increasing personal, interpersonal, or political power so that individuals, families, and communities can take action to improve their situations" (Holcomb-McCoy & Bryan, 2010, p. 262).

Richardson (2012) identified five MI strategies for encouraging positive health changes in interactions with individuals, families, and communities:

1. **Express empathy:** Understand client perspectives
2. **Reduce ambivalence:** Evaluate pros and cons of behavior and change
3. **Develop discrepancies:** Explore conflict between current behavior and important goals and values
4. **Roll with resistance:** Acknowledge feelings, accept ambivalence, stay calm, address discrepancy
5. **Support self-efficacy:** Recognize strengths and support ability to change

These five strategies are consistent with the Stages of Change Model. The example in Table 9.3 illustrates the use of MI strategies with a pregnant adolescent who smokes.

MI is also an effective strategy for community-level interventions. Table 9.4 applies MI strategies in a community-level counseling intervention to address youth depression and the potential for suicide. In this example, the PHN meets with a task force that is addressing the problem of an increased incidence of youth suicide in the community.

It will take practice to develop expertise and comfort with the motivational interviewing process. Pfister-Minogue and Salveson (2010) describe a tool called the Behavior Change Counseling Index (BECCI) that PHNs can use to evaluate interactions to support health behavior change. The tool is an 11-item measure that uses a 5-point Likert scale designed to evaluate practitioner competence in the use of counseling skills. An evaluation of the effectiveness, feasibility, and usefulness of this tool revealed that training PHNs in using the tool helped to increase their communication skills, but they also reported they needed additional training to reach a mastery level in motivational interviewing practice.

### TABLE 9.2 Stages of Health Behavior Change

| Stage | Definition | Change Strategies |
|---|---|---|
| 1. Precontemplation | Has no intention of taking action | Increase awareness of need for change; address specific risks and benefits from client viewpoint |
| 2. Contemplation | Intends to take action but is ambivalent about change | Motivate by encouraging client to make a specific action plan |
| 3. Preparation | Intends to take action and has taken small steps toward change | Collaboratively set gradual goals for a concrete action plan |
| 4. Action | Has made behavior change | Provide feedback, support, and reinforcement |
| 5. Maintenance | Continues to sustain the behavior change | Determine coping strategies, provide reminders, determine alternative actions and strategies to avoid relapses to previous behavior patterns |

*Source:* Rimer & Glanz, 2005

### TABLE 9.3 Application of MI Strategies to Individual Level

| Motivational Interviewing Strategy | Client Statement | PHN Statement |
|---|---|---|
| Express empathy | I started smoking when I was 15. | It can be difficult to stop smoking, because the body is dependent on the nicotine in tobacco. |
| Reduce ambivalence | Smoking helps me relax. | Yes, there are some benefits as well as drawbacks that happen from smoking. |
| Develop discrepancies | I know I should stop smoking. | What have you learned about why it is important to quit smoking during pregnancy or around your baby? |
| Roll with resistance | I don't really think it is so bad. My best friend smoked during her pregnancy, and her baby is fine. | I'm glad to hear your friend's baby is OK. Let's take a look at how smoking might affect your baby's health. |
|  | I just don't know if I can quit. I have so much going on in my life—smoking helps me feel more relaxed. | I would like to hear more about other things that help you relax. |
| Support self-efficacy | I wish I could quit smoking. | It is your choice. What do you think you can do to have a healthy baby? |

### TABLE 9.4 Application of MI Strategies to Community Level

| Action | Example |
|---|---|
| Express empathy | Acknowledge that community organizations serving youth are upset about the increase in incidence of youth suicide. |
| Reduce ambivalence | Discuss the pros and cons of increasing community awareness about youth depression and suicide by using social media. |
| Develop discrepancy | Encourage dialogue about the increasing incidence of youth suicide in the community and its connection to the silence surrounding the occurrence of depression. |
| Roll with resistance | When different viewpoints and strong emotions surface in discussions about responses to youth depression and suicide, listen to everyone's voices, stay calm, and address evidence that supports promotion of community awareness. |
| Support self-efficacy | Work with team/experts to communicate success of strategies in promoting community awareness about youth depression and suicide. |

---

### EVIDENCE EXAMPLE 9.2

**Effectiveness of Motivational Interviewing**

▪ A quasi-experimental study on the use of MI to improve diabetes outcomes in African-American adults demonstrated significant improvements in following recommended physical activity levels, glucose levels, and body mass index in comparison with the usual care group. The experimental group received a maximum of six MI sessions over 3 months (Chlebowy et al., 2015).

▪ A meta-analysis of 119 studies compared the effect of MI with other counseling interventions on outcomes. Authors determined there is a low risk in implementing MI. They found MI was as effective across a range of health problems as with other interventions and was shorter in length (Lundahl, Kunz, Brownell, Tollefson, & Burke, 2010).

## How Do Teaching-Learning Strategies Guide Communication of Health Information?

Teaching-learning principles are useful for making choices about effective methods to deliver health information content to individuals, families, communities, and systems.

PHNs provide health teaching to promote better health for their clients. Their goal is to motivate clients to learn about ways to promote their own health and then act on that knowledge. Teaching/learning principles help you assess how the learner learns so that you can plan the content and teaching method that best fits the client situation (see Table 9.5).

### VARK Theory

Assessing client learning styles helps the PHN develop effective educational strategies. The VARK theory of learning styles identifies four preferred learning styles:

▪ **V**isual
▪ **A**uditory
▪ **R**ead or write
▪ **K**inesthetic (touch and manipulation)

Being aware of individual styles helps the nurse choose teaching methods. PHNs can assess client learning styles using the VARK online learning assessment questionnaire (http://vark-learn.com/the-vark-questionnaire). Many individuals are multimodal and may not have one clear learning style preference. It is also important to realize that a preference for a particular learning style does not necessarily mean that is always the way one learns best, so it is important to incorporate multiple modalities in patient education (Inott & Kenney, 2011).

## TABLE 9.5 Teaching-Learning Principles

| Learning Principle | Explanation |
| --- | --- |
| Preparation | ▪ Target health education messages to the specific audience rather than trying to cover all information.<br>▪ Base content on best evidence: Review literature for most recent evidence-based information. Give credit to information sources.<br>▪ Assess learner readiness: health status, health values, developmental characteristics, prior learning experiences.<br>▪ Evaluate learner motivation: Use life goals, self-concept, responsibility, quality of life, and other factors that can "hook" and are meaningful to the learner.<br>▪ Link information to prior knowledge. |
| Process | ▪ Use learning objectives to guide your teaching plan. Objectives should be Specific, Measurable, Attainable, Relevant/Realistic, Time-bound (SMART).<br>▪ Create a comfortable learning environment that is free from distractions and interruptions. (Ask your client to turn off the TV.)<br>▪ Allow time for interaction to apply information.<br>▪ Send a clear message that is easily understood. Avoid overwhelming the learner with excess materials. Avoid professional jargon. Use short sentences and simple, one- and two-syllable words.<br>▪ When possible, integrate a variety of learning styles to deliver content, making sure to reinforce written materials with verbal messages.<br>▪ Use multiple methods to assess understanding of content, such as questioning and demonstration. |

*Sources:* Braungart, Braungart, & Gramet, 2014; Kolb, 1984, 2005; Lancaster, 2016

## ASSURE Model

The ASSURE Model is a useful guide for planning health teaching interventions (Bastable, 2017). This model has six steps:

1. **A**nalyze the learner
2. **S**tate the objectives
3. **S**elect the instructional methods and materials
4. **U**tilize materials
5. **R**equire learner performance
6. **E**valuate the teaching plan and revise as necessary

See Table 9.6 for additional information on how to implement the steps of the ASSURE Model.

## How Does Health Literacy Affect Client Understanding?

To ensure client understanding, PHNs consider the health literacy of the intended target audience. *Health literacy* is defined as "the degree to which individuals have the capacity to obtain, process, and understand basic health information and services needed to make appropriate health decisions" (Ratzan & Parker, 2000, p. 36). Health literacy is complex, involving not only reading and writing, but also listening, speaking, and math skills. Cultural meaning in the context of healthcare is also an important component of health literacy (Institute of Medicine, 2004).

Individuals with limited health literacy may be less likely to engage in effective self-care and prevention practices, have

**TABLE 9.6  The ASSURE Model for Planning, Implementing, and Evaluating Health Teaching Interventions**

| ASSURE Model | Health Teaching Activities | |
|---|---|---|
| **Analyze the learner** (*Source:* Modified by Patricia M. Schoon (2013) from St. Catherine University, 2008. Developed by Lois Devereaux, Karen Ryan, and Patricia M. Schoon.) | PEEK Learner Readiness Assessment | |
| | 1. **Physical and Developmental Health Status**<br> ■ Cognitive abilities<br> ■ Communication abilities (verbal, nonverbal, written)<br> ■ Developmental level<br> ■ Individual<br> ■ Family<br> ■ Physical environment<br><br>2. **Emotional**<br> ■ Current stress, coping, resilience<br> ■ Motivation for learning<br> ■ Readiness for learning | 3. **Experiential and Social**<br> ■ Culture and language<br> ■ Cultural health beliefs and practices<br> ■ Past experiences with healthcare and specific health topics<br><br>4. **Knowledge**<br> ■ Educational/reading level<br> ■ Language literacy and learning style<br> ■ Present knowledge on topic/past health education<br> ■ Health literacy |
| **State the objectives** SMART (CDC, 2015) | Stated outcomes should be:<br> ■ Specific  ■ Attainable  ■ Time-bound<br> ■ Measurable  ■ Realistic | |
| **Select the instructional methods and materials** | When selecting methods, review teaching-learning principles and consider client learning styles before developing a teaching plan. | |
| **Utilize materials** | Implement the teaching plan<br> ■ Schedule (reasonable time allotted for each activity)<br> ■ Location (distraction-free, adequate room, lighting, comfort)<br> ■ Learner outcomes (achievable and measurable within timeframe)<br> ■ Brief content outline (main topics with learning activities)<br> ■ Teaching-learning strategies (consider learning styles of individual or group)<br> ■ Resources (materials and references)<br> ■ Evaluation (specific and measurable) | |

*(continues)*

**TABLE 9.6  The ASSURE Model for Planning, Implementing, and Evaluating Health Teaching Interventions** *(continued)*

| ASSURE Model | Health Teaching Activities |
|---|---|
| Require learner performance | Design teaching to include learner engagement (Yardley, Morrison, Bradbury, & Muller, 2015). |
| | ▪ Promote client autonomy by offering choices where possible (goals, tools, timing, and method of implementation). |
| | ▪ Promote client competence by providing clear structure and guidance, examples, stories, modeling, and opportunities for goal-setting. |
| | ▪ Promote a positive emotional experience and sense of relatedness by using positive language; acknowledging and addressing concerns; creating communications that are enjoyable, relevant, and helpful to the user; and providing immediate and rewarding feedback. |
| Evaluate the teaching plan and revise as necessary | Questions to ask: |
| | ▪ Were the objectives achieved? |
| | ▪ What strategies contributed to successful achievement of the objectives? |
| | ▪ If the objectives were not achieved, what barriers or factors interfered with learning? |
| | ▪ What could be done differently to achieve the outcomes? |

increased risk for hospitalization, and have worse outcomes than those with higher levels of health literacy (Bastable & Alt, 2014; Berkman, Sheridan, Donahue, Halpern, & Crotty, 2011). Although the public health nursing student may assume that particular patient groups, such as immigrants and the elderly, have more challenges with health literacy, any patient may be overwhelmed with health information during a time of stress (Agency for Healthcare Research and Quality [AHRQ], 2017).

To promote patient understanding and the ability to follow through on health recommendations and treatment plans, providers should communicate with all patients in ways that anyone can understand. The Agency for Healthcare Research and Quality (AHRQ) has developed the Health Literacy Universal Precautions Toolkit to provide evidence-based tools that promote health literacy for all patients. Universal Health Literacy Precautions focus on preventing miscommunication by using clear communication strategies, simplifying navigation of the healthcare system, and supporting client efforts to improve their health (AHRQ, 2017).

Communicating clearly is important to promote client understanding. The AHRQ Toolkit recommends the following strategies for clear communication (AHRQ, 2015):

▪ Welcome patients warmly

▪ Make culturally appropriate eye contact

▪ Listen, pay attention, and be responsive

▪ Use nonmedical language

▪ Use the patient's words

▪ Speak slowly and clearly

▪ Limit information and repeat content

▪ Be specific and concrete

▪ Use simple graphics

▪ Demonstrate how it's done

▪ Encourage questions

▪ Have clients teach back important information

Patients of all health literacy levels rely on healthcare providers to provide and interpret health information. They tend to prefer to receive information directly from their provider (Gutierrez, Kindratt, Pagels, Foster, & Gimpel, 2014). However, as personal health records are increasingly posted to the Internet, patients may need to be able to access health records through an online portal or chart. Those with limited health literacy are more likely to have limited access to a computer and the Internet. They are also more likely to have difficulty navigating an online chart (Sarkar et al., 2010). If the patient does not have sufficient Internet access or health literacy to access and understand online information, the PHN should make sure health information is communicated in ways that are most acceptable to the client.

The Internet is also an important source of health information. However, clients may have difficulty evaluating what is quality information. PHNs can provide information about how to make good choices about online health information. Questions to be asked when evaluating online information include:

▪ Is it up-to-date? Websites and apps will provide a date of release.

▪ Whose name is on it, and who provides it? Sponsors of a site may have interests that conflict with the client.

▪ Is the information accurate? Carefully consider sources, especially if they direct the consumer to a particular product.

▪ Do apps and devices work as advertised? Look for unbiased reviews.

▪ Are the tools easy to use?

## EVIDENCE EXAMPLE 9.3
### Improving Health Literacy for Interpreting a Complex Environmental Message

A partnership was initiated in New Hampshire to communicate the potential health effects of well water to rural residents. The Tuftonboro Conservation Commission (TCC), partnering with state agencies and a college, aimed to increase water testing rates by citizens living in an area with a high number of wells. TCC addressed barriers to health literacy by designing an information campaign that provided stories about local residents who experienced well-water contamination along with clear and simple facts about health effects. TCC also addressed the barrier of inconvenience by providing water testing kits and transporting samples to the lab, which reduced the effort required from citizens to conduct well-water testing. Although there was no follow-up with households, as a result of the initiative, more water tests were done in 1 day at the state laboratory than had occurred over the past 6 years (Paul, Rigrod, Wingate, & Borsuk, 2015).

**TABLE 9.7  Factors Influencing Choice Between Targeting and Tailoring**

| Targeting | Tailoring |
|---|---|
| ■ Behavior is simple | ■ Behavior is very complex, may involve lifestyle changes |
| ■ Resources for high-cost campaign are not available | ■ Resources for high-cost campaign are available |
| ■ There is little variability of behavioral determinants (e.g., diet, physical activity, handwashing, substance use), or determinants are not understood | ■ There is a large variability of behavioral determinants |
| ■ Mechanisms do not exist for individual assessment | ■ Mechanisms exist for assessments of target population |

*Source:* Schmid et al., 2008, p. 8

## EVIDENCE EXAMPLE 9.4
### Targeting a Specific Population

Taxicab drivers in Chicago, Illinois, were targeted for a free influenza vaccination program in airport taxicab lots. The Chicago Department of Public Health provided the vaccine. Experienced volunteers were recruited from the University of Chicago Medicine. The volunteer team included a Spanish translator, and informational materials were available in English, Spanish, and Arabic. The targeted, low-cost campaign reached an underserved, primarily uninsured population. Authors recommended strengthening education initiatives to reduce misconceptions and vaccine hesitancy in the taxicab driver population (Limper, Burns, & Alexander, 2016).

■ Does a tool or resource work with other tools?

■ Is it secure? Does it protect your privacy?

To learn more about evaluating online health information, the PHN student should use resources, such as The National Library of Medicine tutorial, for evaluating for Internet health information (https://medlineplus.gov/webeval/webeval.html).

In Evidence Example 9.3, storytelling motivated citizens to take action. A resource for telling stories to motivate action is the *Toolkit for Developing a Public Narrative: Using Powerful Storytelling to Motivate Action,* found at https://www.rethinkhealth.org/resources/public-narrative-toolkit/. Stories "draw out emotions, build alignment, and motivate stakeholders" (para. 1), which contributes to mobilizing people to take action to improve their health.

## What Is the Difference Between Targeting and Tailoring Health Information?

When targeting audiences, health information is crafted for specific population sub-groups based on characteristics of that population. Tailoring health messages involves customizing health information based on assessment of individuals or a group. Several factors determine whether targeting or tailoring of health information is the preferred method for communicating health information. These factors include resources, the size of the audience, and the complexity of the desired behavior change (Schmid et al., 2008). Table 9.7 contrasts targeting and tailoring approaches to disseminating health communication.

Kreuter and colleagues (2003) discuss targeted and tailored approaches for "cultural appropriateness" in health-promotion programs. Common strategies for moving toward cultural appropriateness when targeting specific cultural groups include:

■ Package the materials to appeal to a cultural group.

■ Present the evidence of the health impact on a group.

■ Make the language accessible to the group.

■ Involve lay community members in planning and decision-making about materials.

■ Integrate social and cultural values of the intended audience.

An assumption in targeting messages is that there is similarity among members of the population since one approach is used to communicate health information. Although culture may be a shared characteristic of the population, individuals within that population may have differing views about their culture. In this case, cultural tailoring can be used to design health-promotion interventions based on individual needs. Many resources for adapting health information are available through the National Culturally and Linguistically Appropriate Services Standards. This government website features information and strategies on cultural and linguistically appropriate services (CLAS) for health professionals (https://www.thinkculturalhealth. hhs.gov/).

---

### EVIDENCE EXAMPLE 9.5
#### Cultural Tailoring

A cognitive-behavioral intervention to reduce the risk of antepartum depression was adapted for African-American, Caucasian, and Hispanic pregnant women who lived in the rural southeastern United States. The intervention, developed based on focus groups with ethnic sub-groups, included psychological and pregnancy-specific information in a manual; recordings of stress-reducing strategies, inspirational music, and motivational messages; and the opportunity for women to record their own responses. The African American women wanted a positive, nonjudgmental facilitator they could trust and access to spiritual-related resources. The Caucasian women asked for educational information and support. The Hispanic women asked for advice on how they could avoid feeling sad and wanted strategies to distract them from problems. Compared with the usual care group, high-risk African-American women who participated in the cognitive-behavioral intervention had reduced symptoms of depression (Jesse et al., 2015).

> *Emily, Hannah, and Darius are ready to design their poster and digital presentation. They learned chlamydia is highest among 15- to 25-year-olds, but incidence has increased across all gender, age, and geographical groups. They realize they need to ask their public health nursing preceptor to evaluate their plan. They are not sure about the reading level of the population group who will be viewing the poster, but know their preceptor is familiar with the population.*

### Activity

Design a layout for the poster on STDs (including chlamydia) for the public health clinic. Consider the following questions:

- How could the students learn more about the population served by the public health clinic?
- Which teaching-learning principles should the students keep in mind as they design the poster?
- Discuss why targeting is a useful approach for designing the poster.

## What Communications Methods Work Best to Reach the Target Audience?

PHNs have a great variety of methods that work well to communicate health messages. Effectiveness depends on many factors, including the size of the audience, client preferences, learning readiness, and the availability of tools and technology. It is a challenge to create simple, accurate, and concise written information. In some settings, PHNs might work with a media or graphic design specialist to communicate clear, captivating, and motivating health messages.

---

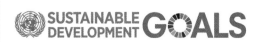 SUSTAINABLE DEVELOPMENT GOALS

**Nurse Family Partnership**

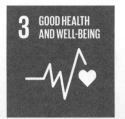 3 GOOD HEALTH AND WELL-BEING

**GOAL 3** Through Nurse Family Partnership (NFP) programs, PHNs provide home visiting, support, and education to low-income mothers. NFP programs have been established across the United States and in other countries. In this example, PHNs provide services to mothers of young children in urban Philadelphia, Pennsylvania. The population receiving services, primarily teen mothers, is African American (73%) or Hispanic (21%) with an average annual household income under US$6,000. The Blue Wedge interventions of health teaching, counseling, and consultation are emphasized in the PHN role in the NFP program (Minnesota Department of Health, 2001). "The expertise that PHNs bring to this intervention is pivotal in gaining the confidence of a new mother. The nurse helps guide first-time mothers through the emotional, social, and physical challenges they face as they prepare for a healthy birth. Prenatal support is the starting point, but the nurse continues to serve her client after she delivers her child, teaching parenting and life skills that foster positive growth for both the mother and child" (International Council of Nurses, 2017).

Often, larger public health departments have a communications specialist whom the PHN can consult for ideas and strategies. Effective messages result from clear and simple writing, a layout that enhances readability, and images that enhance the message. The following list offers tips for designing and formatting written messages, which can take many forms such as pamphlets, handouts, PowerPoint presentations, and online materials.

- Know the intended audience. Use culturally appropriate language, images, and concepts.

- Identify key message(s), and have no more than three or four.

- Write in a conversational style using active voice rather than passive to clearly state actions you want the audience to take. For example, say, "Eat five servings of fruits and vegetables," rather than saying, "Five servings of fruits and vegetables should be eaten."

- Use headings, subheadings, and chunked text.

- Use lists/bullet points to break up text.

- Make sentences simple and relatively short.

- Choose simple words and plain language. Avoid using jargon, acronyms, or abbreviations.

- Explain unfamiliar terms.

- Summarize main points to improve understanding.

- Use large, easily readable font.

- Use boldface to emphasize key points rather than italic, caps, or underlining.

- Avoid large blocks of information. Use white space to provide a more inviting, readable design.

- Ensure that paper and ink contrast.

- Use visuals to support the text. Pictures help grab attention and highlight the key message.

- Include links that clearly explain the content of the web page links.

*Sources:* CDC, 2014; Centers for Medicare and Medicaid Services (CMS), 2012; Office of Disease Prevention and Health Promotion, 2016; PlainLanguage.gov, 2011; U.S. DHHS, 2004

# Using Social Marketing Skills

In the mid-20th century, a question emerged: Is it possible to successfully market positive health behaviors in the same way as commercial products?

By the early 1970s, the answer proved to be yes, and this approach came to be known as *social marketing* (McAlindon, 2017). Keller et al. (2004) define it as the use of "commercial marketing principles and technologies, for programs developed to influence the knowledge, attitudes, values, beliefs, behaviors, and practices of the population

of interest" (p. 456). Programs can address a wide array of health issues, including smoking, obesity, heart disease, sexual behaviors, and violence. Systematic reviews of over 200 studies in the U.S. and globally have demonstrated that social marketing programs can effectively change population behaviors and provide a useful tool for organizations engaged in change work (Firestone, Rowe, Modi, & Sievers, 2016; Stead, Gordon, Angus, & McDermott, 2007).

Successful marketing always has a customer orientation—truly understanding the audience. Audiences are diverse—not all teens are alike, neither are all the elderly. Marketing engages in audience *segmentation*—a process of classifying a population into distinct groups that behave in similar ways or have similar needs (Parvanta, Nelson, & Harner, 2018). Research is used to carefully examine the specific wants, needs, values, resources, and current behaviors of different segments. Segments may be based on identities that transcend race, ethnicity, and gender. For example, Rescue Social Change Group is a national social marketing agency that approaches youth behavior change by focusing on peer crowds they label as hip-hop, preppy, mainstream, alternative, and country (Rescue SCG, 2014).

PHNs, like marketers, use research to customize strategies that best meet the needs and values of different audience segments. Cultural variables—unique health beliefs, values, norms, expectations, and language barriers—influence whether certain health information is even viewed as important (Kreps & Sparks, 2008). To ensure effective communication, involve representatives from the target audience in the communication strategy design and test it for readability, understanding, and appeal. Feedback mechanisms—such as consumer surveys, focus groups, hotlines, and comment cards—can help validate the strategy's effectiveness or weaknesses and provide ideas for improvement.

The key to any successful marketing program is clearly defining the marketing mix, also known as the 4 P's (Weinreich, 2011):

- **Product:** The behavior you want target audience to adopt

- **Price:** What the target audience has to give up to adopt the behavior

- **Place:** Where and how you are going to reach your target audience

- **Promotion:** The message delivered in a creative, relevant, and targeted way

Also, social marketing often includes two additional P's (Luca & Suggs, 2010):

- **Policy:** Changes in organizational or federal policies that support the behavior change

- **Partnerships:** Teaming up with other organizations and stakeholders (e.g., local leaders and elected officials) to address complex societal issues

The following list includes tips for how you can use social marketing effectively:

- Develop a plan that includes attention to all aspects of the marketing mix—product, price, place, and promotion—as well as policy and partnerships.

- Use research throughout the process—careful review of existing literature as well as collecting new data through focus groups, surveys, and observation.

- Involve the target population, including opinion leaders, to actively participate and be co-creators in the development process.

- Locate opinion leaders—people who have social influence and have adopted the desired behavior or attitude—who can be catalysts for behavior change through role-modeling and social relationships.

- Consider socioeconomic factors, cultural beliefs, values, geographic location, and local norms and values.

- Know that exchange theory is fundamental. The target audience must perceive benefits that equal or exceed the perceived costs they associate with performing the behavior.

- Avoid message clutter and information overload.

- Use stories and anecdotes in the presentation of risk data.

- Use multiple approaches (written, oral, visual graphics, electronic) and repetition to maximize your promotion messaging.

- Anticipate and manage the use of controversy and conflict.

- Avoid terminology, phrases, or visual cues that reinforce stereotypes or contradict verbal messages.

- Remember that social marketing is *not* social media marketing. Social media is one valuable channel, but do not neglect other methods, such as radio/podcasts, television, posters, periodicals, and other written material.

Sources: Evans & McCormack, 2008; Lee & Kotler, 2015; Levy-Storms, 2005; Russell, 2009; Weinreich, 2011; Westdahl & Page-Goertz, 2006

**Healthy People 2020**    On the Healthy People 2020 website, go to "Topics & Objectives," and under "H"

**healthypeople.gov**    click "Health Communication and Information Technology." Read the "Overview" and "Objectives." Click "Interventions & Resources" and review evidence on interventions to reduce tobacco use or increase physical activity in communities. Based on the evidence, identify a health communication or information technology strategy for improving community health.

*After reviewing evidence on communicating effective written messages and social marketing techniques, the students decide to make a list of the next steps needed to create the poster as well as the digital presentation to be displayed in the public health clinic.*

### EVIDENCE EXAMPLE 9.6
**Som la Pera ("We Are Cool") Program in Spain**

Som la Pera ("We Are Cool") aimed to increase fruit and vegetable consumption and physical activity while reducing sedentary behavior in low-income neighborhoods of Reus, Spain. At one high school, a peer-led social marketing approach was used to reach high school students, ages 13 through 16. Five adolescents designed and implemented 10 activities as challenges for their 165 school-age peers. The program utilized a variety of methods, including a Facebook page to post "sport selfies" and healthy food plates; playground activities, including food tastings and performing original songs about healthy habits; a contest with a quiz video game about nutritional concepts and myths; as well as a team contest making creative summer recipes covered by local and national television. In a randomized controlled trial, this group was compared with a control group of 223 students at two other local high schools that received no intervention. After 12 months, in the experimental group, 28.9% of students had an increase in eating one or more fruits a day, and 18.5% increased their physical activity 6 or more hours per week (Aceves-Martins et al., 2017).

### Activity

Based on what you have learned about communicating effective written messages and social marketing, answer the following questions:

- What information sources do the students need to access?

- Which principles and tips for communicating written health messages and using social marketing techniques are useful for planning the poster?

- What tips for effective social marketing are useful for creating the digital presentation?

## Using Diverse Technological Tools

National surveys of U.S. adults about the Internet and health found:

- 86% go online

- 77% own a smartphone that connects to the Internet

- 69% use some type of online social media

- 59% looked online for health information

- 35% searched online to figure out what health condition they or someone else might have

*Source:* Pew Research Center, 2013, 2017a, 2017b

## EVIDENCE EXAMPLE 9.7
### Delivering Public Health Interventions Through the Internet

- Rogers, Lemmen, Kramer, Mann, and Chopra (2017) completed a systematic review of 71 meta-analyses of Internet-delivered therapies that represent 1,733 studies and 268 unique randomized control trials (RCTs). Efficacy was demonstrated in managing a wide variety of conditions, primarily substance abuse, mental health (depression, anxiety and panic disorders, and PTSD), chronic pain, insomnia, and childhood health problems, as well as promoting healthier diet and physical activity behaviors. Characteristics of successful Internet-delivered interventions centered on being intensive, interactive, and lasting weeks to months. Interactive elements that prompted personalized feedback and self-monitoring were key. This included assignments that required action while off the Internet, such as tracking sleeping or eating habits or conducting physical activities through the week. Interventions often followed cognitive behavioral strategies and were carefully thought out, progressive models of engagement with multiple layers of targeted approaches. Unfortunately, in most instances, the Internet-delivered interventions were only offered to RCT participants, and websites to deliver the intervention were not maintained after the research study ended. The challenge is to find funding and support to host these evidence-based online programs and promote use to the wider public.

- Eckert et al. (2017) conducted a systematic review of 79 global studies on the use of social media to disseminate health-related communication during a disaster. They recommended that government agencies and healthcare providers should use social media (especially Twitter and Facebook) to address the public and provide accurate, timely, and transparently sourced health information. Additional benefits were the facilitation of peer-to-peer communication and aid, and receiving meaningful, actionable data from affected people on the ground.

The Internet offers an option for broad dissemination to populations in need of health information, provided that they have access. However, information on the Internet can also be overwhelming, sometimes contradictory, and, in the worst-case scenario, inaccurate. One challenge for researchers is to determine the effectiveness of potential Internet interventions for influencing positive behavior change and improving health outcomes.

## Smartphones and Internet-Connected Health Devices

The prevalence of smartphones presents other opportunities for health communication. Both Apple and Android mobile devices have access to over 135,000 apps on each platform that are categorized as either medical or health and fitness; many are free or low cost (AppBrain, 2017; Steel Media Ventures, 2017).

Mobile applications are being used globally to improve the health of mothers and children. These are examples of apps developed to reach pregnant women and mothers:

- **GiftedMom** (http://giftedmom.org) is a mobile app that provides pregnant women and new mothers in Africa with health information to strengthen their connections with antenatal care.

- **MOM Connect** (http://www.askmama.co.za/) aims to register all pregnant women in South Africa for mobile messages, including information about pregnancy and infancy, based on the mother's stage of pregnancy or her infant's age; clinical messages based on care for the mother or baby at different stages of pregnancy or post-delivery; and follow-up notifications of imminent or missed appointments.

- **Back to Work Mom**, #B2Wmom (http://fargond.gov/city-government/departments/fargo-cass-public-health/nutrition-fitness/breastfeeding/for-moms/back-to-work-mom-b-2-wmom), uses text messages to offer supportive tips and resources to promote breastfeeding for moms who return to work/school. The program is funded through the Minnesota State Health Department Maternal and Child Health (MCH) grant. A priority area for MCH grants is to increase the breastfeeding rate at 6 months by offering both support and resources specific to the gestational age or child's age beginning prenatally and continuing until the child's first birthday.

## Evaluation of Mobile Apps

PHNs should research and evaluate apps that might help clients self-manage their own health through data tracking or education. Singh et al. (2016) suggest three criteria for evaluating mobile health applications:

- **Client engagement:** "The ability for apps to enable collaboration, activation and participation, information-sharing, and decision-making in one's one health" (p. 2)

- **Quality:** Reliable information for target population; usefulness that can be recommended

- **Safety:** Response of app to dangerous information entered by client, such as low blood sugar, and commitment to client information privacy and security

### EVIDENCE EXAMPLE 9.8
**Evaluation of Mobile Applications**

Singh et al. (2016) used the criteria of client engagement, quality, and safety to evaluate the effectiveness of 376 iOS and 569 Android patient-focused healthcare apps. Only 43% of the iOS apps and 27% of the Android apps were determined to be possibly useful. The researchers suggested that peer support delivered through social media and ongoing motivational challenges through game-based formats may provide the most engagement for clients.

Singh et al. (2016, p. 3) proposed a framework of client engagement in responding to apps. The lowest level of client engagement is providing information. App designers can increase client engagement levels by adding features such as reminders to users, tracking health information, displaying and summarizing health information, and providing guidance based on information by user. Higher levels of client engagement include communication with providers and caregivers, social network support, and supporting behavior change through rewards.

Be aware that there is a promising surge of Internet-connected health devices and wearables (like smartwatches and fitness trackers) that present new opportunities for health promotion by utilizing the *Internet of Things* (IoT). IoT is machine-to-machine online communication built on cloud computing and networks of data-gathering sensors. Integration through IoT holds promise to make mobile apps, fitness trackers, and new health monitoring devices even more powerful and effective. PHNs should stay abreast of developments in this area that could help clients.

### Social Media

U.S. adults who are online widely use social media platforms, such as Facebook (79%), Instagram (32%), Pinterest (31%), LinkedIn (29%), and Twitter (24%) (Pew Research Center, 2016). Social media offers new opportunities and a wider audience for public health interventions. Early studies show both opportunities and challenges. For example, a clinical trial involving more than 1,500 participants ages 16 to 25 found that exposure to Just/Us, a Facebook page with sexually transmitted infection prevention messages developed with youth input, led to a 12% increase in condom use at two months but made no difference at six months (Bull, Levine, Black, Schmiege, & Santelli, 2012). More research needs to be done to identify which aspects of SMS (short message service) health messages make them more compelling and effective.

### Content Creation Tools

Beyond social media, many free and low-cost content-creation tools available on the Internet allow PHNs to create posters, infographics, videos, podcasts, and more. See Table 9.8. In addition, familiar programs, such as PowerPoint, often have untapped potential for new functionality. Explore how the program can be used to create posters and videos.

> *To create a visually appealing poster, the students decide to use PowerPoint in an innovative but simple way. They change the slide dimensions to 2 x 3 feet under page setup and organize all the content on a single slide, which a local retail printer can produce in full color for $30. Using free online translation tools recommended by Darius, Hannah then translates the poster text into three other languages. Darius emails the poster files in multiple languages to Gail, their preceptor, to review before printing. Gail suggests a few changes to make the English version more accessible to nonprofessionals and has native speakers proof the translated versions. Edits are easy to make electronically. In addition to sharing the physical poster at the clinic, Darius uploads the final version on YouTube, which allows easy connection to other social media sites, such as Facebook and Twitter.*

### TABLE 9.8 Free Content-Creation Tools

| Search Engine Terms | Potential Options |
| --- | --- |
| Free website builder | https://weebly.com |
| | https://wix.com |
| | https://duda.co |
| | https://wordpress.com/ |
| Free brochure templates | https://templates.office.com |
| | *(for both Word and PowerPoint)* |
| | https://canva.com |
| Free screen recorder | https://screencast-o-matic.com |
| | https://flashbackrecorder.com |
| Free digital presentation tools | https://voicethread.com |
| | https://prezi.com |
| | *(Also remember PowerPoint has audio recording and export to video features)* |
| Free PowerPoint poster template | https://posterpresentations.com |
| | https://genigraphics.com |

## How Do PHNs Use Skills in Online Communication?

Communicating effectively online requires a new set of skills for healthcare professionals, commonly referred to as *Netiquette*. Protecting confidentiality and communicating respectfully are essential whenever you communicate online, whether it is through email, social media, websites, blogs, text messages, tweets, or Facebook. Email remains the most commonly used form of electronic communication in professional settings. Tips for professional email communication include:

▪ Avoid cutting, pasting, forwarding, cc-ing, or bcc-ing without the permission of the original sender.

▪ Make sure all written professional communication, electronic or otherwise, is concise and uses the appropriate tone, proper grammar, and spelling.

▪ Avoid use of jargon, unprofessional slang, or (unapproved) abbreviations.

▪ Discuss expected and appropriate response time; absences; the name and contact information of the person (within an agency/organization) who will be available during a vacation, illness, or extended leave of absence; and the use of written informed consent.

Many organizations/agencies use encryption to protect from online phishing and viruses and to ensure receipt of intended email communication. When choosing the appropriate medium, be aware of policies and guidelines regarding online forms of communication and use of social media in your organization, as well as licensing boards, professional insurers, and other appropriate regulatory bodies, because the boundaries may vary depending on your relationship with others.

The exponential growth of social media and online communication offers many benefits to PHNs, including professional networking, improved speed and reach of communication, and dynamic new tools for professional collaboration and client education. However, this growth also brings concerns about confidentiality and privacy for clients. Any online breach of confidentiality or privacy can be instantly and broadly disseminated. The following considerations are ways to avoid problems with social media:

▪ Never disseminate any information or transmit by way of any electronic media information gained in the nurse-client relationship unless legally obligated to do so, or if it is a client care-related need.

▪ Never disseminate or transmit by way of electronic media any images or video gained through the nurse-client relationship. Protection of personal and protected information is your ethical and legal duty. Follow employer policies for taking photographs or videos for legitimate purposes, and use employer-provided devices, not your personal devices.

▪ Never make disparaging remarks about patients, clients, employers, coworkers, or community members, even if they are not identified by name.

▪ Never post content or otherwise speak on behalf of your employer unless you are authorized to do so. If directed to do so, review employer policies regarding communication.

▪ Promptly report any breach of confidentiality or privacy made by you or someone else.

▪ Maintain professional boundaries in the use of electronic media. Online contact with clients blurs the distinction between a professional and a personal relationship. (Refer to Chapter 6 for a discussion of maintaining professional boundaries.)

*Sources:* DeJong, 2014; National Council of State Boards of Nursing, 2011

## How Do PHNs Present Accurate Demographic, Statistical, Programmatic, and Scientific Information?

PHNs also need to develop skills in communicating information about data for making decisions to improve the health of population groups and communities. PHNs might be involved in formal community assessment and conducting surveys and be asked to present that data to identify specific needs of the community. They may be asked to present data to advisory groups, city councils, county boards, health department staff, or other community groups. To make information accessible to the general public, PHNs need to translate information into easily understood and accurate language. To enhance understanding, health data and scientific information need to be reduced and formatted. Earlier sections in this chapter address how to design clear and simple health information.

PHNs review and apply many types of information to their practice, including statistical health data, epidemiology and communicable disease trends, school children's vaccination rates, youth risk surveys, and community health assessments. Some examples of more specific data are the number of motor vehicle deaths and seatbelt and proper car seat use. These are just a few of the different types of data a PHN uses on a regular basis. Knowledge of data is important for determining community health needs and measuring effectiveness of interventions implemented to improve the health of the community.

PHNs can use the following tips identified by Stephanie Evergreen for designing effective presentations:

- **Less is more:** Use text for critical information only.
- **The emotional side:** Use meaningful, relevant visual elements that engage your audience's emotions.
- **Place graphics in the right direction:** Place text and images so that the reader's eyes follow the direction of the graphic toward the text.
- **Add a pop of color:** Minimize cognitive overload and emphasize key content with strategic use of color.
- **Choose the right chart:** Bar and line charts are more effective options than angular pie charts.
- **Use clear data labels and descriptive subtitles:** The easier your data and graph's key points are to digest with properly labeled descriptions, the clearer your data story becomes.
- **Hand it to them:** Use a handout to give your audience just what they need.

*Source:* Evergreen, 2017

---

**EVIDENCE EXAMPLE 9.9**

**Customer Satisfaction Survey**

A metro area public health agency offered an opportunity for nursing students to collect data using a biannual customer satisfaction survey in their mental health clinic. The students assisted the clients in completing a voluntary survey on overall clinic satisfaction. The survey addressed topics such as adequate clinic hours of operation, services, and programs offered through the clinic; ease of transportation for using the services; satisfaction of the staff and client interactions; and the overall physical atmosphere of the clinic. Public health nursing students compiled and analyzed the data to identify emerging trends and client-identified needs in the community. The students discussed the information with the director of the clinic, who then assessed and interpreted the data for quality assurance, staff and client education needs, and gaps in program and services.

Contributed by Carol Roth, PHN, RN, Assistant Professor, Minnesota State University Moorhead

*Gail and Emily discuss creating a 20-minute in-service on sexual health for the public health staff. Because the training room has audiovisual equipment and Internet access, Emily decides to use PowerPoint again to create a multi-slide presentation with graphics and YouTube videos. The students have accumulated a large amount of information on sexual health from journal articles and government websites. However, as Emily is working on the presentation, she becomes perplexed about how to organize the content, how much information to include, and what would be most useful and interesting to staff. Then she remembers that the same principles she had used to guide work on the poster are also applicable to creating effective messages in the PowerPoint presentation.*

**Activity**

- How can the students evaluate the quality of the evidence to include in their presentation? (See Chapter 2.)
- Which principles for creating effective health messages are applicable to the presentation for staff?
- How might students use the tips for presenting data effectively to design the presentation?

---

## Ethical Application

When people communicate with one another, messages might be confusing, misunderstood, or responded to with a high degree of emotion, such as fear or anger. The PHN is accountable to provide professional communication that considers the consequences of this communication for individuals, families, communities, systems, and colleagues. See Table 9.9 on the application of ethical perspectives to communication.

*Gail and the three students meet at the completion of the poster, digital presentation, and staff presentation to evaluate outcomes and their collaborative process.*

**Activity**

- How can the group use the ASSURE Model to evaluate its project effectiveness?
- What questions could the students use to reflect on the effectiveness of their collaborative process? Consider how the tips for effective communication discussed early in the chapter, professional email communication, and ethical perspectives can guide their discussion.

**TABLE 9.9  Ethical Action in Communication**

| Ethical Perspective | Application |
|---|---|
| Rule ethics (principles) | ▪ Maintain the confidentiality of private healthcare information.<br>▪ Ensure the accuracy of health information, because wrong information could result in harm or legal liability.<br>▪ Consider the impact of communication on others in the client's environment—evaluate whether communication could contribute to client harm.<br>▪ When using an interpreter, explain that you expect a verbatim translation to avoid inaccurate or misleading messages.<br>▪ Exercise caution when using social media and electronic communication to avoid harming individuals, families, and communities. |
| Virtue ethics (character) | ▪ When collecting information from individuals and families and developing large data sets, collect only the information needed for decision-making. This approach respects the time of clients and staff.<br>▪ Be respectful of the clients and build on positives if change is needed.<br>▪ In situations of limited time or limited client capability to learn, prioritize the most important health education topics needed to avoid overwhelming the clients.<br>▪ Consider that clients might interpret health education as a criticism of their behavior. |
| Feminist ethics (reducing oppression) | ▪ Create a comfortable, welcoming, and affirming environment for communication.<br>▪ Consider client vulnerability when communicating sensitive information. |

## KEY POINTS

- PHNs need to develop effective communication skills at all levels of practice—with individuals, families, communities, and systems.
- Motivational interviewing is an effective strategy for promoting positive health behavior change.
- Building trust enhances healthy behavior change.
- Health education strategies are based on the characteristics and motivations of learners and on teaching-learning principles.
- Health communication messages are crafted based on the literacy level, cultural inclusiveness, and involvement of consumers in the development of messages.

- PHNs need to become knowledgeable about the use of diverse technological tools for communicating health information to individuals, families, and communities.
- Client engagement, quality, and safety are important criteria for evaluating the use of mobile applications for promoting health behavior change.
- PHNs use social marketing to communicate health messages to targeted population groups.
- PHNs must exercise caution when using social media to deliver health messages to ensure confidentiality and privacy for patients and comply with HIPAA laws.

## REFLECTIVE PRACTICE

Use the ASSURE Model presented in this chapter to design a school campaign to decrease tobacco use among teens.

1. Apply each step of the ASSURE Model to designing the campaign.

2. How will teaching-learning principles guide your campaign design?

3. How will consideration of health literacy influence your plan?

4. With whom will you collaborate to design the campaign?

5. How will you use social marketing principles to design the campaign?

6. What is the key health message that you want to convey to the teen school population?

7. What are some strategies that you can use to involve teens in planning the campaign?

8. How are the Cornerstones of Public Health Nursing reflected in the campaign's design?

## APPLICATION OF EVIDENCE

Gail's public health department has collaborated with the local hospital, county social services, local law enforcement, and school district to establish an opioid prevention hotline. Gail is representing the health department in the Opioid Prevention Coalition that worked to establish the hotline. The coalition is now working on a strategy to publicize the hotline to the community. The coalition members decide that they need to use multiple methods to communicate the availability of this new community resource.

1. How can the coalition members use the evidence on effective communication strategies to reach the community?

2. How should coalition members communicate the availability of the opioid prevention hotline to community members?

3. Which data about opioid use might motivate individuals and organizations in the community to be concerned about opioid use as a health problem? How should these data be communicated?

4. Which tips for effective social marketing should be used to communicate the availability of the opioid prevention hotline?

5. How can the coalition use electronic communication to reach a larger community audience?

## References

Aceves-Martins, M., Llauradó, E., Tarro, L., Moriña, D., Papell-Garcia, I., Prades-Tena, J., … Solà, R. (2017). A school-based, peer-led, social marketing intervention to engage Spanish adolescents in a healthy lifestyle ("We are cool"—Som la pera study): A parallel-cluster randomized controlled study. *Childhood Obesity, 13*(4), 300–313. doi:10.1089/chi.2016.0216

Agency for Healthcare Research and Quality. (2015). *Communicating clearly: Tool #4. AHRQ health literacy universal precautions toolkit* (2nd ed.). Rockville, MD: Author. Retrieved from https://www.ahrq.gov/professionals/quality-patient-safety/quality-resources/tools/literacy-toolkit/healthlittoolkit2-tool4.html

Agency for Healthcare Research and Quality. (2017). *AHRQ health literacy universal precautions toolkit* (2nd ed.). Rockville, MD: Author. Retrieved from https://www.ahrq.gov/professionals/quality-patient-safety/quality-resources/tools/literacy-toolkit/index.html

AppBrain. (2017). Top categories: Most popular Android market categories. Retrieved from http://www.appbrain.com/stats/android-market-app-categories

Bastable, S. (2017). *Essentials of patient education.* Burlington, MA: Jones & Bartlett Learning.

Bastable, S., & Alt, M. F. (2014). Overview of education in health care. In S. B. Bastable (Ed.), *Nurse as educator: Principles of teaching & learning for nursing practice* (4th ed., pp. 3–30). Burlington, MA: Jones & Bartlett Learning.

Berkman, N. D., Sheridan, S. L., Donahue, K. E., Halpern, D. J., & Crotty, K. (2011). Low health literacy and health outcomes: An updated systematic review. *Annals of Internal Medicine, 155*(2), 97–107. doi:10.7326/0003-4819-155-2-201107190-00005

Braungart, M. M., Braungart, R. G., & Gramet, P. R. (2014). Applying learning theories to healthcare practice. In S. B. Bastable (Ed.), *Nurse as educator: Principles of teaching & learning for nursing practice* (4th ed., pp. 63–108). Burlington, MA: Jones & Bartlett Learning.

Bull, S. S., Levine, D. K., Black, S. R., Schmiege, S. J., & Santelli, J. (2012). Social media–delivered sexual health intervention: A cluster randomized controlled trial. *American Journal of Prevention Medicine, 43*(5), 467–474. Retrieved from http://dx.doi.org/10.1016/j.amepre.2012.07.022

Centers for Disease Control and Prevention. (2014). *CDC Clear Communication Index: A tool for developing and assessing CDC public communication products: User guide.* https://www.cdc.gov/ccindex/pdf/clear-communication-user-guide.pdf

Centers for Disease Control and Prevention. (2015). Develop SMART objectives. Retrieved from https://www.cdc.gov/phcommunities/resourcekit/evaluate/smart_objectives.html

Centers for Disease Control and Prevention. (2016). Reported STDs at unprecedented high in the U.S. Retrieved from https://www.cdc.gov/nchhstp/newsroom/2016/std-surveillance-report-2015-press-release.html

Centers for Medicare and Medicaid Services. (2012). *Toolkit for making written material clear and effective.* Retrieved from https://www.cms.gov/Outreach-and-Education/Outreach/WrittenMaterialsToolkit/index.html

Chlebowy, D. O., El-Mallakh, P., Myers, J., Kubiak, N., Cloud, R., & Wall, M. P. (2015). Motivational interviewing to improve diabetes outcomes in African Americans adults with diabetes. *Western Journal of Nursing Research, 37*(5), 566–580. doi:10.1177/0193945914530522

DeJong, S. M. (2014). *Blogs and tweets, texting and friending: Social media and online professionalism in health care.* New York, NY: Elsevier.

Eckert, S., Sopory, P., Day, A., Wilkins, L., Padgett, D., Novak, J., … Gamhewage, G. (2017). Health-related disaster communication and social media: Mixed-method systematic review. *Health Communication, August,* 1–12. doi:10.1080/10410236.2017.1351278

Evans, D. E., & McCormack, L. (2008). Applying social marketing in health care: Communicating evidence to change consumer behavior. *Medical Decision Making, 28*(5), 781–792. doi:10.1177/0272989x08318464

Evergreen, S. D. H. (2017). *Tips for presenting data effectively* [Webinar]. Thousand Oaks, CA: SAGE Publishing. Retrieved from https://us.sagepub.com/en-us/nam/datavisualization?priorityCode=7B0323&utm_source=Adestra&utm_medium=email&utm_content=Readmore&utm_campaign=7B0323&utm_term=

Firestone, R., Rowe, C. J., Modi, S. N., & Sievers, D. (2016). The effectiveness of social marketing in global health: A systematic review. *Health Policy and Planning, 32*(1), 110–124. doi:10.1093/heapol/czw088

Glavin, K., & Saeteren, B. (2016). Cultural diversity in perinatal care: Somali new mothers' experiences with care in Norway. *Health Science Journal, 10*(4), 1–9.

Goto, A., Rudd, R. E., Lai, A. Y., Yoshida, K., Suzuki, R., Halstead, D. D., … Reich, M. R. (2014). Leveraging public health nurses for disaster risk communication in Fukushima City: A qualitative analysis of nurses' written records of parenting counseling and peer discussions. *BMC Health Services Research, 14,* 129. doi:10.1186/1472-6963-14-129

Green, A. (2006). A person-centered approach to palliative care nursing. *Journal of Hospice and Palliative Nursing, 8*(5), 294–301. doi:10.1097/00129191-200609000-00015

Gutierrez, N., Kindratt, T. B., Pagels, P., Foster, B., & Gimpel, N. E. (2014). Health literacy, health information seeking behaviors, and Internet use among patients attending a private and public clinic in the same geographic area. *Journal of Community Health, 39,* 83–89. doi:10.1007/s10900-013-9742-5

Harden, B. J. (2010). Home visitation with psychologically vulnerable families. *Zero to Three, July,* 44–51. Retrieved from https://www.zerotothree.org/resources/1030-home-visitation-with-psychologically-vulnerable-families

Harvard Medical School. (2011). Motivating behavior change. *Harvard Mental Health Letter, 27*(8). Retrieved from https://www.health.harvard.edu/newsletter_article/motivating-behavior-change

Hawkins, R. P., Kreuter, M., Resnicow, K., Fishbein, M., & Dijkstra, A. (2008). Understanding tailoring in communicating about health. *Health Education Research, 23*(3), 454–466. doi:10.1093/her/cyn004

Henry Street Consortium. (2017). *Entry-level population-based public health nursing competencies.* St. Paul, MN: Author. Retrieved from www.henrystreetconsortium.org

Holcomb-McCoy, C., & Bryan, J. (2010). Advocacy and empowerment in parent consultation: Implications for theory and practice. *Journal of Counseling & Development, 88*(3), 259–268. doi:10.1002/j.1556-6678.2010.tb00021.x

Inott, T., & Kenney, B. B. (2011). Assessing learning styles: Practical tips for patient education. *Nursing Clinics of North America, 46,* 313–320. doi:10.1016m.cnur.2011.05.006

Institute of Medicine. (2004). *Health literacy: A prescription to end confusion.* Washington, DC: National Academies Press.

International Council of Nurses. (2017). *Nurse Family Partnership in urban neighborhoods of the USA* [Case study]. Retrieved from https://www.icnvoicetolead.com/case-study/nurse-family-partnership-in-urban-neighborhoods-of-the-usa/

Jesse, D. E., Gaynes, B. N., Feldhousen, E. B., Newton, E. R., Shelia Bunch, S., & Hollon, S. D. (2015). Performance of a culturally tailored cognitive-behavioral intervention integrated in a public health setting to reduce risk of antepartum depression: A randomized controlled trial. *Journal of Midwifery & Women's Health, 60*(5), 578–592. doi:10.1111/jmwh.12308

Keller, L. O., Strohschein, S., Lia-Hoagberg, B., & Schaffer, M. A. (2004). Population-based public health interventions: Practice-based and evidence-supported. Part I. *Public Health Nursing, 21*(5), 453–468.

Kolb, D. A. (1984). *Experiential learning experience as a source of learning and development.* Upper Saddle River, NJ: Prentice Hall.

Kolb, D. A. (2005). *The Kolb learning style inventory. Version 3.1.* Cleveland Heights, OH: Experience Based Learning Systems, Inc.

Kreps, G. L., & Sparks, L. (2008). Meeting the health literacy needs of immigrant populations. *Patient Education and Counseling, 71*(3), 328–332. doi:10.1016/j.pec.2008.03.001

Kreuter, M. W., Lukwago, S. N., Bucholtz, D. C., Clark, E. M., & Sanders-Thompson, V. (2003). Achieving cultural appropriateness in health promotion programs: Targeted and tailored approaches. *Health Education & Behavior, 30*(2), 133–146. doi:10.1177/1090198102251021

Lancaster, J. (2016). Changing health behavior using health education with individuals, families, and groups. In M. Stanhope & J. Lancaster (Eds.), *Public health nursing: Population-centered health care in the community* (pp. 355–376). St. Louis, MO: Mosby Elsevier.

Lee, N. R., & Kotler, P. A. (2015). *Social marketing: Changing behaviors for good* (5th ed.). Thousand Oaks, CA: SAGE Publications.

Levy-Storms, L. (2005). Strategies for diffusing public health innovations through older adults' health communication networks. *Generations, 29*(2), 70–75.

Limper, H. M., Burns, J. L., & Alexander, K. A. (2016). Taxi drivers: A target population for the prevention of transmissible disease? *Journal of Community Health, 41,* 207–210. doi:10.1007/s10900-015-0099-9

Luca, N. R., & Suggs, L. S. (2010). Strategies for the social marketing mix: A systematic review. *Social Marketing Quarterly, 16*(4), 122–149. doi:10.1080/15245004.2010.522767

Lundahl, B. W., Kunz, C., Brownell, C., Tollefson, D., & Burke, B. L. (2010). A meta-analysis of motivational interviewing: Twenty-five years of empirical studies. *Research on Social Work Practice, 20*(2), 137–160. doi:10.1177/1049731509347850

McAlindon, K. (2017). Selling innovations like soap: The interactive systems framework and social marketing. *American Journal of Community Psychology, 60*(2), 242–256. doi:10.1002/ajcp.12157

Miller, W. R. (2004). Motivational interviewing in service to health promotion. *American Journal of Health Promotion, 18,* A1–A10.

Minnesota Department of Health. (2001). *Public health interventions: Application for public health nursing practice.* St. Paul, MN: Author. Retrieved from http://www.health.state.mn.us/divs/opi/cd/phn/docs/0301wheel_manual.pdf

Minnesota Department of Human Services. (2005). Tips for working with interpreters. http://www.dhs.state.mn.us/main/idcplg?IdcService=GET_DYNAMIC_CONVERSION&RevisionSelectionMethod=LatestReleased&dDocName=id_051607

National Council of State Boards of Nursing. (2011). *White paper: A nurse's guide to the use of social media.* Retrieved from https://www.ncsbn.org/Social_Media.pdf

National Council of State Boards of Nursing. (2014). *A nurse's guide to professional boundaries.* Retrieved from https://www.ncsbn.org/ProfessionalBoundaries_Complete.pdf

Office of Disease Prevention and Health Promotion. (2016). *Health literacy online: A guide for simplifying the user experience.* Retrieved from http://www.health.gov/healthliteracyonline

Parvanta, C. F., Nelson, D. E., & Harner, R. N. (2018). *Public health communication: Critical tools and strategies.* Burlington, MA: Jones and Bartlett Learning.

Paul, M. P., Rigrod, P., Wingate, S., & Borsuk, M. E. (2015). A community-driven intervention in Tuftonboro, New Hampshire, succeeds in altering water testing behavior. *Journal of Environmental Health, 78*(5), 30–39.

Pew Research Center. (2013). *The Internet and health.* Retrieved from http://www.pewinternet.org/2013/02/12/the-internet-and-health/

Pew Research Center. (2016). *Social media update 2016.* Retrieved from http://www.pewinternet.org/2016/11/11/social-media-update-2016/

Pew Research Center. (2017a). *Internet/broadband fact sheet.* Retrieved from http://www.pewinternet.org/fact-sheet/internet-broadband/

Pew Research Center. (2017b). *Mobile fact sheet.* Retrieved from http://www.pewinternet.org/fact-sheet/mobile/

Pfister-Minogue, K. A., & Salveson, C. (2010). Training and experience of public health nurses in using behavior change counseling. *Public Health Nursing, 27*(6), 544–551. doi:10.1111/j.1525-1446.2010.00884.x

PlainLanguage.gov. (2011). *Federal plain language guidelines.* Retrieved from http://www.plainlanguage.gov/howto/guidelines/FederalPLGuidelines/TOC.cfm

Ratzan, S. C., & Parker, R. M. (2000). Introduction. In C. R. Selden, M. Zorn, S. C. Ratzan, & R. M. Parker (Eds.), *National Library of Medicine current bibliographies in medicine: Health literacy* (pp. v–vii). NLM Pub. No. CBM 2000-1. Bethesda, MD: National Institutes of Health, U.S. Department of Health and Human Services. Retrieved from https://www.researchgate.net/publication/230877250_National_Library_of_Medicine_Current_Bibliographies_in_Medicine_Health_Literacy

Registered Nurses' Association of Ontario. (2002/2006). *Establishing therapeutic relationships.* Toronto, ON: Author. Retrieved from http://rnao.ca/bpg/guidelines/establishing-therapeutic-relationships

Rescue SCG. (2014, July 21). *Peer crowds: A new approach to youth behavior change (social marketing)* [Video]. Retrieved from https://www.youtube.com/watch?v=V8GDPqU8gPQ&t=9s

Richardson, L. (2012). Motivational interviewing: Helping patients move toward change. *Journal of Christian Nursing, 29*(1), 18–24.

Rimer, B. K., & Glanz, K. (2005). *Theory at a glance: A guide for health promotion practice.* National Cancer Institute. NIH Publication No. 05-3896. Retrieved from https://www.sbccimplementationkits.org/demandrmnch/wp-content/uploads/2014/02/Theory-at-a-Glance-A-Guide-For-Health-Promotion-Practice.pdf

Rogers, M. A. M., Lemmen, K., Kramer, R., Mann, J., & Chopra, V. (2017). Internet-delivered health interventions that work: Systematic review of meta-analyses and evaluation of website availability. *Journal of Medical Internet Research, 19*(3), e90. doi:10.2196/jmir.7111

Russell, E. (2009). *Fundamentals of marketing.* London, UK: Bloomsbury.

Sarkar, U., Karter, A. J., Liu, J. Y., Adler, N. E., Nguyen, R., López, A., & Schillinger, D. (2010). The literacy divide: Health literacy and the use of an Internet-based patient portal in an integrated health system—Results from the Diabetes Study of Northern California (DISTANCE). *Journal of Health Communication, 15*(Suppl. 2), 183–196. doi:10.1080/10810730.2010.499988

Schmid, K. L., Rivers, S. E., Latimer, A. E., & Salovey, P. (2008). Targeting or tailoring? Maximizing resources to create effective health communications. *Marketing Health Services, 28*(1), 32–37.

Singh, K., Bates, D., Drouin, K., Newmark, L. P., Rozenblum, R., Lee, J., ... Klinger, E. V. (2016, February 18). *Developing a framework for evaluating the patient engagement, quality, and safety of mobile health applications* [Issue brief]. The Commonwealth Fund. Retrieved from http://www.commonwealthfund.org/publications/issue-briefs/2016/feb/evaluating-mobile-health-apps

Spiers, J. A., & Wood, A. (2010). Building a therapeutic alliance in brief therapy: The experience of community mental health nurses *Archives of Psychiatric Nursing, 24*(6), 373–386. doi:10.1016/j.apnu.2010.03.001

Stead, M., Gordon, R., Angus, K., & McDermott, L. (2007). A systematic review of social marketing effectiveness. *Health Education, 107*(2), 126–191. doi:10.1108/09654280710731548

Steel Media Ventures. (2017). App Store metrics—Application category distribution. Retrieved from http://148apps.biz/app-store-metrics/?mpage=catcount

U.S. Department of Health and Human Services. (2004). *Making health communication programs work.* Retrieved from https://www.cancer.gov/publications/health-communication/pink-book.pdf

VanBuskirk, K. A., & Wetherell, J. L. (2014). Motivational interviewing with primary care populations: A systematic review and meta-analysis. *Journal of Behavioral Medicine, 37*(4), 768–780. doi:10.1007/s10865-013-9527-4

Weinreich, N. K. (2011). *Hands-on social marketing: A step-by-step guide to designing change for good* (2nd ed.). Thousand Oaks, CA: SAGE Publications.

Westdahl, C., & Page-Goertz, S. (2006). Promotion of breastfeeding—Beyond the benefits. *International Journal of Childbirth Education, 22*(4), 8–16.

Yardley, L., Morrison, L., Bradbury, K., & Muller, I. (2015). The person-based approach to intervention development: Application to digital health-related behavior change interventions. *Journal of Medical Internet Research, 17*(1), e30. doi:10.2196/jmir.4055

Zugai, J. S., Stein, J., & Roche, M. (2015). Therapeutic alliance in mental health nursing: An evolutionary concept analysis. *Issues in Mental Health Nursing, 36*(4), 249–257. doi:10.3109/01612840.2014.969795

# COMPETENCY #8

## Establishes and Maintains Caring Relationships With Communities, Systems, Individuals, and Families

■ **Carolyn M. Porta**
*with Christine C. Andres and Erin Karsten*

" *Susan, a public health nurse (PHN) for several years, has been developing her skills as a family home-visiting nurse. She works with young families whom her supervisor has identified as high risk and has been slowly increasing her caseload. The population that Susan serves is composed of single, young mothers who need support with their parenting skills and identification of normal development for their children.*

*One of Susan's first families was a young mother named Julie with four children. Julie had her first child when she was 16 years old, and then she had two other children before moving to the community where Susan served as a PHN. Julie was not involved in a committed relationship and had no job. She became part of Susan's caseload when a Women, Infants, and Children (WIC) nurse referred her for a PHN baby visit after the birth of her fourth child.*

*During the baby visit, Susan established the foundation for a strong nurse-family relationship. Julie was open about many issues with Susan, including the fact that the two older children were living not with her but with each of their fathers. She told Susan that she was unable to be a "good mother" to them. She was excited about the birth of her new son. Susan explored Julie's strengths and needs with her. It was apparent that Julie could benefit from some parenting information and anticipatory guidance for the 2-year-old and newborn whom she planned to parent. Julie was interested in the program that Susan described, which entailed monthly visits until her newborn turned 3 years old or until she believed she was no longer benefiting from the program.* "

---

### SUSAN'S NOTEBOOK

**COMPETENCY #8** Establishes and Maintains Caring Relationships with Communities, Systems, Individuals, and Families

A. Demonstrates trust, respect, empathy

B. Follows through with commitments

C. Maintains appropriate boundaries

D. Demonstrates tact and diplomacy

E. Seeks assistance when needed in managing relationships

F. Interacts with others in a culturally sensitive manner

*Source:* Henry Street Consortium, 2017

(continues)

## SUSAN'S NOTEBOOK *(continued)*

### USEFUL DEFINITIONS

**Caring:** "Means listening to 'more than what is said'" (Schulte, 2000, p. 7); "facilitates the possibility for a client to feel hope for healing and comfort and/or develop resilience" (Warelow, Edward, & Vinek, 2008, p. 146); "creates a range of possibilities and can be the catalyst of change for the care recipient" (Warelow et al., 2008, p. 147).

**Professional Relationships:** "Key elements include: the need to listen well, establish trust, offer respect and advocacy, avoid power-over interactions and care of self in order to offer care for others" (Jackson, 2010, p. 181).

## Touching Lives Without Stepping on Toes

It is probably not an exaggeration to state that most individuals who choose to become nurses have an inherent desire to care for other human beings. In some ways, caring is synonymous with nursing. As a profession, nursing is a process of assessment, planning, intervention, and evaluation delivered in a context of caring with goals of prevention, healing, recovery, or peaceful transition. As a discipline, nursing is contributing knowledge and advancing science about the complex interplay of health-environment-person-nursing (Fawcett, 2000). Much of this knowledge generation would not be possible in the absence of caring relationships.

PHNs have unique opportunities to develop caring relationships with individuals, families, and groups (e.g., communities and systems). Lillian Wald emphasized caring when she said, "Nursing is love in action, and there is no finer manifestation of it than the care of the poor and disabled in their own homes" (Ridgeway, 2010, p. 1). Although it can be argued that any nurse in any environment can and should establish a caring relationship, many PHNs develop and maintain caring relationships with their clients over weeks, months, and years. This opportunity for lengthy caring relationships is not as common in acute clinical settings but certainly can be observed in nursing care for the elderly (i.e., nursing homes) and the terminally ill (i.e., hospice care) (Olthuis, Dekkers, Leget, & Vogelaar, 2006). Certainly, a meaningful caring relationship can be established regardless of the length of interaction, with thoughtful intentionality. Emotions, in moments of sickness or injury, can be intense for families. Serving a family within an effective caring relationship aids the nurse in considering how best to support the family, and which available programs or resources might be most acceptable and beneficial to the family. This chapter offers strategies for establishing and maintaining meaningful, appropriate, caring relationships in public health nursing and presents challenging situations along with preventive strategies to help you avoid some of these common pitfalls as you launch your nursing career.

To appreciate the nature of a caring relationship, you need to first look at a description of caring. A thorough analysis of caring in the nursing literature has demonstrated five conceptualizations, or expressions, of caring in nursing (Morse, Bottorff, Neander, & Solberg, 1991):

1. Caring as a human trait/state
2. Caring as a moral imperative
3. Caring as an affect
4. Caring as an interpersonal interaction
5. Caring as a therapeutic intervention

In essence, caring is an attribute that, for many, is inherent to who you are as a nurse and human being. In a recent meta-synthesis, caring was explored alongside the art of nursing and being present; caring was defined as "an interpersonal process that is characterized by expert nursing, interpersonal sensitivity and intimate relationships" (Finfgeld-Connett, 2008, p. 528). Caring is also a behavior or emotion that is morally mandated or expected from nurses (Morse, Solberg, Neander, Bottorff, & Johnson, 1990; Shores, 2012). In addition, caring is an action between two or more people, and it is a way to intervene or act to improve the well-being of an individual or community. These last two points—interaction and intervention—in essence reflect a "caring relationship" in nursing because they involve the nurse and another person or group of people.

 **Healthy People** **healthypeople.gov** The Healthy People 2020 website identifies indicators for a variety of public health concerns in the United States, with goals for improvements by 2020. Select a health indicator and develop a public health nursing health-promotion strategy that will include activities at the individual, community, and system levels. Select activities that emphasize establishing a caring relationship with the individual, family, or community. From your perspective, in which activities will it be challenging to establish a caring relationship? Why?

Caring in nursing has been extensively explored, and as a PHN, there is benefit to reflecting on caring, how it is developed in oneself, and how it is expressed to others in meaningful ways. Watson's Theory of Human Caring is a great theory to review and apply to professional caring relationships in public health with individuals, families, and communities. The caritas process (see Table 10.1) has been well described in the literature, and built upon, with measures of caritas being proposed (DiNapoli, Nelson, Turkel, & Watson, 2010).

## Activity

- How much do you agree with the statements regarding caring and nursing? Do you believe that it is possible to be an effective nurse and not care? Why or why not?

- Do you believe it is possible to care too much? If so, how do you determine how much caring is appropriate?

## TABLE 10.1 The Caritas Process

| Stage | Explanation |
|---|---|
| Practice Loving Kindness | Embrace altruistic values and practice loving-kindness with one's self and others |
| Instill Faith and Hope | Instill faith and hope, and honor others |
| Spiritual Beliefs and Practices | Demonstrate sensitivity to self and others by nurturing spiritual beliefs and practices |
| Helping and Trusting Relationship | Develop helping-trusting-caring relationships |
| Promoting Expression of Feelings | Promote and accept positive and negative feelings as you authentically listen to others |
| Decision-Making | Use creative problem-solving strategies to inform caring decision-making |
| Teaching and Learning | Address individual needs and learning styles |
| Healing Environment | Create a healing environment for the physical and spiritual self that also respects human dignity |
| Holistic Care | Assist with physical, emotional, and spiritual needs |
| Miracles | Be open to mystery and allow miracles to enter |

*Source:* Watson Caring Science Institute and International Caritas Consortium, 2013

*Over the year that follows the initial visit, Susan sees Julie and the children monthly. The relationship flourishes as Susan provides Julie with parenting support and information to understand safety and the developmental milestones of her children. Susan works with Julie to access community resources. At times, Julie reveals pieces of her past that includes mental health issues stemming from a childhood of molestation and abuse. Susan always listens without judgment. Susan realizes how much she had come to care about this family and how much Julie trusts her to care for them.*

## Demonstrates Trust, Respect, and Empathy

Relationships exist in every aspect of life: family relationships, casual acquaintance relationships, colleague relationships, distant relationships, and close relationships, to name a few. In public health nursing, relationships can start to build over minutes and often last for years. The variety of settings in which PHNs work is reflected in the diversity of their relationships. For example, a local public health department PHN administering flu shots might spend only 10 minutes with a client, whereas a PHN conducting weekly home visits with a pregnant mom on bedrest might be in that relationship for years. A PHN employed in a jail setting might develop an intermittent relationship with incarcerated individuals who are released and rearrested multiple times over the years. Every relationship a PHN develops, regardless of how long or deep it runs, can be a caring relationship.

A caring relationship can only exist when trust is present. An effective PHN builds trust in verbal and nonverbal ways that reflect awareness of the situation and the needs of the individual, family, or community. Practically, PHNs encourage trust when their actions are consistent, dependable, nonjudgmental, and sensitive to the needs or preferences of the other person. (See Chapter 12 for more information on nonjudgmental nursing.) Professional relationship building is described in the context of a program to prevent teen pregnancy: "The daily presence of the PHN is an important program component for the kind of information nurses provide… as well as relationship building with a professional who can be trusted and is not judgmental about the adolescent's problems and concerns" (Schaffer, Jost, Pederson, & Lair, 2008, p. 308, 310). Often, trust is developed with time and consistency. Diane McNaughton (2005, p. 435) observes that for at-risk pregnant women, multiple nursing visits "were needed for clients to develop trust in nurses, discuss their problems, and utilize the services offered by nurses."

Some PHNs find themselves in situations where they are seeking to create relationships with individuals, families, or communities that might not want the relationship or simply are unsure of what they want, which can occur with vulnerable or stigmatized clients. This challenge to building relationships might occur, for example, when the PHN is working with families involved in child protection situations, necessitating thoughtful intention on the part of the PHN to develop rapport, a necessary precursor (and often the gateway) to developing a caring relationship. Establishing trust is critical, yet doing so can be challenging because many families are vulnerable and powerless (Jack, DiCenso, & Lohfeld, 2005; Porr, Drummond, & Olson, 2012). Often, families trust nurses more readily than they do other professionals (e.g., law enforcement or social workers), although depth of mutual trust takes patience and time and might not be achievable in every situation (Jack et al., 2005).

## EVIDENCE EXAMPLE 10.1

### Exploring the Emotions and Needs of Professionals Working to Keep Children Safe

In this phenomenological (lived experience) study, interviews were conducted with professionals engaged with children and families in high-risk settings (Taylor, Smith, & Taylor, 2017). The purpose of the study was to understand the emotions experienced by these professionals as they work to keep children safe, and how the role they play is supported, or not, by their agencies. The authors identify the need for organizations to recognize the role that providers have in safeguarding children, and particularly the emotions that result from this intensive relationship-based work with families.

## EVIDENCE EXAMPLE 10.2

### Public Health Nursing Practice With "High-Priority" Families: The Significance of Contextualizing "Risk"

A study of PHNs working with high-risk families illustrated how PHNs use critical relational approaches, including providing support, building trust, and applying clinical judgment (Browne, Hartrick Doane, Reimer, MacLeod, & McLellan, 2010). Thirty-two PHNs participated in interviews and focus groups that yielded three themes associated with working with families at risk: contextualizing the complexities of families' lives, responding to shifting contexts of risk and capacity, and working relationally with families under surveillance. PHNs' ability to work with families and recognize the dual influences of risk and capacity is critical to their success in establishing effective working relationships, especially with high-risk or high-priority families.

*After the first year of home visiting, Susan starts to notice a change within Julie: She starts to "care" less about herself and reveals to Susan that she is not happy. Julie reports finding it difficult to get out of bed. Susan notices the environment of the home changing, and Julie begins to miss appointments. Susan decides to have a "heart to heart," or deep, conversation, with Julie, because she believes their relationship is built on trust and honesty. As Susan reveals her observations, stressing the desire to help Julie feel better, Julie states that she doesn't think her depression medication is working anymore. Susan supports Julie and focuses on Julie's strengths, one of which is seeking medical care when appropriate. Susan screens Julie for safety toward herself and the children. They make a plan for Julie to visit her primary care provider as soon as possible.*

*The next week, Julie comes into the office asking for Susan. Susan is immediately concerned. Julie has pink and black hair, a pierced nose and eyebrow, and no children with her. Susan brings Julie into her office to explore her outward changes and her reasons for coming to see Susan. Julie breaks down in tears, saying that she has no energy and is not sleeping and hints that she is cutting herself. Susan has a moment of inward reflection, asking herself how she should respond in a way that will reflect how much she cares, yet also protect Julie and her children. Susan gently explores who is watching the children when Julie has difficulty functioning, knowing that a 3-year-old and a 1-year-old need constant supervision. Julie's answers are vague. Susan has to tell Julie that she is concerned and that if the children are not supervised or cared for, child protection would become involved with her family. This information makes Julie very upset, and Susan, at that point, realizes that she needs to do more. Susan puts herself in Julie's shoes and relies on the trust and strength of the relationship she has with Julie to suggest immediately seeing a crisis mental health nurse working for the county. Julie states she will if Susan believes that it will help. Susan connects them within 15 minutes, and Julie and the mental health nurse initiate a plan of safety and confirm that the children are okay and being cared for by an appropriate person (in this case, a neighbor was watching the children while Julie visited Susan). They also schedule a follow-up appointment within a couple of days with a mental health specialist. This meeting seems to give Julie hope and energy. Susan feels like she has done what she needed to do, but she feels bad about upsetting Julie with her discussion of safety for the children.*

## Activity

- What might you do to encourage a client to feel secure and comfortable during an initial visit?
- How will you acknowledge the client's sense of vulnerability and work with the client to move beyond this vulnerability to establish a trusting relationship?

Respect is an essential component of a caring relationship. Respect in practice is more challenging than most PHNs realize due to the influences of their own cultural beliefs, values, and experiences. According to the Nurses Association of New Brunswick (2015), a therapeutic nurse-client relationship is based on respect for the dignity and worth of a client. It is really difficult, if not impossible, to establish a caring, meaningful relationship with a client or family if respect is absent. Consider how you would feel when receiving service or care for a physical need from someone who is capable of doing the job but does so in a manner that sends the message that you do not deserve the care or that you are not as important as the caregiver. Sometimes nurses send these subtle messages without realizing it; other times, they send the messages intentionally because they have established certain judgments or perceptions about specific client groups or clients with certain characteristics. Effective PHNs critically evaluate personal judgments and consider the extent to which these judgments slip into practice and make it difficult to provide respectful care and establish authentic caring relationships. In addition to reflecting on personal judgments, PHNs can consider the assumptions they are making about clients, families, or communities and avoid doing so by understanding the diversity and differences in people and demonstrating behaviors that appreciate rather than judge or criticize this diversity. Some of these behaviors might include personalizing the care being provided, offering choices regarding care and interventions, and promoting independence to every extent possible when caring for people.

Diane Martins (2008) conducted a phenomenological (lived experience qualitative design) study to explore and understand the experiences of 15 homeless people as they accessed healthcare and highlighted the importance of respect as a value and practice among PHNs caring for all populations, including vulnerable groups such as the homeless. Her recommendations include building on strengths rather than problems and supporting people through practical behaviors, such as recognizing and valuing that they have the right to make informed decisions about their own healthcare. A specific professional development recommendation from the study is to provide continuous education for PHNs, such as interactive lectures and discussions, so that they better understand the needs of the homeless population. Increasing awareness of these needs among PHNs could aid in decreasing the frustrations that can arise when providing care to this population. Finally, Martins also

highlights the essential need for PHNs to advocate at the community and systems levels for social change related to complex social issues such as homelessness. Doing so in a respectful, inclusive way not only could yield positive outcomes for persons experiencing homelessness but could also strengthen individual-level interventions. Caring is the foundation for effective advocacy at community and system levels.

In addition to trust and respect, empathy is foundational to establishing and maintaining a caring relationship. Many people confuse empathy with sympathy, which is problematic, as described by Douglas Chismar (1988, p. 257): "Blurring the distinction between empathy and sympathy has caused us to miss important complexities in human motivation as well as to overlook and fail to develop the unique capacity to empathize." *Empathy* is the ability to respond to someone else's emotional state by experiencing similar feelings, whereas *sympathy* goes a step further by inherently feeling positive and exhibiting lasting concern toward the other person (Chismar, 1988). For example, someone might empathize with a stranger after hearing about the loss of this person's child in a car accident and might express emotions of sadness, including crying. That same person, however, might sympathize with a sibling who has experienced the same loss, not only expressing emotions of sadness and tears but continuing to care and support the sibling over time. Empathy also includes an ability to care generally and specifically about a particular person's situation, while not necessarily agreeing with the other person's perspective. PHNs employed in jails are often asked how they care for criminals who have committed horrible crimes. Empathy enables PHNs in this context to care for and even emotionally mirror the needs of an inmate while not agreeing with or supporting aspects of that individual. Table 10.2 presents distinctions between empathy and sympathy.

Despite the complex conceptualization of empathy in nursing, a scale was developed that could measure a nurse's level of empathic understanding, or ability to understand a client's emotions, feelings, and perspective (Nagano, 2000). The instrument is designed to measure nurse awareness and actions, and research is ongoing to improve its validity and reliability. The 20-item scale includes verbal elements (e.g., "restates important points in own words and confirms with client") and nonverbal elements (e.g., "looks at the client with a warm expression") that in many ways mirror simple yet effective nursing communication strategies.

Judeen Schulte (2000) conducted an ethnographic study exploring the perspectives of PHNs regarding building relationships with clients. These nurses believed that particular actions yielded successes in developing caring relationships, including "being a resource, detecting/asking the next questions, and making informed judgments" (p. 7), because they helped clients believe that they could openly share. Often, the nurses were conducting home visits with no particular disease or problem identified beforehand. Establishing caring relationships was essential for the PHNs to accurately

**TABLE 10.2 Empathy Versus Sympathy**

| Empathy | Sympathy |
|---------|----------|
| Responds to another's perceived emotional state by experiencing feelings of a similar sort | Has a positive regard or a feeling of benevolence for the person |
| Understands but might not agree with the other person's perspective | Agrees with the viewpoint |
| Senses what the other is feeling but without "mutuality" | Offers supportive response to the other's situation |
| Is directed toward anyone, including someone who is not necessarily liked | Is expressed toward those one feels positive about or close to |
| Usually occurs where no prior attachment to the person exists | Usually occurs in the context of a personal relationship or insider (from the community) knowledge |
| Often involuntarily experiences feelings similar to someone else's | Often voluntarily experiences feelings alongside someone else |

*Source:* Adapted from Chismar, 1988

assess and intervene with the families. For the nurses, honesty and directness were important to relationship building, and the nurses described needing to ignore "rude behavior" (2000, p. 7). Schulte shares comments from a participant that summarize the study:

> Felicia's words strongly communicate the link between caring and connections: 'Public health nursing is more than a job… When I'm out there, I care about the people, about what happens to them. I don't think I'd make a really good public health nurse if I didn't care. You get results if they know you care—they're willing to make some change. If they don't think you care at all about them, why should they take a risk for you? I think public health nursing is all about caring about people.' (2000, p. 8)

For the PHNs in this study, caring meant listening to "more than what is said" (Schulte, 2000, p. 7), which is consistent with attention paid in nursing to nonverbal communication and to contextual factors in the family, community, and societal environments.

Although much of what has been discussed thus far in this chapter is specific to nursing care for individuals or families, many of the guiding principles for establishing a caring relationship also apply to relationships at the community or systems levels. At times it can seem (and be) more challenging simply because many other people are usually involved (see Chapter 8 on collaboration). Some literature,

**EVIDENCE EXAMPLE 10.3**

**Negotiating—Experiences of Community Nurses When Contracting With Clients**

Focus groups were conducted with 14 community nurses to explore the issues surrounding negotiating and establishing client care contracts (Duiveman & Bonner, 2012). The nurses' perspectives were represented by three themes: assessment of needs, education toward enablement, and negotiation. Across all themes, it was apparent that for PHNs or community nurses to deliver person-centered care, it is necessary for them to effectively assess and find a balance between the client's needs and the nurse's ability to address them. Doing so appropriately requires meaningful efforts to demonstrate care and establish a caring relationship, which can then result in successfully negotiating a plan for care.

however, does describe community-level caring in public health nursing. PHNs need to consider the importance of caring for communities, as discussed by Kathleen Chafey:

> Nurses must care about what happens to groups of citizens, as well as particular clients… Although proponents of 'caring' seem to have drawn a distinction between an ethic of justice and an ethic of care, this is bipolar, even antithetical. Building the health of communities requires universal application of the principles of justice. It further requires that nurses care enough about their communities and the individuals in them to do battle in political, social, and economic arenas (1996, p. 15).

Betty Smith-Campbell (1999) developed and tested a caring model for communities (see Figure 10.1) because "nurses collectively care with and for communities" (p. 405). In the model, the foundation of caring actions are affect and moral imperative. Interaction is not only with an individual but with the "community," however community is defined. Caring actions result not only from the underlying foundation, interactions, and planning but also from the direct and indirect influences that encompass the community (e.g., economics, policies, politics, and supporting or opposing communities). For example, a parish nurse caring for the congregation will want to plan health-promotion activities with an understanding of the neighborhood and other influences on those whom the PHN is serving. PHNs working in an affluent neighborhood with abundant health-care resources can more easily develop caring relationships that involve extensive health screenings and referrals to outside resources (e.g., services for high blood pressure, weight management, and stress reduction) than PHNs serving a congregation in an impoverished neighborhood with

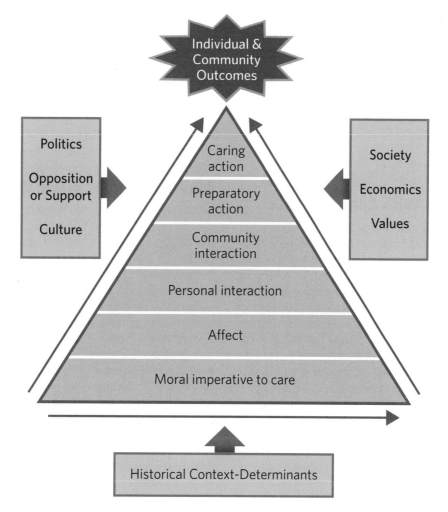

**FIGURE 10.1** Smith-Campbell Caring Community Model (adapted with permission)

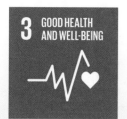

SUSTAINABLE DEVELOPMENT G☉ALS

**PHNs Lead Outbreak Responses Around the World**

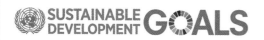

**GOAL 3** Rosa (2016, para. 1) writes, "Public health nurses are at the forefront of this goal, helping to translate the ethic and ethos of human caring to communities and vulnerable populations at large in a way that transforms access to care and provides new opportunities for improved well-being." He goes on, "Public health nurses play a key role in leading research that will contribute to the lessened burden of communicable diseases, guiding policy changes that increase health care coverage for all members of society, and educate the public about the need for medication safety and vaccine scheduling" (para. 2). Public health nurses are on the front line and often first responders to outbreak threats around the world. Nurses in the United States Public Health Service were deployed in response to the 2014 Ebola outbreak (Brown-Stephenson, 2017). Local nurses are in homes and clinics caring for those who are infected and their families, whether the disease is Ebola, Zika, measles, or influenza. Public health nurses care for their communities and are contributing directly to achieving this sustainable development goal.

limited healthcare options. It would be unethical and not very caring for this PHN to proceed with extensive screenings for that congregation without first establishing where they can receive care needed for identified problems. A PHN cannot effectively care for a community unless he or she takes time to understand and appreciate the complexity of factors (e.g., social, economic, political) in and surrounding the community.

## Follows Through With Commitments

PHNs cannot be trusted unless they can demonstrate consistency in care for individuals, families, and communities. Clients for whom PHNs are caring need to know that those PHNs are dependable and reliable in addition to being honest, respectful, and trustworthy. Teri Aronowitz (2005) conducted a grounded theory study to examine the ways in which adolescents develop resilience and change risk behaviors amid environmental stressors in their lives. One of the most important findings from the interviews was that the processes by which the teens felt supported were possible only within the context of a relationship with an adult perceived to be reliable, caring, and importantly, competent. These youths were better able to see a future for themselves when they were feeling competent and had higher expectations for their behavior. These feelings and sentiments were not apparent in the absence of a caring relationship with an adult, and notably, with a reliable adult.

The study highlights ways in which PHNs can support resiliency among at-risk youth—either by being that reliable caring adult or by supporting the development and presence of these characteristics in mentors serving adolescents. At the community level, PHNs can also advocate for strategies that make the community more supportive of at-risk youth (e.g., development of after-school programs, internship experiences, and leadership opportunities). Sometimes PHNs experience conflict in balancing attention toward community-level factors, or population health, versus individual-level care, and the establishment of a caring relationship. Evidence Example 10.4 demonstrates this in the prevention of tuberculosis outbreaks in a population through individual-level care efforts that were sometimes not welcomed (Bender, Peter, Wynn, Andrews, & Pringle, 2011).

## Maintains Appropriate Boundaries

Boundaries can be very challenging, yet they are so important in establishing and maintaining caring relationships. If the PHNs are too personal with and close to a client, they might not garner professional respect, but if they are too distant, the PHNs might not gain the client's trust. With the growing popularity of social media and ease of communication via cellphones, PHNs need to carefully consider how to manage these tools in relationship with clients. An agency might have a policy regarding social media (e.g., Facebook or Instagram) and clients, and likely will have a policy regarding accessibility via professional or personal cellphones. Knowing where boundaries are and when they should be moved or adjusted takes time, experience, and practice. See Table 10.3 for sample warning signs of inappropriate boundaries in a nurse-client relationship. New PHNs can benefit from the insights of experienced PHNs, who undoubtedly have numerous positive and negative examples to share. Refer to Chapter 6 for a more in-depth discussion of professional boundary issues.

When PHNs work in a community where they also live, it is important that they establish appropriate boundaries when they encounter clients in social contexts (Sundelof, Hansebo, & Ekman, 2004). A good time to discuss boundaries in social contexts is at the beginning of the relationship. Accomplishing this comes with experience and the ability to simultaneously achieve closeness and appropriate distance. Setting limits is the nurse's responsibility, not the

---

### EVIDENCE EXAMPLE 10.4

**Welcome Intrusions—An Interpretive Phenomenological Study of TB Nurses' Relational Work**

In a phenomenological (lived experience) study, Amy Bender, Elizabeth Peter, Francine Wynn, Gavin Andrews, and Dorothy Pringle (2011) conducted interviews and observed nurse-client relationships (n = 9 nurses, 24 clients). The nurses were employed in a public health department in Canada and had the challenge of building caring relationships with clients who had tuberculosis while fulfilling surveillance activities to ensure population health. The nurses described experiences that were characterized into an overarching description of "welcome intrusions," with three themes identifying the

relationship process: "getting through the door," "doing TB but more than that," and "beyond a professional" (p.1). The nurses shared stories that demonstrated the tension between establishing and maintaining a caring relationship with TB clients and fulfilling surveillance obligations, which can come across as intrusive and oppositional to a caring relationship. PHNs undertaking these types of core activities need to give focused attention toward establishing caring relationships, particularly when surveillance and reporting requirements are associated with the care being delivered.

client's, and this is particularly important when PHNs are caring for someone with whom they might have had prior personal interactions, such as might often occur in rural communities.

Another element of maintaining boundaries is taking care of yourself to ensure personal safety when you are working as a PHN. Personal safety is important for PHNs, who can often find themselves in vulnerable or potentially harmful situations. This need for caution clearly can slow the development of a caring relationship, but PHNs should never place themselves at risk for personal harm to advance the relationship. Instead, PHNs should creatively explore ways in which relationships can be developed and safety can be maximized. However, note that seeking to be safe does not mean seeking to be comfortable. A home environment might be uncomfortable because of the presence of head lice, cockroaches, or clutter, but PHNs caring for this family need to work amid these factors. In doing so, they gain the family's respect and trust. If the PHNs were to keep the visits short because of their personal discomfort, it might be difficult to reach the level of a caring relationship that can yield positive, lasting results with the family.

In contrast, PHNs might feel unsafe if they observe criminal activities during a visit (e.g., drug use) or if the neighborhood is known for gang violence. Table 10.4 outlines factors influencing safety when conducting home visits. Patricia Fazzone, Linda Barloon, Susan McConnell, and Julie Chitty (2000) conducted a study with PHNs and other home-visiting staff and observed that the staff members believed that risks to their personal safety were high, a finding consistent with additional research on safety for staff providing care in homes, public settings, and communities (Gellner, Landers, O'Rourke, & Schlegel, 1994; Kendra, Weiker, Simon, Grant, & Shullick, 1996; Schulte, Nolt, Williams, Spinks, & Hellsten, 1998). Fazzone et al. found that the staff believed that some personal characteristics were protective in terms of safety, including "self-confidence, self-reliance, self-motivation, flexibility, 'being comfortable with the unknown,' and self-assurance about their personal judgment" (2000, p. 49).

Generally, when students are assigned a public health nursing clinical experience, faculty members ensure that appropriate safety precautions are taken (see Table 10.5). Most clinical sites also review their policies and procedures for safety during orientation with new students. If a student is unsure of what to do or feels concerned about the safety involved in a clinical experience, that student should immediately approach a clinical instructor or preceptor before proceeding. For example, many students do not feel comfortable conducting home visits alone. Although it is becoming more popular to assign students in pairs for home visits or to have students accompany PHNs, many programs continue to encourage students to conduct solo home visits. When a student is uncomfortable making a visit alone, that student needs to talk through the decision

**TABLE 10.3 Sample Warning Signs of Inappropriate Boundaries in a Nurse-Client Relationship**

- Spending extra time with one client
- Doing something for one client that you don't do for others (e.g., attend baby shower, birthday party)
- Changing client assignments to give care to a specific client
- Believing that other members of the team do not understand a specific client as well as you do
- Disclosing personal problems to a client or client's family member
- Thinking about a client frequently when away from work
- Being guarded or defensive when someone questions your interactions with a client
- Spending off-duty time with a client
- Ignoring agency policies when working with a specific client
- Keeping secrets with a client apart from the health team

*Source:* Adapted from Nurses Association of New Brunswick, 2015, Appendix C

**EVIDENCE EXAMPLE 10.5**
**Caring PHN-Family Relationships**

A study was conducted in Manitoba, Canada, to describe the relationships between PHNs and families whose homes they visited as part of an early childhood program (Heaman, Chalmers, Woodgate, & Brown, 2007). Twenty-four PHNs and 20 parents were interviewed. All the nurses had at least a bachelor's degree and on average 14 years of work experience. Both nurses and parents spoke about three phases of the caring relationships: establishing, maintaining, and terminating them. It was clear that the best way to end the relationship was to establish a planned exit that occurred over the last few visits. Key characteristics of caring relationships were described, including respect, support, trust, partnership, and, for the nurses, appropriate levels of supervision and evaluation. A key finding was the maintenance of professional-client boundaries and the need for the PHNs to affirm the professional nature of the relationship. Study findings emphasized the need for the PHNs to put effort into establishing relationships not only with the clients but also with colleagues, such as "home visitors" (e.g., home health aides).

**TABLE 10.4  Factors Influencing Safety When Conducting Home Visits**

| Conditions in/outside the home | Environmental conditions | Organizational factors |
| --- | --- | --- |
| ▪ People loitering around the home or street<br>▪ Known felon in home<br>▪ Verbal, physical, and sexual aggression<br>▪ Gangs and gang activity<br>▪ Police raids and drug busts<br>▪ Weapons and shootings<br>▪ Garbage, debris<br>▪ Poor lighting or ventilation<br>▪ Homes in disarray<br>▪ Pests<br>▪ Pets<br>▪ Secondhand smoke<br>▪ Mental health instability of client/family | ▪ Night travel<br>▪ Traveling in remote areas<br>▪ Increase in number of garage- or home-based methamphetamine labs<br>▪ Domestic and/or neighborhood violence<br>▪ Poverty<br>▪ Lack of cellphone coverage | ▪ Absence or inaccessibility of written policies/procedures<br>▪ Safety policies not enforced<br>▪ Safety policies not relevant to home care issues<br>▪ Staff unfamiliarity with community<br>▪ Lack or delay of security assistance<br>▪ Cellphones not provided for staff<br>▪ Absence of "call-in" or "check-in" systems<br>▪ Lack of or minimal administrative support<br>▪ Staff delay or failure in reporting incidents<br>▪ Staff not always aware of violent or unsafe history with clients or families |

*Source:* Adapted from Fazzone et al., 2000, p. 47

**TABLE 10.5  Safety Suggestions for Student Nurses Conducting Home Visits**

| Suggestion | Tips |
| --- | --- |
| **Know the neighborhood** | ▪ Identify safe and unsafe public spaces.<br>▪ Identify businesses (such as gas stations, restaurants, or grocery stores) in the neighborhood that are safe places to go for help.<br>▪ Know which roads are open and passable.<br>▪ Avoid visits after dark.<br>▪ Park in a location that allows you to leave without being blocked in by others. |
| **Be prepared** | ▪ Make sure your gas tank is full and that your car has appropriate supplies in case you become stranded.<br>▪ If you are taking public transportation, know the transportation schedule.<br>▪ Carry your phone and make sure it is charged.<br>▪ Carry valuables on your person and leave your purse at home.<br>▪ Always let someone know your schedule of visits and changes that occur (e.g., cancellations). |
| **Stay vigilant in the home** | ▪ Know where your exits are.<br>▪ Ensure pets are restrained if necessary prior to entering the space. |

with a preceptor and clinical instructor. Similarly, students might be involved in planning a community health fair but might not feel comfortable attending the fair during evening hours. Students need to address their concerns with a clinical instructor and determine a plan that meets learning goals while maintaining appropriate levels of safety. Remember, too, that feeling uncomfortable in an unfamiliar environment or climate is not the same as feeling unsafe. In many public health nursing clinical experiences, it is common to feel uncomfortable but to learn through reflecting on those feelings and experiences.

## Demonstrates Tact and Diplomacy

In a caring, professional relationship, PHNs act in a tactful and diplomatic manner. Consistent with ethical standards and expectations, PHNs strive to develop caring relationships without consideration for personal or social characteristics, such as income level or social status (Fredriksson & Eriksson, 2006). Effective PHNs are consistent in how they deliver nursing care and services, including the effort they make in seeking and obtaining resources for clients and communities. Beth Crisp and Pam Lister (2004) describe how PHNs who were working with families involved in child protection situations made an effort to see all families so that they avoided the possibility that some families would feel stigmatized. Indeed, sometimes families who receive a visit from a social worker feel stigmatized or think that they are the worst families, however "worst" is defined. When PHNs are addressing sensitive issues with families or communities, acting in a tactful or diplomatic manner enhances the potential for effective impact and enables the PHNs to be viewed as allies.

When PHNs act in a diplomatic manner that is considerate of the opinions, beliefs, ideas, and perspectives of others, they are more likely to be successful in establishing caring relationships. Diplomacy takes time and patience as well as a willingness to listen and truly hear what others are saying. Successful PHNs know this well and protect the time they need to serve individuals, families, and communities in a diplomatic manner. Thomas Gantert, Carol McWilliam, Catherine Ward-Griffin, and Natalie Allen (2009) found that for both clients and their family members, relationship-building is critical to how they perceive the actions of the staff providing care in their home (e.g., PHNs, home health aides). The relationship is not static, but rather fluid, and requires ongoing attention and determination on the part of PHNs. An established caring relationship needs to be maintained, which requires tact, respect, patience, and the ability to perceive/assess the state of the relationship on an ongoing basis. Effective PHNs do not presume that the relationship, once established, is settled and certain. Instead, they regularly take note of the relationship dynamics and make efforts with every interaction to continue to build an optimal caring relationship. In this environment, interventions are successful and lasting, as reflected in both client feedback and observed outcomes.

## Seeks Assistance When Needed in Managing Relationships

Unquestionably, nurses at all levels of experience bring an inherent desire to care and respond to a moral imperative to do so. However, it is also apparent that relationship skills are honed over time as inexperienced PHNs begin to appreciate the daily struggles of clients' lives and learn to judge what does and does not work with increasing refinement (Smith-Battle, Diekemper, & Leander, 2004a, p. 9).

Skills in developing and maintaining caring relationships are built over time; conscientious PHNs early in their careers seek the input and guidance of experienced PHNs as they encounter challenges in developing relationships with clients and communities. Asking busy colleagues to talk through a challenging situation can be difficult, yet this strategy can result in positive results. Supervisors are another great resource, and there is a process referred to

as "parallel process" that new PHNs should know about. It is a process of reflective supervision that encourages "partnership" and models the PHN-client relationship, which in essence provides the new PHN with an interactive role-modeling of what should be occurring with clients in the community (Minnesota Association for Children's Mental Health [MACMH], 2016). This reflective supervision and role-modeling of relationship can be useful to the new PHN not only in relationship with individuals and families, but also in efforts to positively influence parent-child, parent-parent, or similar relationships. Creative solutions or ideas for addressing a barrier in relationship-building often come from talking through the challenge with someone else, such as a colleague or supervisor. More often than not, other PHNs have experienced similar situations and have a variety of strategies they have used to overcome problems and succeed in developing caring relationships.

> *Susan is still not sure of the way she handled the situation with Julie and goes to her supervisor. Her supervisor listens to Susan, and together they explore other options for wordage and interventions. Her supervisor shares some of her experiences and supports Susan's desire to see this family more often to monitor the status of the mother's mental health and the interactions with her children. Susan's supervisor reassures Susan that her caring relationship appears strong and that her actions might have initiated actions by the mother that can improve her quality of life and the family unit's safety.*

Although rare, at times a PHN is unable to establish a caring relationship with a client. In this case, the PHN should bring the matter to a manager as soon as possible so that, if necessary, the client can receive care from another PHN. If this situation occurs, the PHN should not feel ineffective, especially if a solid effort has been made to develop a caring relationship. Sometimes characteristics or experiences beyond the control of a PHN make it difficult for a client to receive care from that PHN. For example, a student who has recently been sexually abused or assaulted might find it difficult to work with a client who has been sexually abused and needs resources to heal. Similar experiences can create a degree of closeness that makes it difficult for the student, or PHN, to remain separate from the client and provide appropriate nursing care.

## Activity

What might be your plan of action in a situation such as the one in which the student has experienced a traumatic event similar to that of the client being served? In whom should the student confide?

More often than not, PHNs experience caring relationships with clients, families, and communities. Over time, they gain experience with each new client. As SmithBattle, Diekemper, and Leander offer, "Cumulative experience provides the foundation for becoming more responsive, for appreciating the strengths as well as the vulnerabilities and suffering of clients, for becoming more open and attentive to clients' needs and concerns" (2004a, p. 9). Cumulative experience develops within each PHN but can also be shared across PHNs, through case reviews or at staff meetings that provide opportunities to express challenges and seek input from peers.

The emphasis here on seeking input from peers is not meant to negate the effectiveness of new PHNs. Indeed, new PHNs often bring passion, energy, excitement, and determination to their roles in ways that can inspire and recharge their more experienced peers. New PHNs also experience success in identifying and addressing client and community needs, sometimes because their optimism levels are high and matched by their willingness to act. The following new nurse's story about identifying an unmet community need through a caring relationship the nurse had with her client is inspiring:

> There was this gentleman who had really bad toenails. And one of the family members asked if I could trim his toenails. I was like, 'Well, I guess I can. I don't know why I can't.' [Laughter] So I did, after soaking his feet. And they were really bad. Turns out that after I trimmed them, he stood up and started tap dancing. And this was a really old guy who had tap danced in another life. Well, of course, word got around. They would call, 'Is the foot lady there?' [Laughter] It was actually kind of a nightmare. All these people needed nail care… [Eventually] we started a foot clinic and got real podiatrists in (SmithBattle, Diekemper, & Leander, 2004b, p. 98).

## Ethical Considerations

Public health nursing often occurs in the places where people live, play, worship, and work, and indeed, health occurs "where we live, work, and play" (Robert Wood Johnson Foundation [RWJF], 2010). These are very personal settings, and PHNs are frequently alone when delivering care. Caring relationships are critical to the success of the public health nursing process that PHNs carry out with their clients. Regardless of how simple or complex the care is, PHNs can accomplish much more in the presence of caring relationships. Among many potentially challenging ethical factors, PHNs can act in a way that optimizes empathetic care. Rosalind Ekman Ladd, Lynn Pasquerella, and Sheri Smith propose ethical ideas for building relationships that are cognizant of "decision-making authority and autonomy, allow the exercise of the nurse's moral rights, and recognize

the patient's relationships to significant others" (2000, p. 103). It is interesting that Ladd et al. realize both the importance of autonomy among clients and the moral rights of the nurses. This recognition is important because it emphasizes that PHNs are not expected to simply go along with everything their clients express to maintain caring relationships. Instead, effective PHNs use judgment in every situation so that they deliver optimal care, encourage autonomy, and respect client morals. At times, this requires PHNs to maneuver between contrasting opinions and preferences among the client and family members or community members. Caring relationships and subsequent interventions are rarely straightforward, but when ethical standards are upheld, the resulting outcomes are worth the invested effort.

Marcellus (2005) has developed a framework for relational ethics (i.e., the ethics of relationships) that gives attention to what the PHN needs to do to establish or encourage the development of a trusting relationship. This framework includes four themes: mutual respect, engaged interaction, embodiment, and creating environment.

***Mutual respect*** is an interesting combination of respect and empathy; it encompasses respect for oneself and for the other, yet it also includes receiving respect from others (Austin, Bergum, & Dossitor, 2003). And, similar to empathy (described earlier in this chapter), mutual respect occurs when the PHN seeks to understand, although not necessarily agree with, the actions or circumstances of the individual, family, or community.

***Engaged interaction*** means being responsive and sensitive in a manner that can counteract, to an extent, the powerlessness that some clients or communities might feel in relationship with a public health professional. This level of interaction can occur only when PHNs are willing and able to truly listen to those whom they are serving. Lee SmithBattle describes this as "listening with caring" (2003, p. 369); similarly, it is important to listen to provide responsive care to clients (SmithBattle, Drake, & Diekemper, 1997). Supporting teen mothers is a common role for PHNs, and listening with care means paying close attention to the context in which the teen mother is living, and supporting her by "validating strengths, joys, difficulties, learning, and development" (p. 369). When PHNs are attuned to the teen mother's situation, needs, and strengths, they can maintain a relationship that facilitates effectiveness in the care they provide. Importantly, this care at times might simply mean being silent and listening to the teen mother. In an engaged, caring relationship, PHNs know when to teach and when not to teach, allowing the relationship to be sustained and preserved.

It is not easy to be attuned to a client's perspectives, beliefs, fears, desires, and needs, but effective PHNs seek to achieve embodiment, the third theme of the relational ethics framework. ***Embodiment*** is demonstrated when a nurse is able to grasp the essence of conversations—not only the mere words but also the intertwined meanings and emotions. In a caring relationship, PHNs need to value authenticity, which requires a willingness to be influenced by the nurse-client relationship.

The fourth element in the relational ethics framework is *creating environment,* emphasizing the need for PHNs to reflect and work through the moral dilemmas and ethical challenges they are going to encounter when establishing and maintaining caring relationships (Marcellus, 2005). PHNs regularly encounter dilemmas that challenge their beliefs, perspectives, and at times their best intentions. In the context of a caring relationship, PHNs use reflection to arrive at the best decision for that moment, recognizing the emotions, needs, and vulnerability of those whom their decision will affect. For example, how do PHNs report child mistreatment while continuing to provide home-visiting services to the family? This is not an uncommon scenario that PHNs face in addition to numerous similar examples of difficult yet surmountable challenges to maintaining caring relationships with individuals, families, and communities. See Table 10.6 for an additional summary of ethical considerations. The following list identifies some useful reflective questions:

- How was I feeling during this experience?
- What does this experience mean for me?
- How can I use what I have learned from this situation as I move ahead?
- Is there another way I can think about this experience?
- What other things can I learn from this experience?
- How might the outcome have been different if I had…?
- What other people were affected by my actions or inactions?

*Susan continues to see Julie and her two children. Julie continues to receive mental health services along with psychological support as she deals with past issues and her newly diagnosed bipolar disease. Julie stabilizes and appreciates the day Susan made her take stronger action for herself. The issue of safety now is part of the family home visits that they share. Susan continues to be committed to the relationship by empowering this mother, building on her strengths, providing her support through education, and, of course, listening. Julie continues to feel that the relationship is beneficial and supportive for her. They both recognize that boundaries must exist in maintaining a caring and ethically strong nurse–family relationship.*

### Activity

Which Cornerstones of Public Health Nursing (see Chapter 1) do you think are consistent with supporting the PHN's interventions in working with Julie and her children?

## TABLE 10.6  Ethical Action in Establishing Caring Relationships

| Ethical Perspective | Application |
|---|---|
| Rule ethics (principles) | ▪ In relationships, realize the autonomy and the authority of individuals, families, and communities to make decisions.<br>▪ Encourage autonomy by asking the primary client which information can be shared with others, including other family members.<br>▪ Encourage shared decision-making (e.g., client and PHN; or client, family, and PHN). |
| Virtue ethics (character) | ▪ Remember that respect is critical to successful caring relationships.<br>▪ Act in a manner that encourages a mutually trusting relationship.<br>▪ Be patient with the development of a caring relationship. |
| Feminist ethics (reducing oppression) | ▪ Respect beliefs, perspectives, feelings, opinions, ideas, cultural traditions, and preferences.<br>▪ Recognize that most clients come to the relationship thinking that they have little power.<br>▪ Encourage shared power in the relationship by practicing mutuality and empathy. |

## KEY POINTS

- Caring relationships are core to effective public health nursing.
- Caring relationships can be established with individuals, families, communities, and systems.
- Caring relationships are built on trust, respect, and empathy.

- A caring relationship will not last if PHNs do not follow through on commitments, maintain appropriate boundaries, and demonstrate tact and diplomacy.
- PHNs need to operate in ways that are safe for themselves and others.
- Establishing a caring relationship might require PHNs to step outside their personal comfort zones.

## REFLECTIVE PRACTICE

These questions provide additional opportunities for reflecting on the challenges a PHN can experience when developing or working in a caring relationship with a client:

1. As you reflect on this chapter, do you believe that a caring professional relationship can also be a friendship? Why or why not? (See Chapter 6 for discussion on professional boundaries.)

2. Describe possible differences in development of a caring relationship if the initial visit with the client is at the clinic versus in the client's home.

3. A PHN has been seeing a family for several visits, and then the family is not home at the next planned visit. How might you address this absence with the family in a caring manner?

4. You are going on your first PHN family home visit. Which aspects of this visit might be uncomfortable for you? How will you deal with these feelings? How are these "uncomfortable aspects" different from "safety issues"?

5. PHNs value authenticity in caring relationships with their clients. How can PHNs better prepare themselves emotionally to be willing to be influenced by the relationship as much as the client is?

6. What are some ways in which trust between PHNs and clients could be threatened?

7. What can PHNs do if trust is broken with the client and the relationship is no longer caring or therapeutic?

8. What are possible implications if PHNs find themselves unable to establish or maintain a caring relationship with a client, and they do not address this concern but continue to provide care?

## APPLICATION OF EVIDENCE

1. Identify the steps you take in your current nursing practice to develop effective caring relationships with clients.

2. Describe three resources available to you in public health nursing practice for difficult caring situations.

3. What are some ways PHNs can assess the extent to which their perceptions of the client–nurse relationship are similar to or different from the client's perceptions?

4. How might you apply the relational ethics framework (refer to the earlier "Ethical Considerations" section) to a specific public health nursing situation, such as needing to do surveillance for tuberculosis?

# References

Aronowitz, T. (2005). The role of "envisioning the future" in the development of resilience among at-risk youth. *Public Health Nursing, 22*(3), 200–208.

Austin, W., Bergum, V., & Dossitor, J. (2003). Relational ethics: An action ethic as a foundation for health care. In V. Tschudin (Ed.), *Approaches to ethics: Nursing beyond boundaries* (pp. 45–52). Woburn, MA: Butterworth-Heinemann.

Bender, A., Peter, E., Wynn, F., Andrews, G., & Pringle, D. (2011). Welcome intrusions: An interpretive phenomenological study of TB nurses' relational work. *International Journal of Nursing Studies, 48*(11), 1409–1419. doi:http://dx.doi.org/10.1016/j.ijnurstu.2011.04.012

Brown-Stephenson, M. (2017). United States Public Health Service nurses: Deployment in global crisis. *OJIN: The Online Journal of Issues in Nursing, 22*(1), Manuscript 6. Retrieved from http://nursingworld.org/MainMenuCategories/ANAMarketplace/ANAPeriodicals/OJIN/TableofContents/Vol-22-2017/No1-Jan-2017/United-States-Public-Health-Service-Nurses.html

Browne, A. J., Hartrick Doane, G., Reimer, J., MacLeod, M., & McLellan, E. (2010). Public health nursing practice with "high priority" families: The significance of contextualizing "risk." *Nursing Inquiry, 17*(1), 26–37.

Chafey, K. (1996). "Caring" is not enough: Ethical paradigms for community-based care. *Nursing and Health Care Perspectives on Community, 17*(1), 10–15.

Chismar, D. (1988). Empathy and sympathy: The important difference. *Journal of Value Inquiry, 22*(4), 257–266.

Crisp, B., & Lister, P. (2004). Child protection and public health: Nurses' responsibilities. *Journal of Advanced Nursing, 47*(6), 656–663.

DiNapoli, P. P., Nelson, J., Turkel, M., & Watson, J. (2010). Measuring the caritas processes: Caring factor survey. *International Journal for Human Caring, 14*(3), 15–20.

Duiveman, T., & Bonner, A. (2012). Negotiating: Experiences of community nurses when contracting with clients. *Contemporary Nurse: A Journal for the Australian Nursing Profession, 41*(1), 120–125.

Fawcett, J. (2000). *Analysis and evaluation of contemporary nursing knowledge: Nursing models and theories.* Philadelphia, PA: F. A. Davis.

Fazzone, P. A., Barloon, L. F., McConnell, S. J., & Chitty, J. A. (2000). Personal safety, violence, and home health. *Public Health Nursing, 17*(1), 43–52.

Finfgeld-Connett, D. (2008). Qualitative convergence of three nursing concepts: Art of nursing, presence and caring. *Journal of Advanced Nursing, 63*(5), 527–534.

Fredriksson, L., & Eriksson, K. (2006). The ethics of the caring conversation. *Nursing Ethics, 13*(1), 138–148.

Gantert, T., McWilliam, C., Ward-Griffin, C., & Allen, N. (2009). Working it out together: Family caregivers' perceptions of relationship-building with in-home service providers. *Canadian Journal of Nursing Research, 41*(3), 44–63.

Gellner, P., Landers, S., O'Rourke, D., & Schlegel, M. (1994). Community health nursing in the 1990s—Risky business? *Holistic Nursing Practice, 8*(2), 15–21.

Heaman, M., Chalmers, K., Woodgate, R., & Brown, J. (2007). Relationship work in an early childhood home visiting program. *Journal of Pediatric Nursing, 22*(4), 319–330.

Henry Street Consortium. (2017). *Entry-level population-based public health nursing competencies.* St. Paul, MN: Author. Retrieved from www.henrystreetconsortium.org

Jack, S. M., DiCenso, A., & Lohfeld, L. (2005). A theory of maternal engagement with public health nurses and family visitors. *Journal of Advanced Nursing, 49*(2), 182–190.

Jackson, C. (2010). Using loving relationships to transform health care: A practical approach. *Holistic Nursing Practice, 24*(4), 181–186.

Kendra, M. A., Weiker, A., Simon, S., Grant, A., & Shullick, D. (1996). Safety concerns affecting delivery of home health care. *Public Health Nursing, 13*(2), 83–89.

Ladd, R. E., Pasquerella, L., & Smith, S. (2000). What to do when the end is near: Ethical issues in home health care nursing. *Public Health Nursing, 17*(2), 103–110.

Marcellus, L. (2005). The ethics of relation: Public health nurses and child protection clients. *Journal of Advanced Nursing, 51*(4), 414–420.

Martins, D. C. (2008). Experiences of homeless people in the health care delivery system: A descriptive phenomenological study. *Public Health Nursing, 25*(5), 420–430.

McNaughton, D. B. (2005). A naturalistic test of Peplau's theory in home visiting. *Public Health Nursing, 22*(5), 429–438.

Minnesota Association for Children's Mental Health. (2016). *Infant mental health: Best practice guidelines for reflective supervision/consultation.* Retrieved from http://www.macmh.org/about-maiecmh/guidelines-reflective-supervision

Morse, J. M., Bottorff, J., Neander, W., & Solberg, S. (1991). Comparative analysis of conceptualizations and theories of caring. *IMAGE: Journal of Nursing Scholarship, 23*(2), 119–126.

Morse, J. M., Solberg, S. M., Neander, W. L., Bottorff, J. L., & Johnson, J. L. (1990). Concepts of caring and caring as a concept. *Advances in Nursing Science, 13*(1), 1–14.

Nagano, H. (2000). Empathic understanding: Constructing an evaluation scale from the microcounseling approach. *Nursing and Health Sciences, 2*(1), 17–27.

Nurses Association of New Brunswick. (2015). *Standards for the therapeutic nurse-client relationship.* Retrieved from http://www.nanb.nb.ca/media/resource/NANB-StandardsNurseClientRelation-E-2015-10.pdf

Olthuis, G., Dekkers, W., Leget, C., & Vogelaar, P. (2006). The caring relationship in hospice care: An analysis based on the ethics of the caring relationship. *Nursing Ethics, 13*(1), 29–40.

Porr, C., Drummond, J., & Olson, K. (2012). Establishing therapeutic relationships with vulnerable and potentially stigmatized clients. *Qualitative Health Research, 22*(3), 384–396.

Ridgeway, S. (2010). Profiles in nursing: Lillian Wald, founded public health nursing. *Working Nurse.* Retrieved from http://www.workingnurse.com/articles/Lillian-Wald-Founded-Public-Health-Nursing

Robert Wood Johnson Foundation. (2010, January 1). *A new way to talk about the social determinants of health.* Retrieved from https://www.rwjf.org/content/dam/farm/reports/reports/2010/rwjf63023

Rosa, W. (2016, May 12). *Public health nursing series: Sustainable Development Goal #3 – Good health and well-being (part 6).* Retrieved from http://www.springerpub.com/w/nursing/blog-public-health-nursing-series-sustainable-development-goal-3-good-health-and-well-being-part-6/

Schaffer, M. A., Jost, R., Pederson, B. J., & Lair, M. (2008). Pregnancy-free club: A strategy to prevent repeat adolescent pregnancy. *Public Health Nursing, 25*(4), 304–311.

Schulte, J. (2000). Finding ways to create connections among communities: Partial results of an ethnography of urban public health nurses. *Public Health Nursing, 17*(1), 3–10.

Schulte, J. M., Nolt, B. J., Williams, R. L., Spinks, C. L., & Hellsten, J. J. (1998). Violence and threats of violence experienced by public health field workers. *Journal of the American Medical Association, 280*(5), 439–442.

Shores, C. I. (2012). Caring behaviors of faith community nurses. *International Journal for Human Caring, 16*(3), 74.

SmithBattle, L. (2003). Displacing the "rule book" in caring for teen mothers. *Public Health Nursing, 20*(5), 369–376.

SmithBattle, L., Diekemper, M., & Leander, S. (2004a). Getting your feet wet: Becoming a public health nurse, part 1. *Public Health Nursing, 21*(1), 3–11.

SmithBattle, L., Diekemper, M., & Leander, S. (2004b). Moving upstream: Becoming a public health nurse, part 2. *Public Health Nursing, 21*(2), 95–102.

SmithBattle, L., Drake, M. A., & Diekemper, M. (1997). The responsive use of self in community health nursing practice. *Advances in Nursing Science, 20*(2), 75–89.

Smith-Campbell, B. (1999). A case study on expanding the concept of caring from individuals to communities. *Public Health Nursing, 16*(6), 405–411.

Sundelof, A. E., Hansebo, G., & Ekman, S.-L. (2004). Friendship and caring communion: The meaning of caring relationship in district nursing. *International Journal for Human Caring, 8*(3), 13–20.

Taylor, J., Smith, P., & Taylor, J. (2017). A hermeneutic phenomenological study exploring the experience health practitioners have when working with families to safeguard children and the invisibility of the emotions work involved. *Journal of Clinical Nursing, 26*(3/4), 557–567.

Warelow, P., Edward, K. L., & Vinek, J. (2008). Care: What nurses say and what nurses do. *Holistic Nursing Practice, 22*(3), 146–153.

Watson Caring Science Institute and International Caritas Consortium. (2013). Caring science theory. Retrieved from https://www.watsoncaringscience.org/jean-bio/caring-science-theory/

# COMPETENCY #9

## Incorporates Mental, Physical, Emotional, Social, and Spiritual Aspects of Health Into Assessment, Planning, Implementation, and Evaluation

■ **Carolyn M. Porta**

*with Christine C. Andres and Renee Kumpula*

> "*Maria has just finished her six-month orientation at a local public health department in the Maternal Child Health division. She received her nursing license just seven months ago after spending a decade in business management as a supervisor of a large customer service and sales department. Maria is concerned about how she can possibly assess all aspects of health in high-risk populations. One weekend, Maria receives a referral from the local hospital involving a child who needs to be seen by a public health nurse (PHN). Maria is excited and nervous about this first case. The only information she receives is that the family has a 2-year-old boy who is being released from the hospital after suffering an asthma attack. Newly diagnosed with asthma, the boy and his family need education and a home assessment.*
>
> *Maria calls the mother to set a time for the visit. While driving to the home, Maria mentally reviews everything she knows about asthma. She anticipates that education will be easy because she has a son with asthma and is familiar with the disease process and management. Upon arrival at the home, she becomes slightly uneasy with the multiple dogs and cats roaming the yard. She knocks several times on the trailer door before a man answers and lets her inside the home. Maria enters the kitchen, and everyone exchanges introductions. Marcus, the boy with asthma, is quiet in his mother's arms. His brothers, 1 and 5 years of age, are running around the kitchen table, trying to open Maria's nursing bag, jumping on her, and attempting to take her pen. It is very chaotic. Maria has to overcome her anxiety as she realizes that completing a nursing assessment is going to be a challenge.*"

---

### MARIA'S NOTEBOOK

**COMPETENCY #9** Incorporates Mental, Physical, Emotional, Social, and Spiritual Aspects of Health into Assessment, Planning, Implementation, and Evaluation

A. Assesses mental, physical, emotional, social, and spiritual health

B. Develops and implements holistic public health interventions that meet the needs of individuals, families, communities, and systems

C. Evaluates the impact of public health nursing interventions on the mental, physical, emotional, social, spiritual, and environmental health of individuals, families, communities, and systems

*Source:* Henry Street Consortium, 2017

*(continues)*

**MARIA'S NOTEBOOK** *(continued)*

**USEFUL DEFINITIONS**

**Assessment:** "Assessment is holistic and conducted with emphasis on fine observation over time in addition to standard tools" (Kemp, Anderson, Travaglia, & Harris, 2005, p. 257). The importance of assessment in terms of culture is summarized in this way: "Accurate assessment of the state of cultural diversity within healthcare organizations and service communities is essential for the development of appropriate culturally congruent care" (Schim, Doorenbos, Benkert, & Miller, 2007, p. 106).

**Environmental Health:** "Environmental health comprises those aspects of human health, including quality of life, that are determined by physical, chemical, biological, social, and psychosocial factors in the environment. It also refers to the theory and practice of assessing, correcting, controlling, and preventing those factors in the environment that can potentially affect adversely the health of present and future generations" —draft definition developed at a WHO consultation in Sofia, Bulgaria, 1993 (U.S. Department of Health and Human Services Environmental Health Policy Committee, Risk Communication and Education Subcommittee, 1998).

**Holistic:** Holistic is defined as "the characteristics of the spiritual self in combination with those of the emotional and physical self-response to situations as a totality" (Labun, 1988, p. 314) or "the interrelationships among the physical, emotional and spiritual aspects of the person" (p. 315).

**Holistic Nursing:** Holistic nursing is defined as "all nursing practice that has healing the whole person as its goal and honors relation-centered care and the interconnectedness of self, others, nature, and spirituality; focuses on protecting, promoting health and wellness..." (Dossey & Keegan, 2016, p. 3).

**Spiritual:** Spirituality is a "fundamental element to the human experience of health and healing, illness and dying" (Hayden, 2011, p. 546). In cases of end-of-life assessment and planning interventions, clients are seeking PHNs to "affirm [their] expressed belief systems" (Ellington et al., 2015, p. 15).

## From the Seen to the Unseen

One of the reasons that nursing is such an exciting profession is the breadth and depth of nursing practice. Nurses work in so many different arenas and engage in a range of health promotion, intervention, and healing or transition-process activities. Public health nursing is no exception, and, to an extent, it sets a precedent for the diversity of nursing practice. PHNs care for people where they work, play, worship, and live. In this space, PHNs are positioned to understand, respect, and support the ways in which individuals and families pursue healing and health for themselves. Consider the breadth of healing practices that fall outside of the traditional Western medicine scope (e.g., aromatherapy, acupuncture, ecotherapy, yoga, Ayurveda, reflexology, herbalism) yet are integral to health and healing for many. PHNs are well positioned to support whole health. An appreciation for the complexity of health informs this public health nursing competency. Indeed, competent PHNs can holistically understand and assess numerous aspects of health and then intervene, support, and evaluate outcomes in creative, meaningful ways. This chapter explores the ninth Henry Street Consortium Competency, with particular emphasis

given to those aspects of health that can be subtle and perhaps more challenging for a beginning PHN. Rather than overwhelm, we hope this chapter informs and encourages you to consider the range of possibilities in public health nursing as viewed through a holistic lens.

## Assessing the Mental, Physical, Emotional, Social, and Spiritual Health of Individuals, Families, Communities, and Systems

Assessment gives PHNs an understanding of what is going on, including what might be contributing to problems or preventing solutions and how they can assist or intervene. In preparation to become a nurse, you spend numerous hours learning and practicing assessments. In a clinical assessment for heart disease, nurses might take a blood pressure, measure cholesterol, run a stress test, and take a verbal personal and family history. In a public health nursing assessment, these objective and subjective types of data are also collected, yet the scope is often broader in that PHNs conduct assessments at the community and systems levels. At all levels, the nurses' emphases on objective and subjective data remain similar. PHNs systematically observe, document, and summarize data to support assessment findings. These data are quantitative (e.g., rates of disease, symptom frequency, number of risks, number of assets, costs) and qualitative (e.g., personal experiences of those affected, expressed opinions, photographs that demonstrate risks/assets). Most important is that an assessment is carefully planned and thoroughly implemented so that results are useful and can be acted upon.

At the individual level, examples of direct care assessment include examining a newborn for signs of healthy development, screening a new mother for postpartum depression, and determining the spiritual state of someone recently diagnosed with terminal cancer. In the home setting, PHNs consider the environment in which a family is living by assessing home safety (e.g., loose rugs that might cause an elderly client to trip or lead paint flakes a toddler could ingest) and the social environment, such as neighborhood safety (e.g., crime levels or access to healthy food sources; see Chapter 5 for more information on environment). In addition, PHNs assess whether clients have sufficient capacity and support for improving health. Although spiritual questions may be associated more with faith community nurses, congregational nurses, and parish nurses, PHNs include spiritual assessment at the individual level. One of the ways PHNs can be more deliberate and intentional about assessing holistic needs is to ask open-ended questions to discover what belief systems may influence the client and family and what values they hold about health and well-being: What faith traditions may be important to them? What spiritual practices may contribute to planning for holistic interventions and care? Where do they go to receive strength and affirmation (i.e., the sources to which they are connected and their network of support)?

Another type of assessment is conducted when individuals are asked how they might be best supported by a PHN. Fifty mothers who had gone through drug dependency court were asked in a study how they could be best supported by PHNs in their treatment and reunification with their children (Somervell, Saylor, & Mao, 2005). In interviews, the mothers suggested they would like PHNs to serve as a bridge of information to them, reporting on the health and well-being of their children while those children were in foster care. This needs assessment provided the PHNs with clarity of what the mothers wanted (and did not want) in services, knowledge that was useful in planning their activities while working with these mothers.

Family-level assessment expands the individual-level focus to the family unit, which is and should be identified by the individual. During the initial relationship-building with the client, the PHN should ascertain from the client the identified "family," living structure, and support system. The family is viewed as an interactional system, with its holistic health determined by such factors as family dynamics and relationships, family structure, and family functioning (Friedman, Bowden, & Jones, 2003). This approach is particularly useful when PHNs try to manage a health condition that is somewhat dependent on the family setting. For example, a school nurse might work with a student to manage asthma, but without adequate family assessment, the nurse might miss risk factors in the home that are aggravating the asthma (e.g., smoking family members, dust, presence of rodents). Assessment of family-level risk behaviors can also contribute to a family-level intervention, such as efforts to increase the activity level of all family members to reduce obesity and risks for diabetes. Holistic public health nursing at the family level might use *family strengths theory*—a theoretical approach that emphasizes building on existing strengths within the family—as a guide to assessment, intervention planning, and implementation (Sittner, Hudson, & Defrain, 2007).

## EVIDENCE EXAMPLE 11.1

### Holistic Public Health Nursing Care for the Family

The following are some helpful clinical examples of holistic public health nursing care for the family unit (Sittner et al., 2007, p. 357):

- Consider assessing a family's strengths when planning nursing care for the family.

- Help families cope with stress and crises effectively by providing consistent information.

- Listen and work toward establishing a trusting relationship with the family.

- Acknowledge the family members' individualized spiritual perspective and implement nursing interventions that promote their spiritual needs.

- Help the family understand that enjoyable time together during an illness is important.

- Encourage the family to be physically close and celebrate occasions.

- Encourage family members to express appreciation for assistance during an illness.

- Help nursing students understand the family strengths perspective.

> *Maria starts with a simple focused assessment of Marcus. He has no temperature and no apparent difficulty breathing. His lung sounds are clear. When she asks about using the nebulizer, his parents respond, "What nebulizer?" Maria calls the hospital triage nurse and, after multiple transfers, reaches a nurse who discovers that the order was never placed but that it would be delivered immediately, with arrival expected later that day. In the meantime, Maria wants to start addressing some of the asthma triggers present in the environment. The floor is coated with food crumbs, and dishes in the sink have flies hovering over them. The windowless room where the boys sleep has three mattresses on the floor with dirty blankets and pillows without coverings. The bathroom has a strong air deodorizer smell; it is also where the parents smoke. Maria starts to feel an itchy sensation on her legs and assesses the children's ankles and legs. They are covered with little red marks, and Marcus's legs feel rough like sandpaper. She mentions the bites on the children, and the mother states that they have a flea problem but have not had the money to do anything about it.*
>
> *As Maria listens, she asks open-ended questions to complete the assessment: When you are in need of help, who do you talk to or where might you go for support? When you are feeling down, describe what you might do that makes you feel better? When your children are sick, what are ways you help them feel better? Other questions Maria might ponder and ask in different ways could be: Where does the family find their strength? What beliefs affect their understanding of health, and what do they embrace regarding wholeness? How do they define "spiritual" and holistic needs? Maria might want to get more information on ways people improve their health, such as yoga, stress relief measures, and prayer. The mother identifies a personal practice of prayer stemming from her religious upbringing and discusses her interest in complementary therapies she heard about on television. She feels anxious and attributes this to the judgment of others on her parenting skills, life choices, and her identifying more with being spiritual than religious. She states that the lack of support or disapproval from relatives within her religious background causes stress. Maria feels overwhelmed. How can she help a family with so many needs?*

Evidence Example 11.2 provides a picture of a unique, holistic approach to assessment at the individual level but focused on past experiences and how those experiences might influence adult health and well-being.

### EVIDENCE EXAMPLE 11.2
#### Department of Health Adverse Childhood Experiences (ACE) Project

In 2011, the Minnesota Department of Health (MDH, 2013) used questions developed by the Centers for Disease Control and Prevention (CDC) to understand the scope and influence of adverse childhood experiences (ACE) on adult health and well-being. The ACE questions focus on exposure to such experiences as emotional, physical, and sexual abuse; substance use; and family disruption. Results of the 2011 survey revealed that many Minnesotan adults report experiencing multiple ACEs in their childhood (before age 18). Many of these adults also reported current social and health problems, including higher rates of chronic illnesses than adults who reported no ACEs in their childhoods. Additional research is needed, but as more researchers utilize ACE questions, there is greater understanding of the influence of ACE on health and well-being into adulthood. Such research strongly supports the need for holistic assessment and health-promotion efforts beginning in childhood; indeed, the Nurse-Family Partnership intervention (https://www.nursefamilypartnership.org/) is an example of positive outcomes from early PHN intervention in the lives of children and mothers (Olds et al., 2007; Olds et al., 2014). The role of resilience in offsetting adverse experiences and promoting well-being despite adversity is also recognized and demonstrated in this research. PHNs have an important role in identifying risk factors as well as protective factors in all aspects of an individual, family, and community.

**Healthy People** The Healthy People 2020 website identifies indicators for a variety of public health concerns in the United States, with goals for improvements by 2020. Select a health indicator and explore how a PHN might work to improve health while paying attention to all aspects of an individual's or community's health. Identify possible collaborators who might work with the PHN to achieve intervention goals and promote health in a comprehensive, holistic manner (e.g., working with a local religious institution or partnering with mental health professionals).

Community assessment broadens the public health nursing perspective to consider the health of a group. Remember that *community* can be defined in many different ways, as a group of people connected by geography, age, ethnicity, spiritual beliefs, or health and risk behaviors. PHNs working with a community need to earnestly examine the strengths and needs in that community before engaging in health-promotion or disease-prevention activities. For example, a faith community nurse might assess the need for a cardiovascular or diabetes screening program and determine the presence of existing resources or gaps in resources in the faith community and surrounding community. The PHN in this case is also going to want to know the extent to which a cardiovascular or diabetes screening program might be a priority health concern for faith community members. A detailed assessment contributes to the increased likelihood of a successful, accepted program.

An occupational PHN might assess the needs and preferences of workers prior to starting a health-promotion intervention. This assessment is necessary because without it, the PHN cannot have a clear picture of the needs and problems and how possible solutions are going to be received. Oxygen delivery drivers might benefit from an intervention that teaches them stretching and ways to prevent repetitive motion injuries, but assessment can inform the PHN whether the drivers have any interest in such a program. Without the drivers' interest or some level of motivation, the intervention could be a significant waste of time, energy, and other resources.

PHNs in local public health departments have often undertaken large-scale geographic community assessments, driving through cities and documenting risks (e.g., crime rates, abandoned buildings, manufacturing plants) and assets (e.g., police presence, recreation areas or opportunities, grocery stores). It is more common in today's environment with constraints on resources (e.g., time, finances) to see PHNs conducting focused or targeted community assessments to inform specific initiatives or activities. However, especially if PHNs are new to a setting, they might benefit from occasional community assessments to inform priorities and goal setting. Often, an assessment helps decision-makers determine how best to use limited funds and resources by prioritizing the greatest areas of need.

The systems level is often more difficult to understand with respect to the nursing process and public health nursing. If you think about the system comprising many of the larger, overarching policies and governmental/societal forces that influence health, then it might be easier to grasp this concept of "system." PHNs employed with the local public health department must work within the guidelines of local-, state-, and federal-level policies, rules, and regulations (see Competency #5, Chapter 7). Assessment at the systems level, then, can be useful when PHNs believe that a particular policy or regulation is needed or should be eliminated. An example of this situation is the assessment that took place across the United States, resulting in indoor antismoking regulations. PHNs worked with many colleagues to assess the potential impact of an indoor smoking ban, including its costs, ethics, and health implications. Systems-level assessment is complex, yet it is so important, because when policies or laws are made, they have the potential for extensive, long-lasting influence.

PHNs can often contribute to the successes of statewide screening programs. When PHNs are directly involved in the assessment, planning, implementation, and evaluation of infant screening programs, they are more likely to be successful (Kemper, Fant, & Clark, 2005). PHNs work directly with infants, parents, and families, and this experience is valuable when large-scale efforts are planned. The PHNs are ideally prepared to develop the screening tools that can be used not only in the home but also in common healthcare settings, such as clinics (Kemper et al., 2005).

Another example is the Follow Along Program (FAP), a Minnesota statewide screening method for young children that is intended to ensure early and continuous screening for health concerns and developmental and behavioral delays. This screening is a cooperative arrangement between the Minnesota Department of Health Children and Youth with Special Health Needs and local FAP agencies, which are typically public health agencies. The PHNs use a computerized tracking program to holistically screen all aspects of a child and to work with families as concerns arise to ensure access to appropriate child and family interventions and support. When the early screening data were evaluated in 1999, the counties with an FAP identified many more children who were eligible for early intervention than those counties that did not have an FAP (MDH, 2009).

See Table 11.1 for an example of a holistic assessment at the individual, community, and systems levels for primary, secondary, and tertiary intervention strategies. Consider which interventions you might explore if you were the PHN addressing this challenge in your community; for example, where might you test a mindfulness intervention, or a restorative justice initiative in the school setting?

### Activity

Using Table 11.1, construct a similar table that is consistent with a holistic approach to addressing a new health problem or condition you have discussed in class or observed in clinical.

**TABLE 11.1 Example of Assessment Addressing Adolescent Substance Use**

| Levels of Assessment and Intervention | Individual | Community | Systems |
|---|---|---|---|
| Primary | Assess risk and protective factors that might influence substance use decision-making. School nurses might screen/survey all students to determine which prevention messages might be ideal based on existing beliefs, assets, and risks among peers, families, and neighborhoods. | Assess community-level attitudes and ideas regarding substance use among adolescents. PHNs might partner with local schools, religious institutions, community parks and playground facilities, and healthcare organizations to conduct focus groups, walk-along interviews, and community assessment to identify key points of intervention—attitudes, behaviors, knowledge, or infrastructure. | Identify the laws and policies that support prevention of substance use among adolescents. PHNs might advocate for stricter penalties for bars selling to underage drinkers if this is a problem in the particular area/city. |
| Secondary | Assess adolescent substance-use behaviors, including risk and protective factors. PHNs might screen a pregnant teen during a home visit to determine substance-use behaviors and plan risk-reduction intervention. | PHNs might assess substance-use behaviors among homeless adolescents to determine incidence and prevalence of drug use and help guide the development of interventions. PHNs might screen homeless youth seeking healthcare and offer cessation programs for those reporting use. | Assess level of substance-use treatment programs available to adolescents in the state. PHNs might work with health insurance providers to ensure that coverage includes adequate time for adolescent participation in a cessation program. |
| Tertiary | Assess adolescent's level of willingness to participate in efforts to reduce risk behaviors during pregnancy. PHNs might provide case management and support for a pregnant adolescent trying not to use during the pregnancy and explore resources with her that promote self-worth, including emotional and spiritual resources. | Partner with community members to assess readiness for change in a community where many adolescents are already using or abusing substances. | Assess the scope of existing resources to serve/treat adolescents who are using/abusing substances. PHNs might collaborate with local community organizations to support or establish treatment centers that can reach and target adolescents. |

## Develops Intervention Plans That Consider Mental, Physical, Emotional, Social, and Spiritual Health

At some point, assessment findings are used to prioritize possible interventions and inform decision-making. The next step, then, is to develop an intervention plan for the target individual, family, community, or systems (see Figure 11.1 for this process). PHNs often work with a family, for example, so that together they consider the findings from the assessment and arrive at a plan to address concerns. Sometimes the intervention plans are very narrow and focused, driven by an assessment that obviously leads to a clear problem and solution. Other times, the intervention plans are broad and encompass several goals and strategies to reach desired outcomes. Regardless of whether the intervention plan is narrow or broad, it can and should be holistic and address multiple aspects of an individual, family, community, or system.

For example, a PHN might conduct home visits with a newborn and mother for the first few postpartum months. Assessment might indicate healthy newborn development but a risk of postpartum depression. The intervention plan is likely to consider all aspects of health for that mom and baby, yielding a multilayered strategy that might include mom breaks (mental), medication for depression or regular walks outside (physical), friend connections (emotional and social), yoga or meditation (spiritual), and housecleaning help (environmental). In this way, a focused intervention to prevent or minimize postpartum depression encompasses, or has the potential to encompass, every aspect of health.

At the community level, the faith community nurse might conclude that a cardiovascular screening program is needed and desired. The resulting intervention plan might include a variety of activities that consider varied aspects of health, including understanding risk impacting heart health (mental), blood pressure or cholesterol measures (physical), stress levels (emotional), relationships (social), and prayer practices (spiritual). In this example, the screening program is holistic and will lead to relevant, individualized interventions.

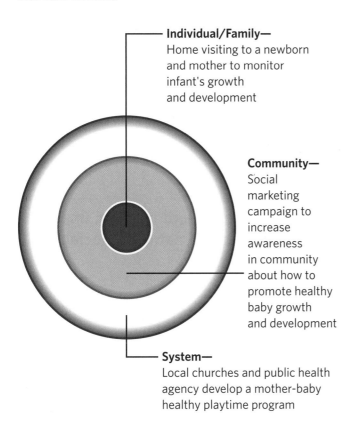

**Individual/Family—**
Home visiting to a newborn and mother to monitor infant's growth and development

**Community—**
Social marketing campaign to increase awareness in community about how to promote healthy baby growth and development

**System—**
Local churches and public health agency develop a mother-baby healthy playtime program

**FIGURE 11.1** Public Health Nursing Process

## EVIDENCE EXAMPLE 11.3
### Listening to Narratives, Understanding the Cycle of Poverty, and Solutions to Inequity

Alicea-Planas (2016) beautifully describes the story of Sammy—a man in poverty who has learned not to trust—in a case study report that exemplifies the importance of a holistic approach to relationship-building and understanding in order to effectively engage with a client. The nurse-client relationship is contextualized in a very challenging environment and is successful because the nurse is willing to listen and the client is willing to be heard. The very real context of poverty and related risk factors is not overlooked or minimized by the nurse, which increases the likelihood that her interactions with the client will yield positive outcomes. Alicea-Planas summarizes, "Although many vulnerable populations live in a perpetual cycle of poverty and poor health, some nurses are able to assess the intricacies of a situation and facilitate understanding, as part of their support, caring, and advocacy for their patients" (2016, p. 162).

In another study, Mabhala (2015) explored the perspectives of public health nurse educators in the UK regarding inequities and the role of public health nurses. The 26 interviews yielded two distinct approaches these educators believe public health nurses should take: (1) an upstream preventive approach focusing on population-level strategies, and (2) directly working with individuals to encourage behaviors that promote health/prevent inequities and poor health outcomes.

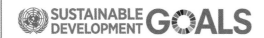

**Reducing Inequality Through Holistic Efforts**

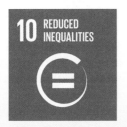

**GOAL 10** This is arguably an aggressive goal, but it is achievable to reduce inequalities. Rather than offer an exemplar project seeking to reduce or eliminate inequality, consider the conclusions of Professor Walter Scheidel on how to reduce inequality, as presented in his text *The Great Leveler: Violence and History of Inequality from the Stone Age to the Twenty-First Century.* Nelson (2017) offers a succinct summary, stating, "After studying thousands of years of human history, Stanford Professor Walter Scheidel identified four indisputable ways to reduce inequality: war, revolution, state collapse, and deadly pandemics" (see https://qz.com/924034/how-to-reduce-inequality-history-suggests-the-only-effective-ways-are-death-and-destruction/).

1. War.    2. Revolution.    3. State Collapse.    4. Deadly Pandemics.

Not on this list are the common interventions encouraged among public health nurses, and others passionate about reducing inequities—interventions such as breaking individual cycles of poverty, improving education among preschool children (and young adults), and implementing policies that encourage economic growth. While reducing inequalities will persist as a goal for many, it behooves you to take note of history and to critically examine what can be done, and where efforts should be directed (such as federal social policy efforts), in the absence of these four dramatic, unfortunate (and temporary) solutions to inequity.

*Maria goes back the next day to review with the family what is important to them and how to prioritize and develop a plan of care. Maria and the parents agree that managing Marcus's asthma is a top priority. Maria completes hands-on education on utilizing the nebulizer. They also agree that the flea infestation and environmental asthma triggers are important, so Maria and the parents plan together how and when they can treat the home to get rid of the fleas, minimize dust, and so forth. Maria addresses some safety issues, such as having the bedroom with no window and hearing Marcus at night if he is having an asthma attack. The father appreciates her help in getting connected to a company that supplies an alarm system.*

A PHN working with the mother and baby in this case study can implement the intervention by carefully discussing the approach with the mother in an empowering manner. It would be overwhelming to recommend and implement every part of the plan immediately. Instead, the nurse and mother could work together to prioritize parts of the intervention and determine achievable goals. For example, access to asthma medication might be an initial goal, and the PHN can help the mother contact and work with her child's primary care provider to arrange a prescription and teach her how to contact the insurance provider to confirm that coverage is available. The PHN can also provide the mother with resources that she feels might be beneficial for her and her family, such as a community center offering yoga classes or a nearby babysitting service that has drop-off

options for moms who need an urgent break. Depending on financial resources, the PHN might explore housecleaning services or might put the mother in touch with youth willing to do this service for needy families at little to no cost. The PHN does not simply give the mother a to-do list but instead works with the mother in a thorough and thoughtful manner to appropriately implement the intervention plan. It is also important to assess the acceptability of the plan to ensure that the mother is not overwhelmed, but rather that she is empowered and building self-efficacy skills to care for herself and her family. A case management intervention, where the PHN intervenes to address many health needs over the course of multiple visits, has been shown to be effective (see Evidence Example 11.4). As explained by the Minnesota Department of Health, "Case management optimizes self-care capabilities of individuals and families and the capacity of systems and communities to coordinate and provide services" (MDH, 2001, p. 93).

## Implements Interventions That Improve Mental, Physical, Emotional, Social, and Spiritual Health

After an intervention plan is identified, the PHN needs to identify resources and arrange the logistics (i.e., details specific to the event) for implementing the plan. This might include collaborating with colleagues, finding community partners, or leveraging financial resources to ensure success. Careful planning is necessary to ensure successful intervention implementation. At times, PHNs have insights and experiences that are also helpful to colleagues working with the family. PHNs are often valuable resources and sources of support to colleagues addressing child protection or abuse concerns with families (Crisp & Green Lister, 2004). The issues surrounding child protection situations are complex and require intention toward understanding multiple factors (e.g., social, emotional, spiritual, and environmental) rather than simply carrying out mandated reporting requirements. Indeed, PHNs have an important role in helping link the public health and child welfare systems so that optimal care is provided to the families in an integrated, comprehensive way (Schneiderman, 2006). When integration occurs, children in the foster care system, for example, can more easily have their healthcare needs met because PHNs can provide a critical link for the families to the healthcare system while being aware of the foster care requirements and restrictions. In another example of prenatal care, PHNs conducted a demonstration project in which they assessed each referred pregnant woman to identify psychosocial risks and to increase her awareness of local community resources available during the pregnancy (Strass & Billay, 2008). The key to the success of this intervention was the effort of the PHNs to assess and consider the diverse psychosocial risks rather than to focus solely on

### EVIDENCE EXAMPLE 11.4
#### PHN Prenatal Care Case Management

A study was conducted to evaluate the effectiveness of case management by PHNs for prenatal care, as compared to programs offering limited prenatal assessment or referral programs (Ricketts, Murray, & Schwalberg, 2005). The PHN prenatal care case management was provided to more than 3,500 women. Key findings for the women receiving the prenatal care case management were that many of them decided to reduce risk behaviors that could lead to poorer birth outcomes. For example, mothers who acted on PHN advice to quit smoking during pregnancy or to gain enough weight had fewer low-birthweight babies than did mothers who did not address these risks. Consistent with case management practices, women who had more than 10 visits were more likely to reduce their risks than those who received fewer visits. The study demonstrated the particular value of PHN case management in helping reduce risks during pregnancy and promoting healthy pregnancy outcomes and the well-being of newborns.

the physical nature of the pregnancy. Healthcare providers making referrals to the PHNs wanted them to continue providing the service—demonstrating support for, and the value of, this public health nursing intervention.

At the community level, a PHN planning a cardiovascular screening program as a faith community nurse needs to organize a team of individuals, depending on the number of people who will be screened and how frequently the screenings will occur. The PHN arranges the logistics, organizes volunteers, and provides leadership for the screening program (see Table 11.2). The most successful intervention is one that is carefully planned and considers all the possible influencing factors for success or failure. Key factors include time of day, day of the week, conflicting local activities (e.g., holidays, meetings), ease of the registration process, adequately trained staff, childcare options, refreshments, signs, presence of multiple events or screenings in one large room, and privacy, to name a few.

## Activity

Reflect on how you might conduct a holistic screening event in your community.

Identify how you would set up the event and which interventions you would offer to address physical, emotional, mental, social, and spiritual needs for a holistic approach.

## EVIDENCE EXAMPLE 11.5
### Community-Based Holistic Care

At the systems level, PHNs can be influential in bringing together community partners to implement interventions that affect the way current healthcare systems function and care for people. Healthcare reform provides the context for new, innovative models of holistic care. For example, in Philadelphia, a PHN led efforts to create a transdisciplinary, nurse-managed health center in partnership with the community, bridging the efforts of the local university and the community (Gerrity, 2010). The underserved community desired a "place of their own where healthcare was delivered in response to their identified needs" (p. 62). The center's holistic approach to create health includes primary care by nurse practitioners, integrated behavioral health, dental care, chronic disease management, health promotion, and wellness services, including a variety of complementary integrative therapies. PHNs can be involved in many aspects of this intervention as they advocate for new healthcare systems to support the development of healthy communities. Creating and implementing this healthcare system change to improve health outcomes requires trust between the community and providers and support from government agencies, as well as collaboration between many community partners.

*Maria develops a strong relationship with this family, especially the mother and children, over the next year. She spends time following up on past referrals and interventions. Maria monitors the emotional, physical, environmental, and spiritual health of this mother through tough times that include multiple housing moves, relationship issues, and a period of homelessness. The mother ends her marriage in a bitter divorce that results in many crises for this family. Despite the tension that was created for the mother and her extended family during this period, the client feels support and acceptance because of Maria's ongoing assessment and affirmation of the mother's belief system, use of her support system, and spiritual practices such as prayer to maintain well-being. Throughout, Maria helps the mother monitor Marcus's asthma. As Maria continues to monitor the children's development, she becomes concerned about the youngest son and helps the mother access local services, including early childhood education and parenting groups.*

## Activity

Reflect on the ways in which Maria has provided a holistic case management intervention for this family and the benefits of this strategy as compared to one or two home visits only.

## TABLE 11.2  Setting Up a Screening Clinic

### In Advance

- Assess risk to determine the need for a screening clinic.
- Identify screeners (e.g., determine whether you will use volunteers, paid staff, people from the community or outside the community). Conduct interviews/application process as needed. Note that screeners might need criminal background or reference checks, depending on their activities.
- Train screeners (e.g., screening equipment, process).
- Establish protocol and schedule for screening, referrals, and follow-up.

### Day of the Event

- Focus on logistics (i.e., details specific to the event, such as signage, refreshments and supplies, and the staffing schedule).
- Offer childcare options.
- Convey a clear communication and decision-making structure.
- Plan for adequate, supportive, and thorough follow-up and referrals.

# Evaluates the Impact of Public Health Nursing Interventions on Mental, Physical, Emotional, Social, and Spiritual Health

As the intervention plan is being implemented, PHNs begin to evaluate the impact it is having on the target individual, family, community, or system. It is true that some outcomes might not be realized in the short term, yet PHNs need to pay careful attention to how the intervention is influencing aspects of health right away. Evaluating the impact of a PHN intervention can be complex. Generally, PHNs need to evaluate the intervention process, such as how it went, whether implementation was successful, and how future interventions could be improved. PHNs also need to focus on the impact of the intervention, as determined by the outcomes in the short-, mid-, and long-term. Has the intervention contributed to health? How so? PHNs then return to the assessment strategies that identified the need for the intervention to reassess the situation. This return is a good way to determine whether changes have occurred and to complete a cycle of assessment, planning, intervention, and evaluation.

Entry-level PHNs are expected to have an understanding of what impact evaluation is and how to determine the value and impact of interventions (see Chapter 14 for further discussion of program evaluation and quality improvement). Most commonly, terms such as "continuous quality improvement" are used to capture the scope of evaluation beyond the intervention outcomes themselves to also include performance outcomes by the healthcare team, and factors such as cost effectiveness. The Minnesota Department of Health has developed a toolkit that includes numerous valuable resources to guide processes of evaluation for a variety of purposes. The toolkit can be found at http://www.health.state.mn.us/divs/opi/qi/toolbox/. New public health nurses should see evaluation and continuous quality improvement as important opportunities for skills development and leadership growth and should be confident these skills will be valuable for numerous activities including grant-seeking, collaboration projects within and across health systems, improving departmental value, and meeting accreditation requirements as an organization.

At the community level, a child-obesity surveillance program implemented in numerous Canadian public health clinics with more than 7,000 participants was evaluated (Flynn et al., 2005). In addition to such outcomes as rates of childhood obesity, parent satisfaction was evaluated because the authors of this study believed that one measure of the program's success was the extent to which the parents participating were content with their experience. PHNs administered the obesity surveillance program with families; among those who completed the evaluation survey

## EVIDENCE EXAMPLE 11.6
### Evidence for Home Visits With Mothers and Children

One of the most exemplary studies evaluating the effectiveness of public health nursing interventions is an original randomized controlled trial that measured outcomes of public health nursing visits to 743 mothers and children (Olds et al., 2007). Numerous aspects of health were evaluated over 9 years, including the economic, social, physical, and educational health of the mothers and the physical and educational health of the children. Importantly, children receiving the PHN home visits were less likely to die between birth and 9 years of age and more likely to report higher grade point averages and reading scores than those who did not receive PHN visits. Mothers who received home visits from PHNs were more likely to wait longer to become pregnant with their second child and to maintain longer relationships with their partners, and they reported less use of economic assistance (e.g., welfare assistance or food stamps) than mothers who did not receive home visits from PHNs. The findings from this study have informed national initiatives across the United States to implement PHN home visiting programs for at-risk first-time mothers, and importantly, have been replicated in additional longitudinal randomized trials with similar positive outcomes for the children and the mothers (see Eckenrode et al., 2010 and Olds et al., 2014).

A qualitative approach can also be used to evaluate the effectiveness of the nursing process (see Evidence Example 11.7). In another example of qualitative evaluation, essays written by 62 clients who received PHN home visits in Alaska to help prevent child abuse and neglect were analyzed (DeMay, 2003). Some clients received "intense" services and about twice as many home visits as those assigned to receive "standard" home visit services. The evaluation, however, was not focused on whether one group showed greater benefits compared to the other but instead focused on the extent to which the essays about the PHN visits reflected the PHNs' perspectives about the visits. Interestingly, parents in both groups wrote in their essays about the trusting relationships developed with their PHNs and the importance of these positive relationships. It was noted that those receiving more visits (the intense group) wrote much longer essays than those in the other group, possibly reflecting the depth of relationship that can be built when more home visits are involved.

about the program, more than 98% indicated being "very happy" or "happy" with the information received. The PHNs' confidence in conducting obesity screenings, providing education, and making referrals for follow-up was also assessed in questions posed to the PHNs who participated in the screening pilot project. This assessment is important because the success of any nursing intervention depends not only on the nurses' abilities but also on their confidence in those abilities. Study results indicated that after participating in this screening program, the PHNs had increased confidence in their abilities to screen children accurately for weight and obesity risks and to provide parents with information they could use to improve their children's health.

---

### EVIDENCE EXAMPLE 11.7
**PHN Home Visits to Elderly Clients**

A qualitative approach was used to evaluate the impact of PHN home visits to elderly clients after they had been hospitalized (McKeown, 2007). In interviews, the older people shared that the PHNs helped meet many, but not all, of the needs they experienced following hospitalization (e.g., access to services, social aspects, home environment safety). In this study, it appears that only one home visit was provided, which certainly could be important in interpreting the findings specific to unmet needs. The study is helpful in that it shows the importance of evaluating PHN services to identify (a) what has been successful and (b) what is lacking or could be strengthened. It is very likely that with increased visits and support, these older adults would have shared different experiences in their interviews.

In another study, researchers identified the significance of spiritual conversations that were naturally occurring in the home environment with clients who were receiving end-of-life (EOL) and hospice care (Ellington et al., 2015). Researchers explored the nurse-client or family dyad over 33 home visits with seven client or spouse pairings. Recordings provided insight that critical and deeply personal conversations with spiritual exchanges occurred frequently but were of short duration. The study demonstrated the importance of PHNs opening a dialogue about spiritually relevant concerns. PHNs used approaches such as disclosure of personal EOL life experiences (e.g., what happened with their own loss of a mother), asking open-ended questions, and recommending practical help for the family. Although the study had limitations due to sample size, PHN presence was shown to help provide meaning for clients and families, which in turn provided a sense of support, "spiritual strength," and increased client and family resilience (Ellington et al., 2015, p. 14).

An evaluation of services delivered via a public health nursing sexual health clinic also yielded valuable information about the PHNs' roles and successes. Surveys and semi-structured interviews were conducted with 166 at-risk young people to learn their perspectives toward the services they received from the PHNs (Hayter, 2005). In the interviews, participants reported having confidence in the PHNs' ability to provide services in a confidential manner. Other abilities and attributes of the PHNs were assessed via the survey, and the majority of respondents indicated feeling comfortable talking with the PHNs (84%) and perceiving the PHNs as good listeners (more than 90%). These findings led to the conclusion that PHNs were successfully delivering sexual healthcare to at-risk, marginalized young people in a manner that was acceptable and welcoming to the youth. These data were important because they informed program planning about how to staff and continue the sexual health clinic.

These types of evaluations, including not only the participants but also the PHNs delivering the interventions, require more time and economic resources, yet they yield more holistic information that can be useful in determining whether an intervention is effective and efficient. In today's world, interventions need to be cost-effective and efficient (e.g., with respect to staffing), or they will not be sustained over time. Evaluations that include data to justify the value and efficiency of an intervention are critical.

> *Time passes. Maria has not seen this family for a while since they have moved out of the county. She receives a phone call from the mother to update her on the family's situation, including that she and her boyfriend are expecting a baby. Maria asks how Marcus is doing with his asthma. His mother states that he has not had any episodes for six months and takes his medication every day. They discuss the development and successes of all the children. The mother calls again prior to the birth of her baby to tell Maria she is being induced the following day at a local hospital. Maria states that she might be able to stop by and see her and her new baby. The mother is very excited. Maria enters the hospital room and is greeted by the mother nursing her newborn. No concerns or crises arise during this visit. Maria leaves with tears in her eyes. This is the beginning of a new "family," and they will be residing in another county. Therefore, Maria has to accept that she can no longer serve this family she has become part of for the past three years. She reflects on the journey from that first flea-infested day to the sharing of this birth. Maria has addressed many mental, emotional, environmental, and spiritual issues with this family.*

## Ethical Considerations

PHNs must conduct assessment, planning, implementation, and evaluation in an ethical manner. PHNs should engage with individuals, communities, and systems in ways that demonstrate respect, a willingness to listen and learn, and a desire to come alongside rather than dictate or demand. The way a PHN conducts an assessment directly informs the type of intervention that he or she develops and implements. If the assessment focuses only on problems or risks, the intervention might not build on existing strengths or assets. This approach can lead to dependency rather than autonomy or capacity building. Instead, PHNs' assessments should be holistic, focused on strengths and weaknesses, assets and risks. Interventions should not be dictated but collaboratively designed, with input from those who are receiving the intervention. This collaboration should enhance the potential that the intervention will be welcomed or adhered to, which will increase its likelihood of success. When evaluating the impact of an intervention, PHNs will find it most useful to include multiple sources and types of data. When PHNs ensure that the public health nursing process is holistic and inclusive, they gather the ingredients for successful health promotion and disease prevention. And when they adhere to ethical ideals, PHNs are doing what is needed to yield healthy, sustainable outcomes. See Table 11.3 for an application of ethical perspectives to the holistic nursing process.

### TABLE 11.3  Ethical Action in Holistic Assessment, Intervention, Planning, and Evaluation

| Ethical Perspective | Application |
| --- | --- |
| Rule ethics (principles) | ▪ Understand that the goal of a holistic public health nursing process should be beneficence or the promotion of good (improvement in health status).<br>▪ Encourage autonomy by ensuring that those being affected, including children, have input in determining interventions to improve health. |
| Virtue ethics (character) | ▪ Be respectful when conducting an assessment and carrying out an intervention.<br>▪ Be persistent in obtaining what is needed to successfully intervene based on what the assessment reveals.<br>▪ Be patient when it takes time for an intervention to bear fruit or to be acceptable to those it is for (e.g., a family or a community). |
| Feminist ethics (reducing oppression) | ▪ Ensure that assessment includes strengths and assets in addition to the risks, problems, or challenges.<br>▪ Respect everyone.<br>▪ Emphasize strengths and assets when developing an intervention.<br>▪ Advocate for individuals and community groups that have less power.<br>▪ Evaluate using qualitative and quantitative approaches that consider the broad ways in which an intervention has or has not been effective. |

## KEY POINTS

▪ The public health nursing process of assessment, planning, intervention, and evaluation is an ongoing cycle.

▪ Thorough assessment is critical to the success of the other nursing process phases.

▪ Assessment should include consideration of mental, physical, emotional, social, and spiritual assets and risks.

▪ Successful interventions build on strengths and are implemented with the collaboration and support of those being served.

▪ Evaluation of interventions should be planned before the intervention is initiated.

▪ Thorough evaluation should include qualitative and quantitative strategies.

▪ PHNs are uniquely positioned to collaborate with many different agencies in promoting the health and well-being of individuals/families, communities, and systems.

## REFLECTIVE PRACTICE

Conducting a blood pressure screening clinic in a church with a Spanish-speaking congregation takes thoughtful planning. Faith community nurses need to carefully assess congregational needs and readiness for screening activities. They also have to thoughtfully address many logistical aspects. Realizing that holistic assessment, planning, implementation, and evaluation processes are complex, consider how you might answer the following questions:

1. What might Maria need to consider in planning a health-promotion activity in the neighborhood near the family she has been visiting?

2. Where might Maria go to find out whether the needs she is observing in one family are common to others in the neighborhood?

3. Who would be potentially valuable partners to Maria when she decides that a health-promotion/nutrition screening fair might be of benefit to the neighborhood?

4. How will Maria know whether the health-promotion fair has been successful?

5. What will Maria want to know following this health fair before she organizes another one?

6. How might Maria self-reflect on the process to realize the holistic nature of the screening and to encourage even more effective public health nursing in her future work?

7. Refer to the Cornerstones of Public Health in Chapter 1. Which of these Cornerstones supports efforts to be holistic in conducting PHN interventions or assessments?

## APPLICATION OF EVIDENCE

1. When PHNs conduct a neighborhood needs assessment, where will they find data, and whom might they want to speak with about the community?

2. To enhance the potential for the nutrition health fair to be successful, who are the people/agencies PHNs will want to partner with in planning, implementing, and evaluating the fair and its outcomes?

3. What are the differences in home safety checklists that PHNs might provide to families with young children, families with adolescents, or families with elderly members?

4. What are some qualitative and quantitative ways to assess the successes of public health nursing programs or interventions?

## References

Alicea-Planas, J. (2016). Listening to the narratives of our patients as part of holistic nursing care. *Journal of Holistic Nursing, 34*(2), 162–166.

Crisp, B. R., & Green Lister, P. (2004). Child protection and public health: Nurses' responsibilities. *Journal of Advanced Nursing, 47*(6), 656–663.

DeMay, D. A. (2003). The experience of being a client in an Alaska public health nursing home visitation program. *Public Health Nursing, 20*(3), 228–236.

Dossey, B. M., & Keegan, L. (2016). *Holistic nursing—A handbook for practice* (7th ed.). Burlington, MA: Jones & Bartlett Learning.

Eckenrode, J., Campa, M., Luckey, D. W., Henderson Jr., C. R., Cole, R., Kitzman, H., … Olds, D. (2010). Long-term effects of prenatal and infancy nurse home visitation on the life course of youths: 19-year follow-up of a randomized trial. *Archives of Pediatric and Adolescent Medicine, 164*(1), 9–15.

Ellington, L., Reblin, M., Ferrell, B., Puchalski, C., Otis-Green, S., Handzo, G., … Clayton, M. (2015). The religion of "I don't know": Naturalistic pilot observations of spiritual conversations occurring during cancer home hospice nurse visits. *Journal of Death and Dying, 72*(1), 3–19.

Flynn, M. A., Hall, K., Noack, A., Clovechok, S., Enns, E., Pivnick, J., … Pryce, C. (2005). Promotion of healthy weights at preschool public health vaccination clinics in Calgary: An obesity surveillance program. *Canadian Journal of Public Health, 96*(6), 421–426.

Friedman, M. M., Bowden, V. R., & Jones, E. G. (2003). *Family nursing: Research, theory, and practice* (5th ed.). Upper Saddle River, NJ: Prentice Hall.

Gerrity, P. (2010). And to think that it happened on 11th Street: A nursing approach to community-based holistic care and health care reform. *Alternative Therapies in Health and Medicine, 16*(5), 62–67.

Hayden, D. (2011). Spirituality in end-of-life care: Attending the person on their journey. *British Journal of Community Nursing, 16*(11), 546–551.

Hayter, M. (2005). Reaching marginalized young people through sexual health nursing outreach clinics: Evaluating service use and the views of service users. *Public Health Nursing, 22*(4), 339–346.

Henry Street Consortium. (2017). *Entry-level population-based public health nursing competencies.* St. Paul, MN: Author. Retrieved from www.henrystreetconsortium.org

Kemp, L., Anderson, T., Travaglia, J., & Harris, E. (2005). Sustained nursing home visiting in early childhood: Exploring Australian nursing competencies. *Public Health Nursing, 22*(3), 254–259.

Kemper, A. R., Fant, K. E., & Clark, S. J. (2005). Informing parents about newborn screening. *Public Health Nursing, 22*(4), 332–338.

Labun, E. (1988). Spiritual care: An element in nursing care planning. *Journal of Advanced Nursing, 13*(3), 314–320.

Mabhala, M. A. (2015). Public health nurse educators' conceptualisation of public health as a strategy to reduce health inequalities: A qualitative study. *International Journal for Equity in Health, 14,* 1–11.

McKeown, F. (2007). The experiences of older people on discharge from hospital following assessment by the public health nurse. *Journal of Clinical Nursing, 16*(3), 469–476.

Minnesota Department of Health. (2001). *Public health interventions: Applications for public health nursing practice.* St. Paul, MN: Author. Retrieved from http://www.health.state.mn.us/divs/opi/cd/phn/docs/0301wheel_manual.pdf

Minnesota Department of Health. (2009). Early identification of young children with special health care needs. *Minnesota Department of Health fact sheet: Title V (MCH) block grant children and adolescents with special health care needs.* St. Paul, MN: Author.

Minnesota Department of Health. (2013). *Adverse childhood experiences in Minnesota.* Retrieved from http://www.health.state.mn.us/divs/cfh/program/ace/content/document/pdf/acereport.pdf

Nelson, E. (2017). The Great Leveler. Throughout history, the best ways to reduce inequality have been disease and destruction. Retrieved from https://qz.com/924034/how-to-reduce-inequality-history-suggests-the-only-effective-ways-are-death-and-destruction/

Olds, D. L., Kitzman, H., Hanks, C., Cole, R., Anson, E., Sidora-Arcoleo, K., … Bondy, J. (2007). Effects of nurse home visiting on maternal and child functioning: Age-9 follow-up of a randomized trial. *Pediatrics, 120*(4), 832–845.

Olds, D. L., Kitzman, H., Knudtson, M. D., Anson, E., Smith, J. A., & Cole, R. (2014). Effect of home visiting by nurses on maternal and child mortality: Results of a 2-decade follow-up of a randomized clinical trial. *Journal of the American Medical Association Pediatrics, 168*(9), 800–806. doi:10.1001/jamapediatrics.2014.472

Ricketts, S. A., Murray, E. K., & Schwalberg, R. (2005). Reducing low birthweight by resolving risks: Results from Colorado's Prenatal Plus Program. *American Journal of Public Health, 98*(11), 1952–1957.

Schim, S., Doorenbos, A., Benkert, R., & Miller, J. (2007). Culturally congruent care: Putting the puzzle together. *Journal of Transcultural Nursing, 18*(2), 103–110.

Schneiderman, J. U. (2006). Innovative pediatric nursing role: Public health nurses in child welfare. *Pediatric Nursing, 32*(4), 317–321.

Sittner, B., Hudson, D., & Defrain, J. (2007). Using the concept of family strengths to enhance nursing care. *MCN: American Journal of Maternal/Child Health Nursing, 32*(6), 353–357.

Somervell, A. M., Saylor, C., & Mao, C. L. (2005). Public health nurse interventions for women in a dependency drug court. *Public Health Nursing, 22*(1), 59–64.

Strass, P., & Billay, E. (2008). A public health nursing initiative to promote antenatal health. *Canadian Nurse, 104*(2), 29–33.

U.S. Department of Health and Human Services Environmental Health Policy Committee, Risk Communication and Education Subcommittee. (1998). An ensemble of definitions of environmental health. Retrieved from https://health.gov/environment/DefinitionsofEnvHealth/ehdef2.htm

# COMPETENCY #10

## Demonstrates Nonjudgmental/ Unconditional Acceptance of People Different From Self

■ **Carolyn M. Porta**

*with Christine C. Andres, Carol J. Roth, Kelly Zaiser, and Renee Kumpula*

> " *Josie is a public health nursing student completing her final clinical hours before graduating. She and a classmate have been volunteering in a school-based clinic. The school nurse has invited Josie to join her on a home visit to check up on a student who has just given birth. Josie uses the GPS on her smartphone to find the apartment; it is located in a part of the city she normally avoids. She carefully locks her car and joins the school nurse in the apartment lobby. The client answers the buzzer, and they are invited upstairs to the apartment. The unfamiliar hallway lighting and smells cause Josie to proceed cautiously. She hopes to focus on what the school nurse accomplishes rather than on her own feelings of discomfort.* "

## JOSIE'S NOTEBOOK

**COMPETENCY #10** Demonstrates Nonjudgmental/Unconditional Acceptance of People Different from Self

A. Listens to others in an unbiased, respectful manner

B. Promotes the expression of diverse opinions and perspectives

C. Identifies the role of diverse factors when selecting or designing public health interventions tailored to specific individuals, communities, or systems

D. Interacts respectfully, sensitively, and effectively with individuals, families, and communities

*Source:* Henry Street Consortium, 2017

### USEFUL DEFINITIONS

**Acceptance:** "To consider their patients' culture and incorporate it in care" (Cioffi, 2003, p. 305) and the "respect of another's individual person and self-defined reality" (Porr, 2005, p. 189).

**Nonjudgmental:** "Being open to understanding cultural uniqueness and respect for individuals" (Pasco, Morse, & Olson, 2004, p. 239). A nurse describes being nonjudgmental as she sought to "establish a... communion into which I enter having cleansed myself of harmful bias through honest self-reflection; and, in which I exude humility and openness" (Porr, 2005, p. 195).

**Unconditional:** "A form of respect that involves profoundness of feeling, treasuring, warm regard, [and] solicitous concern" (Dillon, 1992, p. 120).

## Activity

Consider the following questions about Josie's situation:

▪ What are some of the fears or worries Josie might be experiencing in this or other situations that are different for her?

▪ What are some things that might have helped Josie prepare for the "discomfort" that can often be experienced during home visits?

▪ What does Josie need to know or understand to help her work with clients who do not have similar lifestyles and cultural habits?

## They Do Not Live Like I Do

Public health nursing is similar to other areas of nursing when it comes to valuing the ability to deliver nursing care in a nonjudgmental, accepting manner. A public health nurse (PHN) is often a guest, invited into the client's space, such as in the home, and this situation provides endless opportunities for a nurse's acceptance of others to be tested, confirmed, or challenged. A PHN might work with a faith community to offer blood pressure screening that might require the nurse to work alongside others with different values or beliefs. It is important to recognize that some people or populations, due to their past experiences, have a heightened level of *stigma consciousness* (i.e., perception or awareness of being stigmatized) and expect to be judged, which can present a challenge for nurses (Porr, Drummond, & Olson, 2012). Similarly, nurses might also have past experiences that have contributed to their development of biases or prejudices that need to be addressed in order to provide nonjudgmental or unconditional care. This chapter explores the ways in which a PHN can demonstrate nonjudgmental or unconditional acceptance of people. It also provides examples of how PHNs have worked to develop acceptance for individuals, families, and communities across difficult situations. Finally, the chapter concludes with suggestions for assessing your own acceptance of others and ways to develop yourself as a nonjudgmental person and a nurse.

A nurse can be nonjudgmental yet at the same time disagree with something that is observed or said. This distinction is subtle but important; a nurse should be able to discern whether a behavior is healthy or harmful yet should also be able to make these assessments in a manner that is nonjudgmental. For example, it is important to note that there are instances when a nurse must act on a duty to report apparent abuse that might be "acceptable" in that personal or cultural context by the individual or family, but violates a law in the United States. In these very difficult situations, the effective nurse will carefully intervene, realizing at the time that the interventions might not appear to be nonjudgmental. In attitude and behavior, the nurse can strive to be as accepting as possible, even in difficult situations that must balance legal and ethical obligations to individuals/families and society. A PHN caring for someone who has committed a violent crime is likely to feel strongly about the crimes that have been committed. This nurse will regularly face the challenge to provide nursing care that is not conditionally based on what the person has done or not done. The nurse's clients will perceive the care being provided as nonjudgmental and unconditional when the nurse demonstrates a sincere desire to learn more about the client through respect, openness, and unbiased listening and asking of questions.

Another example in which PHNs might be confronted with a challenge of being nonjudgmental is when they are providing nursing care to a generation very different from their own. This challenge is often encountered within the context of changing cultural trends. For example, a current cultural trend seen in late adolescence and young adults is expression through the form of body tattooing. Nurses displaced by several decades from this population group might have negative perceptions of tattooing. Those PHNs have the challenge of trying to "fit" into this generation and to understand the current trends and values and their importance. PHNs can be more successful in building nonjudgmental, ongoing relationships when they respect possible cultural generational differences. In the case of tattooing, respecting differences might mean not addressing the issue of whether someone is getting a tattoo but rather promoting safe tattooing practices.

Diversity is reflected in numerous ways, which might include:

▪ Culture
▪ Ethnicity
▪ Lifestyle preferences
▪ Gender roles
▪ Family styles
▪ Religion
▪ Spiritual beliefs
▪ Socioeconomic position
▪ Age
▪ Race
▪ Physical appearances
▪ Sexual orientation
▪ Education level
▪ Neighborhood
▪ Geographic region
▪ Language use
▪ Immigration status
▪ Health status
▪ Beliefs
▪ Values

It is increasingly important to be aware of diversity, because the U.S. population will shift to a multiracial/multiethnic majority in the next few decades (see Table 12.1).

This population transformation will occur in some areas of the country sooner than others. Figure 12.1 demonstrates state and regional differences.

Some of the ways that nurses demonstrate nonjudgmental and unconditional public health nursing might include:

▪ Listening to others in an unbiased manner
▪ Respecting others' points of view
▪ Promoting the expression of diverse opinions and perspectives

■ Identifying the role of cultural, social, spiritual, religious, and behavioral factors when selecting or designing public health interventions

■ Interacting respectfully, sensitively, and effectively with diverse persons (e.g., diverse by culture, socioeconomic position, educational level, race, ethnicity, gender, sexual orientation, religious background, health status, age, or lifestyle preferences)

## Listening to Others in an Unbiased Manner

Have you watched yourself in a mirror to observe your non-verbal cues and signals when you are reacting to what someone else is saying? Do you smile? Do you nod cautiously or in positive support for the other person? Do you scowl quickly when something you do not agree with is said?

Effective listening is a combination of verbal and non-verbal responses to the person with whom you are talking.

**TABLE 12.1 U.S. Population, Actual and Projected: 2005 and 2050**

|  | 2005 | 2050 |
|---|---|---|
| Population (in millions) | 296 | 438 |
| **Share of total** | | |
| Foreign born | 12% | 19% |
| Racial/Ethnic Groups | | |
| White | 67% | 47% |
| Hispanic | 14% | 29% |
| Black | 13% | 13% |
| Asian | 5% | 9% |
| Age Groups | | |
| Children (17 and younger) | 25% | 23% |
| Working age (18–64) | 63% | 58% |
| Elderly (65 and older) | 12% | 19% |

Note: All races modified and not Hispanic; Americal Indian/Alaska Native not shown. See "Methodology."

Source: Passel & Cohn, Pew Research Center, 2008

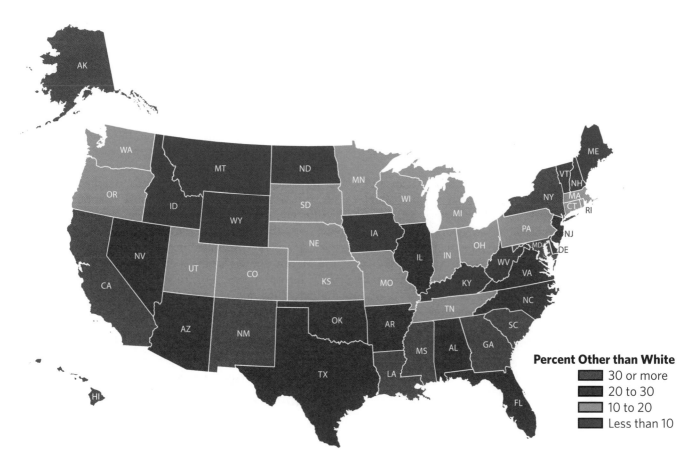

**FIGURE 12.1** Population Percent Other Than White by State: 2000 Census
*Source:* U.S. Census Bureau, 2013

**TABLE 12.2 Nonverbal and Verbal Listening Cues**

| Nonverbal | Verbal |
|---|---|
| ▪ Eye contact (not too little, not too much) | ▪ Supportive sounds (uh huh, ah) |
| ▪ Facial expressions (smile, stare, frown, grimace) | ▪ Timing and pace (responding quickly might indicate active listening rather than distraction but too quickly might indicate lack of listening and readiness with your preconceived point) |
| ▪ Gestures (head nod, hand motions) | |
| ▪ Intensity (the amount of energy you exude to the other person can support or bother that individual) | |
| ▪ Movements and posture (leaning toward someone indicates interest) | ▪ Voice tone (calming with lower and softer tones) |
| ▪ Space (closeness and proximity to the other person/people) | ▪ Silence (can facilitate or hinder conversation) |
| ▪ Touch (hand on shoulder, hug) | |
| ▪ Attire (balance and awareness to avoid being underdressed or overdressed, or in another way culturally offensive) | |

Note: Use of an interpreter will require careful attentiveness and listening to nonverbal and verbal cues among all involved participants.

*Source:* Adapted from Segal, Smith, & Jaffe, 2013

Another concept that is growing in popularity is that of *deep listening,* which is a process of listening to learn (Center for Spirituality and Healing [CSH], 2013). When you listen deeply, you do not generate what your response is going to be to what is being said or relayed nonverbally. Instead, deep listening is reflective listening in which you listen to learn, you listen for understanding rather than agreement, and you ask powerful questions (CSH, 2013). Listening in an unbiased manner takes effective listening to a higher level, because it requires you not only to listen in a way that helps people who are talking believe that they are being heard, but also to listen in a manner that expresses acceptance for those people.

As with most communication attributes (see Chapter 9), verbal and nonverbal listening cues can vary by individual, developmental age, culture, and other factors. Therefore, you need to know the clients you are working with and understand what conveys listening and support to them. Do not presume to know. Table 12.2 includes broad categories that serve as examples of the many ways in which you can express listening, support, inattention, or boredom.

You must adequately prepare for interactions with clients and families so that your nonverbal actions are consistent with their cultures. Learning about your clients' beliefs and value systems, as well as their preferred learning style, through open-ended questions will support your knowledge of appropriate interactions. For example, in some cultures it is not appropriate to pat a child on the head, and in others it is not acceptable to look people in the eye. Importantly, remember that differences often exist within a cultural "group" as well, so awareness of a nonverbal behavior that is acceptable or not to some people in a culture should not be automatically assumed as universal to everyone in that cultural group.

## Respecting Others' Points of View

Are you quick to defend your own views or beliefs? Is it hard for you to listen to someone argue for a value that is not your own? It can be difficult to respect others' points of view when they do not naturally align with your own. However, respect is critical to being a nonjudgmental nurse. The key is demonstrating respect for another point of view regardless of whether you concur. You can express respect verbally and nonverbally. For example, when a PHN visits a mother who has recently delivered her fifth child, the nurse is likely to explore birth control or child spacing plans with the mother. If the mother expresses a view that opposes family planning or use of birth control, the nurse needs to respect that view. Alternatively, a PHN might not personally endorse certain treatment strategies but would need to support the preferences of a client. One way you can show respect is through offering relevant information in an unassuming manner and choosing to respect the client's autonomy for maintaining a different perspective. This respect can be particularly difficult when you perceive client, family, or community views as unhealthy, but it is important.

## Promoting the Expression of Diverse Opinions and Perspectives

Do you seek others' opinions before making a decision? Do you welcome multiple perspectives, or do you find them annoying? Nurses are often in situations that require advocacy for families and communities, and each family and community includes multiple perspectives and opinions. Effective PHNs can assess the situation and intervene in a

**EVIDENCE EXAMPLE 12.1**

**Impacts of PHN Interventions Within a Context of Nonjudgmental Relationships**

One qualitative study reported women's perceptions of the effectiveness of PHN nursing interventions on their own parenting skills and choices for nurturing children from birth to 5 years old. The study was conducted to understand how PHN interventions worked in home visits and what was needed for the maternal and early childhood program to be successful. When discussing their relationship with the nurse, 24 of 28 participants used descriptors for the PHN such as "very friendly," "very nice," "straightforward," and "nonjudgmental" (Zapart, Knight, & Kemp, 2016). The mothers reported how PHNs supported both their overall well-being and emotional well-being. Moreover, participants identified how PHNs conducting a developmental assessment on a child provided them with feelings of confidence and reassurance along with validating their child's developmental benchmarks. Two areas were highlighted as long-term impacts after PHN interventions within a context of nonjudgmental relationships. Mothers (1) identified using continued services as a result of positive outcomes in the short term and stated they (2) applied the new parenting skills to other children in the family, thereby enhancing the impact for the long term (Zapart et al., 2016). The education and support provided by PHNs was reported to be valued by mothers; this flowed from the PHN establishment of a "respectful, nonjudgmental relationship" that undergirded the PHN-client connection for interventions (Demay in Zapart et al., 2016).

manner that helps everyone express an opinion. For example, a PHN visiting a family with a hospice client might encounter many opinions from that family about how to best help their loved one go through the dying process. It is very helpful when the nurse can learn who is the spokesperson for the family or community, if one has been identified and agreed upon. Even though it might be impossible to act upon each opinion, the nurse can assist family members in expressing their perspectives and, ultimately, in coming together to make many difficult decisions.

not proactive. For example, in some immigrant communities, the community leaders are consulted by their members about issues of concern. Effective PHNs assess the extent to which these cultural patterns exist within a community and act in accordance with the sociocultural norms to gain entry and intervene. Similarly, PHNs, including those who serve as faith community nurses, carefully consider the religious or spiritual implications of certain interventions. For example, PHNs might need to schedule a health-promotion intervention around certain holidays or celebrations so that attendance and involvement are optimal.

## Identifying the Role of Cultural, Social, Spiritual, Religious, and Behavioral Factors When Selecting or Designing Public Health Interventions

Have you thought about how a nursing action might look differently if you are caring for someone with a lot of money versus someone with very little? Do you enjoy learning about other cultures? Throughout this book, you have been reminded that PHNs consider multiple factors when providing care for individuals, families, and communities. Nonjudgmental PHNs carefully consider the particular clients being served when they are planning specific interventions. For example, when PHNs implement a childhood-obesity prevention program, they need to consider the cultural perceptions that might impede or support the program. A recent refugee population might view additional weight on a child as a positive, healthy attribute because they are comparing this to the poverty and malnourishment experienced by many children in their home country. Sociocultural expectations can also influence the success of public health nursing interventions if PHNs are

## Interacting Respectfully, Sensitively, and Effectively With Diverse Persons

Are you comfortable having a conversation with an individual who is homeless? Do you enjoy learning about cultures different from your own? Do you believe you are deserving of good things, maybe more so than other people? Do you see the person serving you in a store or a restaurant, or do you see through them?

Ultimately, your success as a PHN depends on your ability to establish a meaningful relationship with the individual, family, or community you are serving. You cannot establish that relationship unless you can interact with diverse people in a nonjudgmental and accepting manner. You are going to find it easier to be nonjudgmental toward some people more than others, and you should engage in learning activities or reflective exercises to help yourself recognize and address preconceived stereotypes you might have about certain groups of people. Certainly, your worldview provides, in essence, a cultural filter for how you view and interact with others. Over time and with experience, you will learn more about yourself, including your reactions to those who are different from you. You might find that you are very accepting toward certain people and communities, whereas with others you struggle to be accepting. Becoming nonjudgmental is a process that takes a long time and is constantly evolving as you encounter new situations that challenge what you believe or feel about the world and those around you.

Practically, you can begin to implement behaviors helpful in your development toward being a nonjudgmental and accepting nurse: understanding specific personal beliefs and values; being respectful to everyone; interacting in a sensitive, responsive manner (rather than an overbearing, assuming one); and developing effective verbal and nonverbal communication skills. For example, you might reflect on what you choose to wear in your professional role as a PHN and how others might view your attire; this perception is particularly important because PHNs generally dress in business casual attire or in casual clothing in a way that is respectfully consistent with the population being served. You can practice these behaviors in a variety of settings and begin to learn about the environments, situations, or moods that make being accepting more difficult for you. Most important are your willingness to learn, your reflections on personal behavior and thinking, and your attempts at new skills that enhance your acceptance of others.

You can also explore ways in which you can develop cultural humility (Gallardo, 2014; Tervalon & Murray-Garcia, 1998). Cultural humility is a concept that has gained popularity as discourse has matured beyond discussion of cultural competence "skills" and whether it is possible to "achieve" these skills and turned instead toward self-reflection (and attention toward personal biases) that can then inform appreciative, respectful openness informed by desire for equity. *Cultural humility* has been defined as a humility that "incorporates a lifelong commitment to self-evaluation and self-critique, to redressing the power imbalances… and to developing mutually beneficial and non-paternalistic clinical and advocacy partnership with communities on behalf of individuals and defined populations" (Tervalon & Murray-Garcia, 1998, p. 117). Tervalon and Murray-Garcia (1998) identify three ways in which cultural humility is encouraged:

1. Lifelong learning and critical self-reflection
2. Recognition and challenging of power imbalances for respectful partnerships
3. Institutional accountability

PHNs can play a significant role in developing cultural humility and promoting cultural humility within their organizations and with stakeholder partners.

Empathy is an important attribute that can contribute to a PHN's ability to practice in a nonjudgmental manner (Porr et al., 2012). In essence, *empathy* is an ability to accurately perceive the emotions, feelings, and thoughts of others. Often, people can express empathy more easily when they have experienced something similar to what is causing another person's current emotions, feelings, or thoughts. A nurse's ability to express empathy can encourage a client to feel cared for, heard, and accepted rather than judged. Similarly, the concept of *mutuality,* or the ability to get into someone else's "shoes," is valuable. This sense of mutuality encourages empathy, because the nurse purposefully works to understand as closely as possible what the client is experiencing. Mutuality is a skill that can be developed as you regularly take the time to reflect on what you would be feeling or thinking if you had just experienced what the other person has had happen. Challenge yourself to try this exercise in work and personal settings and reflect on how your ability to connect with, respond to, or support that other person strengthens with greater levels of mutuality and empathy.

It is interesting to look back in history and examine how some people worked to encourage nonjudgmental attitudes, particularly in such eras as the early 1970s, which followed the civil rights efforts in the 1960s. Remember that "becoming nonjudgmental is hard work and a lifetime process" (Goldsborough, 1970, p. 2,340). Steps you can take to work toward becoming nonjudgmental are (Goldsborough, 1970):

1. Recognize judgmental feelings. (Becoming nonjudgmental begins with openness to yourself, even though it might be painful to acknowledge your judgmental feelings.)

2. Accept your judgmental feelings for what they are. (Without acceptance, you will be unable to move toward changing the feelings.)

3. Explore the origin of the judgmental feelings, maybe with a friend or colleague. (Where did these feelings come from?)

4. Take steps to change. (Realize that there will always be another person and another judgment to work through over the course of your life and nursing career.)

---

### Activity

- Have you ever experienced someone acting judgmental toward you? How did you feel? How did you react?

- What do you wish you would have done differently?

- What could that person have done to express his or her opinion or beliefs in a nonjudgmental manner?

- Do you believe that a person can change from being judgmental to become nonjudgmental? How do you think this change happens? How can you encourage this process in your life and in the lives of those around you?

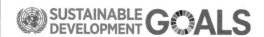

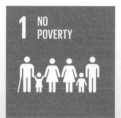

**Public Health Nursing and the Myths of Poverty**

**GOAL 1**  Amanda Redhead (2016) provides a powerful essay in the Huffington Post, titled "Public Health Nursing and the Myths of Poverty" accessed at https://www.huffingtonpost.com/amanda-redhead/ public-health-nursing-and_b_9182900.html. She demonstrates honesty about her own misconceptions and her naiveté when she started out as a PHN. She challenges the reader to see poverty, to face the feelings of helplessness, and to do something. She writes hopefully about those she visits in their homes, that they are able to " see that I will not judge you and truly only want to help. To see that I will do everything I can to leave your family in a better place than where I found you" (para. 17).

---

*Josie and the PHN enter the apartment and find they are in a cheery, well-decorated but modest home for the teen, her newborn daughter, and the teen's mother. Josie continues to absorb the surroundings as she hears the school nurse ask the teen about her baby and her healing body. She is surprised that the apartment is so clean and organized. She considers her reaction and tunes out the conversation.*

*"Why am I surprised this apartment is so nice? Do I expect that if you are poor, you are dirty or unkempt? Where is this opinion coming from? Did my facial expressions portray discomfort when I walked through the door?" Josie reflects on her reaction and compares it to that of the PHN, who appears to be at ease and enjoying her interaction with the new mom and baby. At this point in the visit, Josie is questioning her reaction and the judgments her thoughts have revealed. This reflection is critical to growing toward an unconditional acceptance of others. It is an example of mindful nursing practice, which is simply being aware, present, and in the moment with those you are serving or caring for.*

**Healthy People**

**2020**

healthypeople.gov

The Healthy People 2020 website identifies indicators for a variety of public health concerns in the United States, with goals for improvements by 2020. Select a health indicator and develop a public health nursing health-promotion strategy that will include activities at the individual, community, and system levels. Identify activities that will emphasize nonjudgmental acceptance of others and will minimize the barriers that various groups often encounter. What are some things the PHN can do when working with populations that are different from his or hers?

## Evidence-Based Practice for Acceptance of Others in Public Health Nursing

A logical question, now, is where in public health nursing practice can you observe acceptance of others and how this improves outcomes for individuals, communities, or systems? In the following sections, we explore the existing research at these three levels of care delivery for public health nurses.

### Individual

Much of the research supporting the need for PHNs to be nonjudgmental and accepting when working with individuals, families, or communities focuses heavily on relationship building. This focus makes sense because, in essence, when a nurse is nonjudgmental and accepting, the client-nurse relationship is likely to be positive and healthy, which leads to more successful interventions and more meaningful interactions for everyone. Evidence Example 12.1 demonstrates positive results experienced by PHNs working with new moms.

Few scenarios can demonstrate the challenges that a PHN might face in providing nonjudgmental and accepting nursing care better than poverty. Caroline Porr (2005) is a PHN who reflected on her interactions with clients in poverty and specifically challenged herself to answer the following question:

> By all accounts I was thorough, or was I? I certainly "dealt with" Karen and her family in scrupulous fashion but did I adequately "dwell with" Karen; that is, did I understand her lived experience as a lone parent enduring the margins of society due to poverty?. (p. 190)

## EVIDENCE EXAMPLE 12.2
### Nurse-Mother Relationship—What Moms Want and Nurses Can Offer

In a qualitative study, moms and nurses were interviewed to understand how the nurses engage the mothers in a way that is empowering so that the mothers can more effectively bear and raise children (Aston, Meagher-Stewart, Sheppard-Lemoine, Vukic, & Chircop, 2006). In this study, a researcher observed the interactions between the PHN and the mother during a home visit with the new mom (baby born 2–3 weeks prior). Following this observation, the researcher interviewed the mother and PHN to talk about how the home visit had gone. This information helped identify key themes in the relationship, many that are directly relevant to the PHN's ability to be accepting and nonjudgmental. For example, the mothers identified key attributes of the PHNs that made them feel comfortable, at ease, and positive toward the nurses, including being "full of confidence… gentle… quiet" (Aston et al., 2006, p. 63). The nurses also talked about the importance of their actions in encouraging the moms to feel comfortable and competent, including "respect, trust, listening, confidence, and communication" (p. 63). At a time when women feel incredibly vulnerable and incompetent, these nurses were able to express acceptance in a way that facilitated feelings of confidence in the new moms.

## EVIDENCE EXAMPLE 12.3
### Quantitatively Assessing Empathy

A scale was developed to assess the level of empathic understanding that a nurse has demonstrated (Nagano, 2000). Although the scale is intended to provide an opportunity for a client to give feedback about a nurse, it can also be useful in self-reflection by the nurse regarding verbal and nonverbal behaviors. Examples on this scale include the following:

- "The [nurse] summarizes the client's emotions or feelings by saying, 'It seems that you are feeling this…'
- The [nurse] looks at the client with a warm expression (eyes, facial expression).
- The [nurse]'s voice and rate of speaking are calm, slow, and relaxed.
- The [nurse] faces the client and shows interest in the client" (pp. 26–27).

thus could never appreciate the uniqueness of her human existence and of her experiences in the world" (2005, p. 194).

A variety of tools have been developed to measure empathy. Jolliffe and Farrington (2006) developed an empathy scale for adolescents that could be adapted to other populations. Evidence Example 12.3 describes the development of a tool that clients could use to assess the level of empathy they perceive from the PHNs caring for them; this was done nearly two decades ago but is shared here because it was explicitly designed for the nurse-client relationship and client perceptions of nurse empathy.

## Community

Culture is an area in which many PHNs are regularly faced with opportunities or challenges to be nonjudgmental and unconditionally accepting. Realizing that every PHN has a distinct cultural and ethnic background is fundamentally important when engaging with diverse communities in health promotion or disease-prevention activities. In nursing, much time is spent examining culture in the context of providing care, but what exactly is culture? *Culture* refers to "the learned, shared, and transmitted values, beliefs, norms, and lifeways of a particular group that guides their thinking, decisions, and actions in patterned ways" (Reynolds & Leininger, 1993, p. 19). This definition presents some challenges, because any cultural group, or community, always has a range of "patterned ways" that are not necessarily consistently similar. So, on the one hand, culture might cause a community to share some behaviors or norms that are distinct from other groups, but on the other hand, culture is colorful and inherently diverse, which requires commitment and time to gain understanding. Effective PHNs

Poverty is something that every PHN is going to encounter when serving individuals and families in a variety of contexts (e.g., home visits, food shelves, community gardens, homeless shelters).

How PHNs respond to a family in poverty influences the relationship and, subsequently, the outcomes of the care provided. Without reflection, PHNs might consider the poverty as more central to the problems and solutions than the individual or family living in poverty perceives it to be. PHNs therefore need to seek to understand how the individual or family perceives the experience of poverty and their broader values. After gaining this understanding, PHNs can then effectively support and accept the individual or family. Rather than focusing simply on the reason for the visit (e.g., a home visit to provide education), nonjudgmental and accepting PHNs can dig deeper and appreciate the clients simply for who they are, not as they exist within in the narrow context of their situations (e.g., poverty). Similarly, PHNs need to identify and examine the strengths in the situation within the individual, the family, and potentially the community, and in doing so, practice cultural humility. As Porr concludes, "I had once thought that client assessment and intervention were sufficient until I became curious about *who is* the Other sitting across from me. It was then that I realized that I did not know this mother and

working with communities understand that effective interventions begin with investments of time and themselves.

For example, a PHN might have opportunities to promote the health of individuals and families who are part of a religious community. Often, the support of religious and spiritual leaders can foster trust of the PHN among the community members. However, if the leaders are not supportive of the PHN's specific priorities, this situation can be challenging, especially if the religious and spiritual leaders are primary decision-makers and members do not have high levels of autonomy. The PHN in this case needs to respectfully and carefully work with the religious leaders to achieve mutual goals related to health promotion or disease prevention.

The culture of the poor, those in economic poverty or homeless, provides an example of how PHNs rise to provide respectful, quality care amid differences. Public health nursing research on providing care to the poor can be traced back to the first year, 1984, that the *Public Health Nursing* journal was published. A multidimensional model of poverty was developed that considers individual/group and environmental factors influencing the person experiencing poverty (Pesznecker, 1984). In this model, a person in poverty is cared for with careful consideration of how that person is dealing with his or her specific situation and how he or she is feeling about it (e.g., depressed, powerless, incapable).

---

### Activity

As a new PHN, you need to learn to carefully reflect on why people might be reacting the way they are when you are trying to intervene. What are they going through? How are they handling their situations?

When the response you are receiving is cautious or unwelcoming, how can you determine whether it is because of the situation and not necessarily specific to you?

Consider how you might incorporate strategies into your practice that convey the message to those you are serving that you come open-minded and open-handed.

---

Certainly, PHNs are in a work environment that values nursing efficiency. Yet many of those that PHNs serve have overarching values that prioritize building relationships and taking time to do so rather than rushing through an appointment. For example, in the culture of generational poverty, time might be valued differently than in a culture of economically secure people. Poverty often necessitates that people view the present time (i.e., in the moment) as most important and make decisions based on immediate feelings or survival needs, whereas those in stable economic situations often value future time as most important and make their decisions with more consideration of future ramifications (Payne, DeVol, & Smith, 2001). PHNs who clearly understand this distinction allow some flexibility

in scheduling visits or appointments. You might view an efficient nurse as one who has carefully planned the week with full days of scheduled, often back-to-back, appointments. However, this efficiency might be challenged as the week unfolds and the PHN finds that several of the clients are not home at their scheduled visit times. How can the PHN incorporate and respect the time value for this poverty culture and still implement effective nursing interventions? The PHN might incorporate some time in the schedule each week for same-day home visits or might have a time each week when families can "drop in" for in-office visits. This aspect of scheduling can be very distressing to new PHNs, as many view such client behavior as a sign of disrespect or a lack of desire to see them. This perspective often changes as the PHN gains more experience and has a deeper appreciation, understanding, and acceptance of the unique value of time for each person or family. Working hard to understand and respect clients' sense of time will make you a more relevant, respectful, and effective PHN.

### Systems

At the systems level, demonstration of acceptance of others is most often reflected in policy or program-level strategies. When home visiting agencies put extensive constraints on their PHNs, the nursing staff subsequently experience challenges as they face choices that differ in benefiting their employer, themselves, or their clients. Evidence Example 12.4 exemplifies this struggle for home visiting nurses in Norway.

Commonly, there can be challenges in achieving continuity of care across organization systems, such as collaboration across clinical care and community-based care settings (e.g., hospital or clinic care transferred to a PHN agency). PHNs need to be aware of the diversity of perspectives that can emerge due to the setting in which they work. As described by Helleso and Solveig Fagermoen (2010), a nurse's assessment and the information obtained for a patient are influenced extensively by the patient's situation, the context in which the nurse works, and the nurse's character. Being aware of differences can enhance nonjudgmental exchanges across organizational systems to improve the continuity of care of populations. In addition to differences across various healthcare organizations, multigenerational conflict can arise among healthcare professionals within and across these organizations. Multigenerational conflict occurs when the values and practices of healthcare professionals vary across the different generations (i.e., the new PHNs versus the "old guard" PHNs; Kupperschmidt, 2006). Key to addressing or minimizing multigenerational conflict is a commitment to respecting one another and exhibiting that respect within and across healthcare organizations.

Policies that support interpreter services for those who do not speak English well are an ideal example of system-level strategies to support service delivery to diverse clients. Much research has shown that the quality of healthcare is

## EVIDENCE EXAMPLE 12.4
### Efficiency Requirements, Community Health Nurses, and Emotional Labor

In a qualitative inquiry, 19 community health nurses participated in semi-structured interviews designed to obtain "information about how nurses perceived differences or similarities in the way they provided care to ethnic minority patients, compared with ethnic Norwegians, which situations they found particularly challenging, and how they understood the situation of ethnic minority patients" (Debesay, Harsløf, Rechel, & Vike, 2014, p. 76). Thematic content analysis yielded important themes about the struggles experienced by these nurses as they sought to provide excellent care for their clients. Notably, the time needed for PHNs to provide care was often longer than the agency parameters for length of visits. This tension of time allotted and time needed resulted in dissatisfaction with the visit because topics were not covered adequately or at all, and notably, no space was available for informal conversations the nurses felt were critical to relationship-building and subsequent intervention outcomes. The limited flexibility resulted in nurses feeling inadequate and not perceiving themselves as having autonomy in their community health nursing roles. This was particularly obvious when the nurses were working with clients from other cultural backgrounds and required more time than was allotted. The result was an emotional struggle for these nurses as they made choices about their use of time, and did so feeling pressure from their employing organization. The authors importantly conclude, "The point here is not to suggest that nurses cannot provide extra efforts despite institutional and social barriers, but rather that such an involvement is often regarded primarily as an individual obligation, not a collective responsibility" (p. 78). There is little question that home visiting nurses are positioned to be most successful when the institution demonstrates support for autonomy and decision-making that prioritizes the needs of the client and the nurse-client relationship, not simply efficiency.

---

better when interpreters are available for Limited English Proficiency (LEP) persons. Pam Garrett (2009) has proposed a cultural empowerment model for an interpreter service policy that can serve as a guide for healthcare organizations that need to implement such a policy. The model identifies key attributes that promote cultural empowerment, including: (a) facilitating language; (b) negotiating family involvement; (c) understanding patient beliefs, experiences, and constructions; (d) compassionately respecting patient and human rights; (e) negotiating the care partnership; and (f) providing systems so that providers can be competent. These types of models can be useful when organizations are not sure where to begin creating their own policies.

The use of cultural brokers, or community health workers, in providing health education, outreach, support, and resources to others in their community is another example of systems realizing the need to provide culturally relevant care and outreach (Mack, Uken, & Powers, 2006; O'Brien, Squires, Bixby, & Larson, 2009). PHNs can delegate appropriate activities or tasks to paraprofessionals, such as community health workers. In many situations, community health workers can be important liaisons for families navigating the complex U.S. healthcare system. It is important to note, though, that PHNs can serve diverse cultural groups and effectively care for those who are different from them. This is the essence of this competency—namely, realizing that PHNs need to develop acceptance of others, which can go far in reaching clients and communities. Policies that support unconditional PHN care, such as approaches using community health workers when appropriate, can promote optimal delivery of nursing care.

The following example illustrates the impact that can be made when a policy does not exist to support particular activities and when a policy is changed without considering its impact on others. In a community with a large population of African immigrant families, Personal Care Attendants (PCAs) were providing care for men who lived alone. As part of their home care, the PCAs were cooking meals because the men had no knowledge or experience preparing meals. The law changed with respect to the PCAs' scope of practice, preventing them from preparing meals for these clients. No organizational policy was in place to support this informal job duty the PCAs had been performing. As a result of this change, the community had to generate creative options to address the gap in care. Although the community did come up with alternative solutions (e.g., cooking classes for the men, a meal delivery service), in the short term, the men lost valuable care and services because a reimbursement law had changed.

It is important to recognize the societal practices, values, and standards that influence the delivery of public health nursing care in an accepting manner. Society is always changing, and with these changes come challenges or solutions that support or impede what you are trying to do. For example, many groups in the United States have endured societal oppression that directly and indirectly influences how they receive services, such as public health nursing care. Being respectful of where people have been or come from (i.e., their lived history), and what they have experienced in the past, or recently, is imperative to being a successful PHN. Even if you are a very accepting person, you are going to have barriers to overcome if you are providing care to someone who has experienced discrimination or judgments from a person who looks or acts in ways that are similar to your own. You need to maintain awareness of the societal climate, federal and state policies, and local sentiments within which you are working as a PHN. When you do this, your care is going to be attuned, aware, and, ideally, effective and meaningful.

## Intra-Agency

Finally, PHNs must also demonstrate acceptance of each other and of their colleagues in the workplace. This can be difficult but is critical as workforce diversity expands in healthcare, nursing, and public health. Coworkers might experience differences in work ethics, time management, and opinions concerning how a nursing procedure should

be done. Experiences in practice or in the field certainly contribute to opinions regarding how things should be done in PHN practice, and it is not uncommon for two experienced nurses to differ in their opinions about what should or should not be done. Knowledge of best practices continues to grow. An evidence-based practice framework could be used to minimize differences across professions.

Some studies addressing healthcare work environments offer relevant research findings. For example, although it was conducted with nursing assistants rather than PHNs, an important study examined organizational respect and emotional exhaustion, or burnout (Ramarajan, Barsade, & Burack, 2008). Organizational respect was measured using such statements as "staff members respect each other," "cultural diversity of staff is valued," and "staff members are treated with dignity." Not surprisingly, when nursing assistants reported higher levels of organizational respect the first time they were interviewed, when they were later re-surveyed, they were less likely to report feeling emotional exhaustion than their colleagues who had initially reported feeling that organizational respect levels were low. PHNs need to be in a work environment that respects and values them. This respect is very important because without it, a PHN might be less satisfied with work, might be more emotionally exhausted, and might choose to leave public health nursing. Because the need for PHNs is so great across the United States, workplace environments need to be supportive and accepting. If you feel judged by coworkers, consider the following strategies:

- Confront the person making you feel this way. Explore with that person why the differences exist. (Are you from different generations, cultures, experiences?)
- Reflect on the situation with your supervisor (or another appropriate person) to clarify your feelings and actions that you should take.
- Approach human resources staff for assistance.

Similarly, new PHNs need to be in an environment that supports their learning and growing in new roles and experiences. Experienced nurses might find it difficult to adapt to the next generation of PHNs, but they need to make the effort to understand each other and grow together. In this way, the public health nursing workforce can remain strong and express acceptance of one another and of clients being served.

Some specific techniques to gain trust at the individual, community, systems, and intra-agency levels are included in Table 12.3. Regardless of the level, keep in mind three overarching strategies to establishing trust (Falk-Rafael & Betker, 2012): (1) Ensure clear boundaries for the relationship and comfort among all with these boundaries, (2) be authentic, and (3) create an optimal environment for interactions (i.e., comfortable, safe, relaxed).

---

## EVIDENCE EXAMPLE 12.5
### Development of Nonjudgmental Behaviors

A grounded theory study, based on social and critical theory, explored how nurses negotiated structural constraints and learned to mobilize resources in order to value different cultural perspectives and convey nonjudgmental attitudes across all practice settings. Nurse participants identified challenges such as a lack of time for providing quality care, language issues impeding understanding of client needs, and an imposed agency agenda that sometimes prohibited client-centered interventions (Garneau, Pepin, & Gendron, 2017). In particular, some nurses articulated how they used their own cultural background and "intercultural reality" to be more nonjudgmental and competent with clients. Others reported how seeing cultural insensitivity in a colleague's behavior prompted them to use individual agency to change their attitudes and practice to that of acceptance (Garneau et al., 2017). In addition, nursing student participants reported increased understanding of how culture affects nursing interventions and how multiple realities exist in client situations; they also reported gaining cultural sensitivity when working with diverse clients (Garneau et al., 2017). The findings indicate that participants, whether nurses or students, found themselves responding to structural constraints by choosing to assert individual autonomy and create opportunities for social and cultural engagement, which, in turn, led to more informed and nonjudgmental practice.

## TABLE 12.3 Techniques to Gain Trust at Individual, Community, Systems, and Intra-Agency Levels

### Individual Level

Find a commonality with which you can connect to the individual or family. Approach the client with an openness to learning about them. Apply the four A's: Acknowledge, Awareness, Ask, and Act.

#### Acknowledgeness and Awareness

■ Respect the client's time schedule and availability. For example, clearly state your intended length of visit at the time you set the appointment, or upon arrival, so that you provide an opportunity for the client to make any necessary adjustments. This practice builds trust through mutual investment in the commitment.

■ Respect the client's "home rules" that might be different from your own, such as shoe removal, where to park, or which door to use to enter the home. If you are not sure, ask.

■ Whether you are seeing a specific client or an entire family, include and interact with additional family members present at the home visit. This inclusion allows you to develop a trusting atmosphere that expresses the understanding that they function within the context of their family unit.

#### Ask

■ Ask easy, open-ended questions on the telephone or at initial home visits with a genuine interest, allowing the client/family to share information. This action is essential to developing a trusting, nonjudgmental relationship. Recognize that a trusting relationship might not develop until the client sees that you keep your word and maintain confidentiality and trust, which might require many visits to demonstrate.

■ Initially, focus on positive aspects and strengths of the client or family unit. Until you establish a trusting relationship, interventions are going to be less effective when they lack emphasis on assets and focus solely on problems to be addressed or fixed.

■ Ask whether you can share information prior to providing it. This approach allows respect and trust to develop.

#### Act

■ Communicate with language that avoids medical or technical language/terms.

■ Avoid using a laptop or a tablet in the home if it is apparent that the client/family do not trust that data will not be shared (because of prior experiences they might have had with others).

■ Position yourself in a physically respectful space (e.g., sit at similar eye level, if possible).

### Community Level

Find a fit with the members' goals (e.g., working with faith communities).

■ Invest time in building professional relationships with key community members and in understanding the goals and missions of other agencies that are serving the community. This outreach can lead to the establishment of trusting collaborative efforts to serve community population segments.

■ Be honest and provide accurate, consistent messages to the community about health-related situations that might arise (e.g., a pertussis outbreak).

### Systems Level

Ensure that policies are accepting and do not ostracize.

■ Implement policies and programs that meet the needs of the population being served. For example, if women utilizing the Women, Infants, and Children (WIC) program (a supplemental nutrition program) are surveyed in the community and 25% indicate that they could only come to the office to receive their food vouchers between 4 and 6 p.m., it would be appropriate to have some evening hours available and to establish a policy supporting this within the agency. This act displays openness and acceptance to the needs of this WIC population segment.

■ Use community-based participatory research methods so that communities have a voice and an opportunity to participate in planning, implementing, and evaluating interventions or policies.

**Intra-Agency Level**

**Show acceptance of coworkers within and across disciplines.**

- ▪ Openly share and discuss evidence-based nursing practice in a nonthreatening way that encourages group reflection. This approach can lead to a more unified nursing workforce based on mutual respect and trust in research and in each other's nursing practice.

- ▪ Engage in reflective supervision or reflective practice groups. This process goes beyond reflection and journaling and has become increasingly popular in evidence-based home-visiting protocols/models. Simply, reflective supervision provides PHNs with feedback to help them examine the patterns they might be using in caring for their clients and to readjust patterns that are not optimal.

**TABLE 12.4  Ethical Action in Providing Nonjudgmental and Unconditional Care**

| Ethical Perspective | Application |
|---|---|
| Rule ethics (principles) | ▪ Nonjudgmental public health nursing should simultaneously encourage beneficence and promote the good of families and communities. <br> ▪ Encourage autonomy by listening respectfully and showing verbal and nonverbal respect for the opinions of those being cared for. |
| Virtue ethics (character) | ▪ Be respectful in actions and words. <br> ▪ Be persistent in showing tolerance and creatively promoting health. <br> ▪ Be accepting and aware of how responses and actions can promote or discourage those being served. |
| Feminist ethics (reducing oppression) | ▪ Conduct assessments in a manner that appreciates strengths while also identifying areas for intervention. <br> ▪ Respect everyone. <br> ▪ Advocate for individuals and community groups that might have less power because they are regularly judged (e.g., homeless youth). |

## Ethical Application

Feminist and virtue ethics provide excellent principles with which to examine this competency. Feminist ethics emphasizes that actions should not oppress others. This competency focuses on accepting others and not being judgmental. By respecting the clients with whom you are working, you demonstrate acceptance, and you do not oppress others. Similarly, virtue ethics emphasizes tolerance and justice as two leading principles. When you are tolerant of others' experiences, beliefs, or perspectives, your actions reflect an ethical mindset acting as an ethical nurse. Finally, when you act in a just manner, you express to other people that they have worth and dignity.

Imagine the positive influence you, the PHN, can have in the diverse lives and communities you serve when you ethically provide care. This positive influence might come from something as simple as maintaining appropriate confidentiality, facilitating a nonjudgmental environment in a home visit or a community screening event, or expressing acceptance in verbal and nonverbal ways. With regard to the importance of maintaining appropriate confidentiality, PHNs care for clients in vulnerable states and complex situations. PHNs, therefore, need to be very conscientious to respect their clients and the confidentiality of the nurse-client relationship by refraining from talking about clients to other people beyond what is necessary for care coordination purposes. In the case study included in this chapter, you have observed Josie addressing many preconceptions regarding the client she is visiting. You have noticed how easy it can be to make judgments and how challenging it can be to provide nursing care in a nonjudgmental manner. Yet, when nursing care is nonjudgmental, it is much more likely to be effective and promote lasting change (see Table 12.4).

## KEY POINTS

- Even the most experienced PHNs can struggle with being nonjudgmental and accepting of other people.

- People and communities can be different from each other on multiple levels, including social, economic, geographic, religious, behavioral, age, ethnicity, race, or sexual orientation.

- Acting in a nonjudgmental manner does not mean that PHNs are accepting of everything.

- PHNs can increase the potential for program or intervention success by carefully examining the key cultural or social beliefs or practices within a community.

- Reflecting on your own reactions toward those who are different from you is a critical starting point toward achieving this competency.

- Remember that policies can promote acceptance or judgment of people or groups and that they should be made with input from diverse stakeholders.

## REFLECTIVE PRACTICE

Considering what you have learned in this chapter, identify what Josie might do next to act on her reflections during the home visit and her realization that her preconceived judgments are not only inaccurate but also not helpful in providing optimal care for the teen and her new baby.

1. What does Josie need to understand about being nonjudgmental and accepting?

2. What are some additional reflective questions that Josie needs to ask herself, and which information sources might be useful to her in growing more accepting of others?

3. How will Josie know that her efforts to be increasingly accepting of diverse people and communities are successful?

4. How might the Cornerstones (see Chapter 1) inform Josie's efforts to be accepting and nonjudgmental?

## APPLICATION OF EVIDENCE

1. Which ethical considerations are important to think about when responding to individuals, families, and communities in a nonjudgmental manner?

2. How might you work with colleagues to process judgmental feelings and work toward becoming more nonjudgmental?

3. What might you do to contribute to a work culture that supports nonjudgmental and unconditional acceptance of people?

## References

Aston, M., Meagher-Stewart, D., Sheppard-Lemoine, D., Vukic, A., & Chircop, A. (2006). Family health nursing and empowering relationships. *Pediatric Nursing, 32*(1), 61–67.

Center for Spirituality and Healing. (2013). Deep listening. Retrieved from https://www.csh.umn.edu/education/focus-areas/whole-systems-healing/leadership/deep-listening

Cioffi, J. (2003). Communicating with culturally and linguistically diverse patients in an acute care setting: Nurses' experiences. *International Journal of Nursing Studies, 40*(3), 299–306.

Debesay, J., Harsløf, I., Rechel, B., & Vike, H. (2014). Dispensing emotions: Norwegian community nurses' handling of diversity in a changing organizational context. *Social Science & Medicine, 119*, 74–80.

Dillon, R. (1992). Respect and care: Toward a moral integration. *Canadian Journal of Philosophy, 22*(1), 105–132.

Falk-Rafael, A., & Betker, C. (2012). The primacy of relationships: A study of public health nursing practice from a critical caring perspective. *Advances in Nursing Science, 35*(4), 315–332.

Gallardo, M. (2014). An invitation to dialogue and reflection. In M. E. Gallardo (Ed.), *Developing cultural humility* (pp. 1–25). Thousand Oaks, CA: SAGE Publications.

Garneau, A. B., Pepin, J., & Gendron, S. (2017). Nurse-environment interactions in the development of cultural competence. *International Journal of Nursing Education Scholarship, 14*(1). doi:10.1515/ijnes-2016-0028

Garrett, P. (2009). Healthcare interpreter policy: Policy determinants and current issues in the Australian context. *Interpreting and Translation, 1*(2), 44–54.

Goldsborough, J. D. (1970). On becoming nonjudgmental. *American Journal of Nursing, 70*(11), 2340–2343.

Helleso, R., & Solveig Fagermoen, M. (2010). Cultural diversity between hospital and community nurses: Implications for continuity of care. *International Journal of Integrated Care, 10,* e036.

Henry Street Consortium. (2017). *Entry-level population-based public health nursing competencies.* St. Paul, MN: Author. Retrieved from www.henrystreetconsortium.org

Jolliffe, D., & Farrington, D. P. (2006). Development and validation of the Basic Empathy Scale. *Journal of Adolescence, 29*(4), 589–611.

Kupperschmidt, B. R. (2006). Addressing multigenerational conflict: Mutual respect and carefronting as strategy. *Online Journal of Issues in Nursing, 11*(2).

Mack, M., Uken, R., & Powers, J. (2006). People improving the community's health: Community health workers as agents of change. *Journal of Health Care for the Poor and Underserved, 17*(1), 16–25.

Nagano, H. (2000). Empathic understanding: Constructing an evaluation scale from the microcounseling approach. *Nursing and Health Sciences, 2*(1), 17–27.

O'Brien, M. J., Squires, A. P., Bixby, R. A., & Larson, S. C. (2009). Role development of community health workers: An examination of selection and training processes in the intervention literature. *American Journal of Preventive Medicine, 37*(6), s262–s269.

Pasco, A. C. Y., Morse, J. M., & Olson, J. K. (2004). The cross-cultural relationships between nurses and Filipino Canadian patients. *Journal of Nursing Scholarship, 36*(3), 239–246.

Passel, J., & Cohn, D., Pew Research Center. (2008). *U.S. population projections: 2005–2050.* Retrieved from http://www.pewhispanic.org/files/reports/85.pdf

Payne, R. K., DeVol, P. E., & Smith, T. D. (2001). *Bridges out of poverty: Strategies for professionals and communities.* Highlands, TX: aha! Process, Inc.

Pesznecker, B. L. (1984). The poor: A population at risk. *Public Health Nursing, 1*(4), 237–249.

Porr, C. (2005). Shifting from preconceptions to pure wonderment. *Nursing Philosophy, 6*(3), 189–195.

Porr, C., Drummond, J., & Olson, K. (2012). Establishing therapeutic relationships with vulnerable and potentially stigmatized clients. *Qualitative Health Research, 22*(3), 384–396.

Ramarajan, L., Barsade, S. G., & Burack, O. R. (2008). The influence of organizational respect on emotional exhaustion in the human services. *Journal of Positive Psychology, 3*(1), 3–18.

Redhead, A. (2016, February 8). Public health nursing and the myths of poverty. *The Huffington Post.* Retrieved from https://www.huffingtonpost.com/amanda-redhead/public-health-nursing-and_b_9182900.html

Reynolds, C. L., & Leininger, M. (1993). *Madeleine Leininger: Cultural care diversity and universality theory.* Thousand Oaks, CA: SAGE Publications.

Segal, J., Smith, M. A., & Jaffe, J. (2013). *Nonverbal communication skills: The power of nonverbal communication and body language.* Retrieved from https://www.helpguide.org/articles/relationships-communication/nonverbal-communication.htm

Tervalon, M., & Murray-Garcia, J. (1998). Cultural humility versus cultural competence: A critical distinction in defining physician training outcomes in multicultural education. *Journal of Health Care for the Poor and Underserved, 9*(2), 117–121.

U.S. Census Bureau. (2013). *Demographic trends in the 20th century.* Retrieved from https://www.census.gov/prod/2002pubs/censr-4.pdf

Zapart, S., Knight, J., & Kemp, L. (2016). 'It was easier because I had help': Mothers' reflections on the long-term impact of sustained nurse home visiting. *Maternal Child Health Journal, 20,* 196–204.

# COMPETENCY #11

## Shows Evidence of Commitment to Social Justice, the Greater Good, and the Public Health Principles

■ **Patricia M. Schoon**
*with Noreen Kleinfehn-Wald and Colleen B. Clark*

> *Erica is a new public health nurse (PHN) in a large urban county where 40% of the children live in poverty. During Erica's home visit to a young family, the mother states that the 2- and 3-year-old children have become "slow to get things and were tripping and falling more than usual." A year ago, the family had moved from a newer apartment building into a 70-year-old building when the husband lost his job. Erica notices paint chips on the floor and is concerned that they are from lead-based paint. She advises the mother to have her children's blood lead levels checked. The mother says she does not have health insurance and cannot afford a trip to the doctor. Erica tells the mother the paint should be replaced, but the mother is concerned that the landlord will not listen to her. Erica consults with her public health nursing supervisor about what else can be done.*

## ERICA'S NOTEBOOK

**COMPETENCY #11 Shows Evidence of Commitment to Social Justice, the Greater Good, and the Public Health Principles**

A. Applies principles of social justice to promote and maintain the health and well-being of populations

B. Understands the impact of the social determinants of health on vulnerable and at-risk populations

C. Advocates for the disadvantaged and underserved

D. Participates in collaborative social actions to reduce health disparities and inequities

*Source:* Henry Street Consortium, 2017

### USEFUL DEFINITIONS

**Advocacy:** Actions to ensure that individuals or populations have basic human rights and justice: "Advocacy pleads someone's cause or acts on someone's behalf, with a focus on developing the community, system, individual, or family's capacity to plead their own cause or act on their own behalf" (Minnesota Department of Health [MDH], 2001, p. 263).

**Charity:** Giving of oneself (volunteering) or of one's resources to those in need.

**Civic Engagement:** Working with community members to improve the civic life of the community through social and political actions based on an understanding of the community, its diversity, assets, and problems (Gehrke, 2008).

**Ethnicity:** A collective group of individuals with presumed common ancestry sharing cultural symbol and practices. Individual identification of ethnicity may be voluntary and self-defined (Ford & Harawa, 2010; Lee, 2009).

*(continues)*

## ERICA'S NOTEBOOK

COMPETENCY #11 *(continued)*

**Health Disparities:** Preventable, population-specific differences in health and disease (incidence and prevalence), health outcomes, or access to care that place some populations at greater risk than others and that are primarily the result of the social determinants of health.

**Health Equity:** "When every person has the opportunity to realize their health potential—the highest level of health possible for that person—without limits imposed by structural inequities. Health equity means achieving the conditions in which all people have the opportunity to attain their highest possible level of health" (MDH, 2014, p. 11).

**Human Rights:** Individual and family rights to live an independent, fulfilling, healthy life and earn a living wage for food, clothing, housing, and a safe environment; self-determination and autonomy. Human rights are rights inherent to all human beings. They are universal and inalienable, interdependent and indivisible, equal and nondiscriminatory, entailing both rights and obligations (Office of the High Commissioner for Human Rights, n.d.).

**Institutionalized Racism:** Historical and systematic discrimination that results in normalization and acceptance of differences in how minority populations of race and ethnicity are perceived and treated that results in educational, social, economic, and health inequities (Blodern, O'Brien, Cheryan, & Vick, 2016; Feagin & Bennefield, 2014; Gordon-Burns & Walker, 2015).

**Market Justice:** Personal resources and choices provide the basis for use and distribution of healthcare services based on concepts of individualism, self-interest, and individual effort; no collective obligation of society or government exists to provide for healthcare (Budetti, 2008).

**Race:** A social construct rather than a biological construct that is consistent with historical racial and ethnic population histories as opposed to specific genetic differences; different from ethnicity although frequently combined in healthcare practice; may be considered part of ancestral background (Frank, 2008; Jaja, Gibson, & Quaries, 2013; Lee, 2009).

**Racialization:** A process in which racial, ethnic, and cultural descriptions of groups of people in combination with statistical data combines to create distinct and different categories of people who are identified as having common risk factors and behaviors. This process leads to stereotyping groups of people with the tendency to see people as part of a specific group rather than as individuals (Cloos, 2015; Smedley & Smedley, 2005). This phenomenon is part of institutionalized racism.

**Social Determinants of Health:** The social determinants of health are the circumstances in which people are born, grow up, live, work, and age, as well as the systems put in place to deal with illness. These circumstances are in turn shaped by a wider set of forces: economics, social policies, and politics (World Health Organization [WHO], n.d.).

**Social Justice (syn., distributive justice):** The concept that individuals have the right to receive resources based on their needs and that a collective social obligation exists to provide for basic human needs, including health services (Budetti, 2008).

## Taking Action for What Is Right—Applying Principles of Social Justice

Professional nurses have a social contract with their clients and the public to ensure that the healthcare needs of individuals, families, populations, and communities are met in a caring, nonjudgmental, just, and equitable manner. Nurses as professionals and as private citizens are guided by the rule of law that protects basic human rights and by ethical principles that undergird basic human rights and social justice, a core principle of public health. Nurses in public health are confronted with ethical issues or moral challenges surrounding human rights and social justice on a daily basis. *Moral challenges* are situations in which a nurse's ethical beliefs are challenged and require critical thinking to arrive at a solution that protects the rights of individuals, families, and communities. The integration of caring (a core component of nursing) and social justice (a core component of public health), in conjunction with the moral challenge resulting when PHNs witness their clients experiencing health disparities and social injustice, propel PHNs to become involved in social and political advocacy (Falk-Rafael & Betker, 2012).

As students, you will be challenged and at times conflicted by the decisions you face that require choosing between two important and good things. For example, do you decide to respect individual autonomy and confidentiality, or do you find it necessary to enforce a public health law? This chapter provides guiding principles for social justice, information about population health disparities that confront PHNs, and a framework for public health advocacy interventions to help prepare you for the difficult situations you may encounter as a student and as a professional nurse.

## Guiding Principles for Taking Actions for What Is Right

Matwick and Woodgate (2016) report that social justice is considered a core value of nursing present since the late 19th century and evident in the actions of public health nursing leaders such as Nightingale and Wald. It is central to the practice of public health nursing. The two key attributes of social justice in nursing practice are *equitable distribution of resources* and *helping relationships* that occur when those with social advantage and power help those with less social advantage and power. Matwick and Woodgate believe that in order to practice social justice, nurses need to recognize and acknowledge social oppression and inequities, which then lead nurses to take caring actions toward social reform. They propose the following definition of social justice (p. 182):

> Social justice in nursing is a state of health equity characterized by both the equitable distribution of services affecting health and helping relationships.

Principles of social justice and human rights provide a framework for the ethical principles of public health practice. The principles of *social justice* that are key to the health and well-being of populations include:

- Collective social responsibility for community members
- Responsibility of government to ensure the basic human rights and healthcare needs of its citizens
- Equitable allocation of healthcare resources based on need
- Protection of the rights of individuals and families to live safe, healthy, and fulfilling lives

The United Nations published *The Universal Declaration of Human Rights* detailing 30 articles defining human rights (UN, 1948). The Preamble states, "Whereas inherent recognition of the inherent dignity and of the equal and inalienable rights of all members of the human family is the foundation of freedom, justice, and peace in the world… a common understanding of these rights and freedoms is of the greatest importance." Articles 1 and 25 provide an international standard for health as a basic human right.

### TABLE 13.1 Selected Human Rights From the UN's *Universal Declaration of Human Rights*

**Article 1.** All human beings are born free and equal in dignity and rights. They are endowed with reason and conscience and should act towards one another in a spirit of brotherhood.

**Article 25.** (1) Everyone has the right to a standard of living adequate for the health and well-being of himself and of his family, including food, clothing, housing, and medical care and necessary social services, and the right to security in the event of unemployment, sickness, disability, widowhood, old age or other lack of livelihood in circumstances beyond his control. (2) Motherhood and childhood are entitled to special care and assistance. All children, whether born in or out of wedlock, shall enjoy the same social protection.

*Source:* United Nations, 1948

Article 25 also speaks to many of the social determinants of health that have both societal and individual origins (see Table 13.1).

Respect for human rights is a basic tenet of ethical nursing practice (American Nurses Association [ANA], 2015, 2016; Fowler, 2015). The International Council of Nurses (ICN, 2011) views healthcare as a basic right for all individuals; they state that nurses are obligated to provide fair and equal treatment and have a responsibility to safeguard client rights at all times and are held accountable for both their actions and their inactions. The ANA Code of Ethics identifies the obligations of nurses to support both human rights and principles of social justice for all:

> A fundamental principle that underlies all nursing practice is respect for the inherent dignity, worth, unique attributes, and human rights of all individuals. The need for and right to health care is universal, transcending all individual differences. Nurses consider the needs and respect the values of each person in every professional relationship and setting; they provide leadership in the development and implementation of changes in public and health policies that support this duty (ANA, 2015, p. 1).

In addition, the ANA code stipulates that nurses are obligated as individuals and as a profession to act at the community and systems levels of practice to reduce health disparities.

- Provision 8: "The nurse collaborates with other health professionals and the public to protect human rights, promote health diplomacy, and reduce health disparities" (p. 31).
- Provision 9: "The profession of nursing, collectively through its professional organizations, must articulate nursing values, maintain the integrity of the profession, and integrate principles of social justice into nursing and health policy" (p. 35).

For example, at the *individual/family level* of practice, a PHN would arrange to have an interpreter present when providing health education and counseling to an immigrant family who cannot speak English. At the *community level,* PHNs could create a social marketing campaign to help the community understand and respond to the challenges English language learners have in understanding English language signage posted throughout the community. At the *systems level,* PHNs could work with interprofessional teams to improve access to healthcare services for immigrants and English language learners. Figure 13.1 depicts the three levels of practice.

Nurses have a social contract with the public. The American Nurses Association *Guide to Nursing Social Policy Statement* (Fowler, 2015) outlines the social contract that nurses have with the public. The contract involves 16 elements of reciprocal expectations between nursing and the public (p. 19). The ninth expectation, *Promotion of the Health of the Public,* stipulates that nurses have a social responsibility to address health disparities at all levels of society:

> Promotion of the Health of the Public: It is expected that nurses will address the problems faced by individual patients including issues of health disparities and that nursing will be involved with and lead in health-related issues important to society. In some instances, nursing will be in the vanguard of emerging health-related issues. Nursing will participate in the promulgation of healthcare policy at regional, state, national, and global levels. Protection of the public through advocacy also includes whistleblowing (p. 21).

The World Health Organization (WHO) considers the human right to healthcare from a very holistic perspective (2015).

The right to the highest attainable standard of health requires a set of social criteria that is conducive to the health of all people, including the availability of health services, safe working conditions, adequate housing, and nutritious foods (WHO, 2015, para. 1). Achieving the right to health is closely related to that of other human rights, including the right to food, housing, work, education, nondiscrimination, access to information, and participation. The right to health includes both freedoms and entitlements.

- **Freedoms** include the right to control one's health and body (e.g., sexual and reproductive rights) and to be free from interference (e.g., free from torture and from nonconsensual medical treatment and experimentation).

- **Entitlements** include the right to a system of health protection that gives everyone an equal opportunity to enjoy the highest attainable level of health.

WHO also identifies principles and standards of human rights that provide guidance to address the causes of human

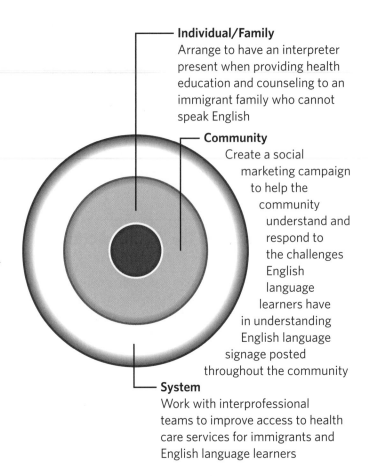

**Individual/Family**
Arrange to have an interpreter present when providing health education and counseling to an immigrant family who cannot speak English

**Community**
Create a social marketing campaign to help the community understand and respond to the challenges English language learners have in understanding English language signage posted throughout the community

**System**
Work with interprofessional teams to improve access to health care services for immigrants and English language learners

**FIGURE 13.1** How a PHN Can Practice at All Three Levels

rights inequities. These principles and standards are outlined in Table 13.2 (2015, para 7).

These human rights, especially those emphasizing access to living conditions that encourage health, guide much of the work that PHNs do. Sometimes advocating for the human rights of individuals and concurrently advocating for social justice for vulnerable individuals, families, or populations results in ethical conflicts. Nurses have ethical responsibilities to protect the rights of individuals and to protect the health and welfare of the community. Consequently, some actions, such as mandated reporting of specific communicable disease incidents, require nurses to identify an ethical rationale for whether they choose to protect the individual or the community when protecting both simultaneously is not possible. Public health professionals have a code of ethics (Public Health Leadership Society, 2002) that directs them to act to protect vulnerable and at-risk populations and to work to eliminate health disparities. (See Table 13.3 for principles and examples of PHN actions.)

## TABLE 13.2 Human Rights-Based Approaches

**Nondiscrimination:** The principle of nondiscrimination seeks "…to guarantee that human rights are exercised without discrimination of any kind based on race, colour, sex, language, religion, political or other opinion, national or social origin, property, birth or other status such as disability, age, marital and family status, sexual orientation and gender identity, health status, place of residence, economic and social situation."

**Availability:** A sufficient quantity of functioning public health and healthcare facilities, goods and services, as well as programs.

**Accessibility:** Health facilities, goods, and services should be accessible to everyone. Accessibility has four overlapping dimensions: nondiscrimination; physical accessibility; economic accessibility (affordability); information accessibility.

**Acceptability:** All health facilities, goods, and services must be respectful of medical ethics and culturally appropriate as well as sensitive to gender and life-cycle requirements.

**Quality:** Health facilities, goods, and services must be scientifically and medically appropriate and of good quality.

**Accountability:** States and other duty-bearers are answerable for the observance of human rights.

**Universality:** Human rights are universal and inalienable. All people everywhere in the world are entitled to them.

*Source:* WHO, 2015

PHNs have both a moral and a legal obligation based on human rights to secure and provide public health services to those who need them. However, because resources are finite, PHNs are faced with the difficult situation of setting priorities to determine which at-risk populations and who among these populations will receive services. PHNs employed by governmental agencies work with community partners to identify need, available resources, and service gaps. A human rights approach presented by Gruskin and Daniels (2008, p. 1573) provides a framework for these decisions:

- Direct concern with equity in the utilization of resources.
- Examination of the factors that may constrain or support planned interventions, including the legal, policy, economic, social, and cultural context.
- Participation and negotiation between all stakeholders, even as primary responsibility rests with government officials to facilitate these processes and to determine which interventions may have the biggest impact on health.
- Government responsibility and accountability for the manner in which decisions are made, resources are allocated, and programs are implemented and evaluated, including the impact on these decisions on health and well-being.

## TABLE 13.3 Ethical Principles That Guide Public Health Professionals in Confronting Health Disparities

| Principles | PHN Practice Examples |
|---|---|
| Public health should address principally the fundamental causes of disease and requirements for health, aiming to prevent adverse health outcomes. | ▪ Focusing on primary prevention with individuals, families, and communities<br>▪ Assessing the social determinants of health as part of the community assessment process<br>▪ Sharing the data on the social determinants of health that adversely affect the health of community members |
| Public health should advocate and work for the empowerment of disenfranchised community members, aiming to ensure that the basic resources and conditions necessary for health are accessible for all. | ▪ Targeting services to vulnerable and at-risk populations experiencing the greatest levels of health disparities<br>▪ Advocating through the political process for funding and services for vulnerable and at-risk populations<br>▪ Using an assets-based approach to collaborate with community members to empower them to manage their own healthcare needs |
| Public health programs and policies should be implemented in a manner that most enhances the physical and social environments. | ▪ Providing services to the uninsured and underinsured in homes and in community and mobile clinics<br>▪ Creating and providing culturally sensitive services<br>▪ Collaborating with community organizations that provide safety-net services |

*Source:* Public Health Leadership Society, 2002

## EVIDENCE EXAMPLE 13.1

### Social Justice and Human Rights Issues Identified by Practicing PHNs

A focus-group process was used to identify social justice and human rights issues that cause staff PHNs to confront ethical dilemmas on a daily basis. Sixteen nurses working in a suburban-rural county public health agency used storytelling to draw out examples of the social justice issues and human rights principles that were being violated which resulted in negative health outcomes. All four examples identified resulted in reduced health outcomes for individuals and families.

**Right to self-determination (human right)**—Clients are in need of services but do not qualify for existing programs. For example, an elderly person may need personal care attendant services but does not qualify for medical assistance, so the client remains at risk for placement in a long-term care facility.

**Right to a standard of living adequate for the health and well-being of individuals and families (human right)**—The working poor often work in entry-level jobs and earn salaries that make them ineligible for public services, even though their income is not enough to adequately support their families.

**Autonomy (human right) versus greater good (social justice)**—A client with a communicable disease chooses to break home isolation and exposes many people by going out in public. Parents choose not to vaccinate their child, who then becomes ill with pertussis and exposes an entire classroom of children, including one child who is immune-compromised.

**Inequitable distribution of power, money, and resources (social justice)**—Legal immigrants arriving in the state have received no health examination in their home country and are not provided with a health screening upon arrival in the United States. Other foreigners seeking admission to the country as refugees have a health examination and have a health screening upon arrival in their county of residence.

*Source:* Kleinfehn-Wald, 2010

## Market Justice Versus Social Justice

Globally, healthcare systems vary but are generally based on principles of market justice, social justice, or a combination of the two. The U.S. healthcare system, like the rest of the U.S. economy, is based on free enterprise and the principles of market justice. An alternative healthcare system, based on social justice, is embodied in the nonprofit and governmental healthcare systems. See Chapter 7 for a discussion of the U.S. healthcare system. Advocates of *social justice* believe that the government has a role to play in the provision of and assurance of basic health services to its citizens. Advocates of *market justice* believe that individuals and the private sectors are better prepared to meet the healthcare needs of private citizens. Social justice requires that the government be responsible and accountable for the health and well-being of its citizens. Market justice requires that individuals be responsible for their own health and well-being. Table 13.4 compares the concepts of market and social justice relative to healthcare.

The United States has a dominant and enduring cultural value of *individualism*—a belief that individuals are able to create their own destiny and that individual rights are more important than society's rights (Ludwick & Silva, 2000). This cultural belief presents a significant barrier to the development of a social justice model of healthcare. It is important for nurses in the United States to understand the cultural values of our society to determine how health equity might be achieved.

## Social Determinants of Health

Social determinants of health are the conditions and circumstances that vulnerable populations experience over their life span in their homes, neighborhoods, work places, schools, and the larger community. The social determinants of health include access to healthcare and the systems put in place to deal with their ongoing health status and illness. These circumstances are in turn shaped by a wider set of economic, social, and political forces at the local, national, and global levels (WHO, n.d.). These social determinants of health have a significant impact on the health status of populations—often a negative one. Research has shown that interventions that address social determinants of health well in advance of identified health problems or concurrently with medical care improve health and reduce health disparities (Williams, Costa, Oduniami, & Mohammed, 2008). The social determinants of health (social and economic factors and physical environment) account for 40% of the health determinants that influence health outcomes, as illustrated in Figure 13.2.

Examples of social determinants of health identified by Healthy People 2020 are outlined in Table 13.5. Both the categories of social determinants and physical determinants in the table are considered social determinants of health.

Healthy People 2020 has identified objectives for the social determinants of health in the following categories: economic stability, education, neighborhood and built environment, and social and community context (HealthyPeople.gov, n.d.).

## TABLE 13.4  Market Justice Versus Social Justice in the United States

| Market Justice | Social Justice |
|---|---|
| People are entitled only to those valued ends, such as status, income, and happiness, that they acquire by individual efforts, actions, or abilities. The focus and beliefs include: | People in society receive benefits by belonging to a community, and the burdens and benefits of society should be fairly and equitably distributed. The focus and beliefs include: |

| Market Justice | Social Justice |
|---|---|
| ▪ Individual rights and responsibility | ▪ Individual rights as members of the community |
| ▪ Death and disability as individual responsibilities and problems | ▪ Death and disability as collective responsibilities and problems |
| ▪ Minimal collective action | ▪ Collective action for the common good |
| ▪ Freedom to act with minimal obligations for the common good | ▪ General obligation to protect individuals against disease and injury |
| ▪ Respect for the rights of individuals | ▪ Quality of life; stewardship of future |
| ▪ Individuals and the local private and public sector having responsibility and control over health and healthcare | ▪ Private business's obligation to the community as a whole |
| ▪ Local short-term goals that are treatment-oriented | ▪ Global, long-term goals that are prevention-oriented |
| ▪ Government infringement on individual rights, its inefficiency, and mistrust of it | ▪ Government obligation and responsibility to protect citizens and trust that it will do the right thing |
| ▪ Support for the medical model of healthcare | ▪ Support of a universal or single-payer model of healthcare |

*Sources:* Based on work by Keller, 2010, & Beauchamp, 2013

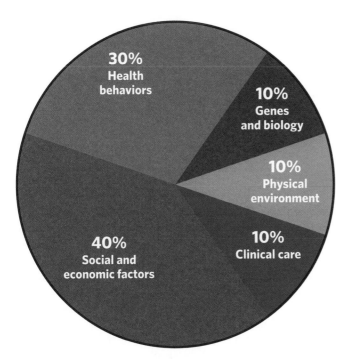

**FIGURE 13.2** Determinants of Health
*Source:* MDH, 2014, p. 12

It is important to note that the list of the social determinants of health does not include culture or ethnicity. Nor is the category of race considered a health determinant that results in poorer health outcomes. In order to organize public health data in a way that identifies populations with poorer health outcomes and health disparities, governmental agencies report health outcomes by specific categories of people (grouping people by a set of defined biological, cultural, and ethnic characteristics). The purpose of this categorization is to identify and target specific population groups for specific interventions to reduce health disparities (Cloos, 2015; Smedley & Smedley, 2005). This categorization is referred to as *racialization* in that these categories lead to stereotyping individuals by racial, ethnic, and cultural categories. PHNs must be careful that, when developing interventions for specific population groups (immigrants, Native Americans, etc.), they are able to set aside data-driven stereotypes and develop services that meet the needs of unique individuals.

**TABLE 13.5 Healthy People 2020 Social Determinants of Health**

| Social Determinants of Health | Examples |
|---|---|
| Social | ■ Availability of resources to meet daily needs (e.g., safe housing and local food markets) |
| | ■ Access to educational, economic, and job opportunities |
| | ■ Access to healthcare services |
| | ■ Quality of education and job training |
| | ■ Availability of community-based resources in support of community living and opportunities for recreational and leisure-time activities |
| | ■ Transportation options |
| | ■ Public safety |
| | ■ Social support |
| | ■ Social norms and attitudes (e.g., discrimination, racism, and distrust of government) |
| | ■ Exposure to crime, violence, and social disorder (e.g., presence of trash and lack of cooperation in a community) |
| | ■ Socioeconomic conditions (e.g., concentrated poverty and the stressful conditions that accompany it) |
| | ■ Residential segregation |
| | ■ Language/literacy |
| | ■ Access to mass media and emerging technologies (e.g., cellphones, the Internet, and social media) |
| | ■ Culture |
| Physical | ■ Natural environment, such as green space (e.g., trees and grass) or weather (e.g., climate change) |
| | ■ Built environment, such as buildings, sidewalks, bike lanes, and roads |
| | ■ Worksites, schools, and recreational settings |
| | ■ Housing and community design |
| | ■ Exposure to toxic substances and other physical hazards |
| | ■ Physical barriers, especially for people with disabilities |
| | ■ Aesthetic elements (e.g., good lighting, trees, and benches) |

*Source:* HealthyPeople.gov, n.d.

## Impact of Social Determinants of Health

In the United States, the social determinants of health of social status (e.g., education, income, place of residence, historical discrimination based on perceptions of race and ethnicity) and the ability to control one's life and health have a significant impact on health outcomes of both individuals and populations.

A comparison of life expectancy among different social groups in the United States illustrates both health disparities and health inequities. For example, the gap in life expectancy between the rich and the poor and those with more education versus those with less education is widening (Isaacs & Choudhury, 2015). Although gaps in life expectancy might be partially explained by lifestyle decisions and biological factors, societal factors also play a role. Those who are poor or live in poor neighborhoods have less access to healthy food, parks and public spaces, jobs, and education

(California Newsreel, 2008, p. 2). Children from low-income families are about seven times as likely to be in poor or fair health compared to children in the highest-income families (p. 1). In a study of 40,000 children, obesity rates for all U.S. children ages 10 to 17 increased 10% from 2003 to 2007, while the rate increased 23% for low-income children (Singh, Siahpush, & Kogan, 2010). Social determinants of health have a significant impact on early childhood development that persists into adulthood. Poverty, language differences, and vocabulary skills all have an effect on high school graduation rates, which have an impact on adult earning potential and health status across the life span (Robinson et al., 2017).

Infant mortality rates are considered a gold standard of health worldwide. The U.S. infant mortality rate, estimated at 5.80/1,000 live births for 2017, ranks 170th globally (Central Intelligence Agency [CIA], 2017). Education, income, and access to prenatal care are all causative factors. A review of African-American infant deaths in Milwaukee from 2008 to 2010 demonstrated that many of the mothers received late or no prenatal care (Salm Ward, Mazul, Ngui, Bridgewater, & Harley, 2013). Infant mortality rates in the U.S. continue to decrease, but significant gaps among racial groups are noted in Figure 13.3 (Matthews & Driscoll, 2017).

Life expectancy trends, although improving, also demonstrate health disparities, with Black males consistently having the lowest life expectancy over a 14-year period from 1999 to 2013 (see Figure 13.4).

Although Figure 13.4 only includes the racial categories of Black and White, there are data of years of potential lives lost before age 75 (death of individuals before their expected life span) that demonstrate disparities across multiple racial categories from 1990 to 2015 (see Table 13.6).

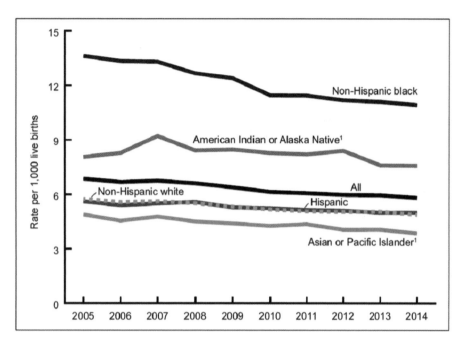

**FIGURE 13.3** Infant Mortality in the United States, 2005–2014
*Source:* Matthews & Driscoll, 2017

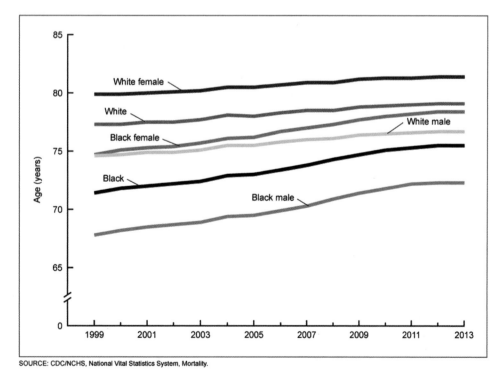

SOURCE: CDC/NCHS, National Vital Statistics System, Mortality.

**FIGURE 13.4** U.S. Life Expectancy by Race and Sex, 1999–2013
*Source:* Kochanek, Arias, & Anderson, 2015

It is important to note that health disparities represented by racial comparison mask the actual causes of the health disparities. Race is primarily a social construct rather than a genetic marker. So, although health data comparisons by racial categories historically and socially defined in the United States demonstrate correlation, these data do not demonstrate causation. Structural (e.g., income, education, housing, employment, social power, and opportunity) and spatial (e.g., geographic locations within neighborhoods, cities, counties, states, and areas of the country and concentration of poverty and race in specific neighborhoods) social determinants are the major causes of health disparities.

Institutionalized racism is a significant social determinant of health that provides multiple and complex pathways to poor health (Ramaswamy & Kelly, 2015). PHNs need to be educated about the social determinants of health embedded in society in order to advocate effectively to reduce the effects of institutionalized racism and work to change the systems that perpetuate it. An explanation of the multiple and often hidden causes of institutionalized racism that result in health disparities for African Americans is illustrated in Figure 13.5.

Progress is being made in reducing the health disparities between identified racial groups in the United States, but gaps do remain. The gap in life expectancy between African Americans and Whites is decreasing; however, the remaining gap is most pronounced between Black and White males. The reduction of the gap for Black males was related to decreased death rates for cancer, HIV, and unintentional injuries. For Black females, the reduced gap was due to decreased death rates for heart disease, HIV, and cancer.

The burden of excess deaths of the five leading causes of death (heart disease, stroke, chronic respiratory disease, cancer, and unintentional injury) is greater for those who

**TABLE 13.6 U.S. Years of Potential Life Lost Before Age 75 by Sex, Race, and Hispanic Origin, 1990 & 2015 (Age adjusted per 100,100 under age 75)**

| Category by Race | 1990 | 2015 |
|---|---|---|
| All | 9,085.5 | 6,757.7 |
| American Indian or Alaskan Native | 9,506.2 | 7,176.2 |
| Asian or Pacific Islander | 4,705.2 | 3,049.7 |
| Black (non-Hispanic) | 16,583.0 | 9,702.3 |
| Hispanic or Latina | 7,963.3 | 4,750.4 |
| White | 8,159.5 | 6,514.8 |

*Source:* National Vital Statistics System (NCHS), 2016

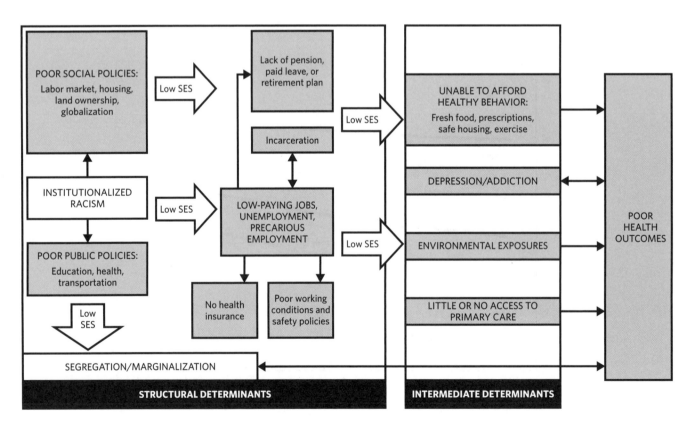

**FIGURE 13.5** Impact of Institutionalized Racism on Health Outcomes of African Americans
*Source:* Doede, 2015, p. 152

live in rural areas than in urban areas (Garcia et al., 2017). The excess death rate for unintentional injury was 50% higher in rural versus urban populations.

## Health Equity and Health Disparities

A major goal of public health is to achieve health equity; *health equity* exists when all people have the right and ability to reach their health potential regardless of their social positions or social circumstances (Brennen Ramirez, Baker, & Metzler, 2008). Reutter and Kushner (2010, p. 272) outline the requirements of health equity as follows:

- Resources should be allocated equitably and fairly.

- Human rights perspective includes the right to health and its prerequisites, the right to participate fully in society, and the right to nondiscrimination.

- Access to healthcare and the social determinants of health (social, economic, material, cultural, and political structures) should be equitable.

- Health equity is shaped by politics and achieved through the political process.

- Achieving health equity requires an intersectional approach (beyond the healthcare sector).

Many initiatives across the United States focus on developing solutions to health inequities at the local and state levels. The National Academy of Science in partnership with the Robert Wood Johnson Foundation (2017) published a report detailing how communities working collaboratively with diverse partners could identify and implement solutions to achieve health equity. The initiatives described in this report are based on several beliefs (National Academies of Sciences, Engineering, and Medicine, 2017):

- Health equity is crucial for the well-being and vibrancy of communities.

- Health is a product of multiple social, economic, environmental, and structural factors.

- Health inequities are mainly a result of poverty, structural racism, and discrimination.

- Communities have the ability or agency to promote health equity.

- Supportive public and private policies and programs at all levels facilitate community action.

- Collaboration and engagement of new and diverse (multi-sector) partners is essential to promoting health equity.

Their report provides a roadmap for community-based solutions.

Another initiative, A *Triple Aim of Health Equity,* was established by the Association of State and Territorial Health Officials (ASTHO) to empower state and territorial health agencies to develop policies, develop cross-sector collaboration, and implement programs to promote health equity at the state and local level (see the upcoming Figure 13.6). The idea is to move from a fragmented planning approach to an integrated approach that deals with all of the factors that can improve population health status: implementing policies that can improve health across all health, political, economic, and social sectors; developing an understanding of what health is and valuing it; and empowering communities to have the capacity to improve the health of their citizens (ASTHO, 2016).

Nurses represent the largest segment of healthcare professionals with more than 3.6 million nationwide. The Gallup annual honesty and ethics survey has recognized the nursing profession as the most trusted profession for the last 16 consecutive years (Brenan, 2017). With this acknowledgement comes privilege: advantages, power and authority, and a mandate to promote health equity and social justice by taking actions to reduce health disparities (Reutter & Kushner, 2010). *Health disparities* are preventable, population-specific differences in health and disease (incidence and prevalence), health outcomes, or access to care that place some populations at greater risk than others and that are primarily the result of the social determinants of health. PHNs know from experience that the populations they serve experience different levels of health status and have differing abilities to achieve their health potential. These disparities in health status are often the result of social determinants of health that negatively affect individual and family health outcomes and are not within the control of individuals and families to change. PHNs work to eliminate the social determinants of health that lead to health inequalities or health inequities:

- *Health inequalities* are differences in health disparities based on social conditions that reflect the level of deprivation of one group versus another group.

- *Health inequities* are systematic disparities in health and in the major social determinants of health between diverse populations with different social positions that persist over time (e.g., race; class; and advantages or disadvantages such as wealth, power, and prestige).

The Commission on the Social Determinants of Health, established by the WHO in 2005, recommends that the focus be on creating the conditions in which health and well-being can flourish (Baum, Gollust, Goold, & Jacobson, 2007). The Commission made three recommendations for action: (1) improving daily living conditions in which people are born, grow, live, work, and age; (2) tackling the inequitable distribution of power, money, and resources; and (3) measuring and understanding the problems of health inequities and assessing the impact of action (Baum et al., 2007). In 2015, the UN General Assembly adopted resolution *70/1. Transforming Our World: The 2030 Agenda for Sustainable Development* (2015). This resolution addresses the social determinants of health at a global level and sets out an action plan for people, the planet, prosperity, peace, and partnership. This action plan identifies 17 Sustainable Development Goals (SDG) (see Chapter 1).

## EVIDENCE EXAMPLE 13.2
### Food Insecurity

*Food insecurity* refers to the USDA's measure of lack of access, at times, to enough food for an active, healthy life for all household members and limited or uncertain availability of nutritionally adequate foods. Food-insecure households are not necessarily food insecure all the time. Food insecurity may reflect a household's need to make trade-offs between important basic needs, such as housing or medical bills, and purchasing nutritionally adequate foods. The lack of access at times to enough food to provide for a healthy, active life for all family members is a significant health determinant risk in the United States. In 2015, 42,238,000 people were identified as food insecure. Of these people, 26% were above the 185% of poverty level ($45,510 annual income for a family of four), which made them ineligible for almost all governmental nutrition assistance programs. In some states, the Supplemental Nutrition Assistance Program (SNAP) has raised the eligibility to 200% of poverty (Feeding America, 2017).

SNAP uses the Thrifty Food Plan (TFP) to calculate the cost to provide a nutritious diet that meets minimum daily dietary requirements as a means to determine the amount of SNAP family cash food benefits. A systematic review of market basket surveys (MBS) using actual grocery store food prices was conducted by Horning and Fulkerson (2014). They found that SNAP cash allotments based on TFP calculations may not be sufficient to meet a nutritious family diet based on the actual cost of groceries. The ability of low-income families to change their behaviors to eat a healthier diet may be cost prohibitive. Nurses need to advocate for increases in food assistance and the affordability of healthy foods.

---

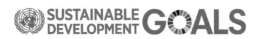 SUSTAINABLE DEVELOPMENT **G✪ALS**

**Native Diabetes Wellness Program**

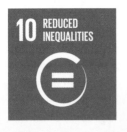

**GOAL 10** Poverty and food insecurity have been identified as risk factors for obesity and diabetes in Native Americans. The Native Diabetes Wellness Program (NDWP) was established in 2004 to reduce health inequities in tribal communities. Principles of practice included cultural humility and community-led participation. The *Eagle Books* series for young children, highlighting the wisdom of traditional ways of health, and a K–12 curriculum, Health Is Life in Balance, were instituted in 2006. The interactive Diabetes Education in Tribal Schools curriculum included engagement, exploration, explanation, elaboration, and evaluation. The Traditional Foods Project for American Indian and Alaska Native Communities was instituted by the CDC in 2008. The project included sustainable, ecological approaches to traditional foods and physical activity, increased access to local foods, and revived and shared stories of healthy traditional practices. Community members were engaged to track the progress of the project. In 2012 and 2013, Traditional Foods Project partners and NDWP staff were invited to present to the CDC Tribal Advisory Committee, which recommended continuing the Traditional Foods Project for a year beyond the 5-year cycle. Partners applied for a sixth year of funding for 2014 by demonstrating their evaluation results and plans to sustain their native food systems. Factors identified as important for the success of the program included: the significance of land; interest in Native American food pathways and food sheds; respect for traditional knowledge; consistency with traditional values; the role of elders as teachers of traditional knowledge fostered intergenerational relationships; traditional foods facilitate dialogue about health; emphasis on planning; the importance of community-driven planning; and sustained efforts beyond the project's end (CDC, 2016).

---

## Advocacy: PHN Advocacy for Population Health

Advocacy is considered a fundamental basis of nursing (Curtin, 1979; Gadow, 1999; MacDonald, 2006), while social justice is considered the fundamental basis of public health. The ANA (2013) directs PHNs to advocate for the protection of the health, safety, and rights of populations (Standard 16). In public health nursing, a primary focus of advocacy is health equity.

PHNs most often work with vulnerable individuals and families—those who are oppressed, marginalized, disenfranchised, or underserved and therefore at greater risk for disease, disability, and premature death. Although it is possible to improve the health status of individuals and families one by one, it is more effective, when possible, for PHNs to take actions to improve the health status of vulnerable populations as a whole.

## The Journey to PHN Advocacy

Caring leads to advocacy, and PHNs care passionately about those experiencing health disparities. PHNs enter into the practice of "critical caring" when they recognize health disparities in individuals and families and work to change the context of people's lives to improve their health (Falk-Rafael, 2005a). It is not always easy to advocate for clients, either at the individual or the population level of public health practice. Social justice dilemmas are part of the everyday lives of nurses. What is different for PHNs is that they often have to confront and resolve these dilemmas when they are out in the community by themselves. In an acute care setting, ethics committees can usually help resolve ethical issues related to autonomy, rights to self-determination, rights to refuse treatment, and rights to a safe and comfortable death. In the home and community setting, PHNs are often practicing alone, although they consult with other health team members when faced with challenging situations. Sometimes ethical decisions related to social justice and human rights need to be made during a home visit, such as reporting unsafe "garbage" homes to the county sanitarian, contacting animal control about a client's pet that has just bitten a young child, or requesting court-ordered Directly Observed Therapy (DOT) for a client with active TB who is not adhering to the medication regime. Sometimes PHNs carry out advocacy interventions by themselves, and sometimes they are part of a group advocating for change.

The pervasive barriers to advocacy are economic, political, and public opinion obstacles. Shankardass, Lofters, Kirst, and Quinonez (2012) believe that political will is shaped by public awareness and opinion. The ability of PHNs to create awareness of health inequities in their communities at the local or national level is key to influencing the health equity agenda of both the public and the politicians. Advocacy messaging generally needs to be tailored to the specific human rights or social justice theme and tailored to the targeted audience. The key messaging themes that should be considered when developing an advocacy message include: health as a value and social justice; human rights and governmental policies; environmental sustainability; economic cost of health inequities; and self-interest, in that inequities may lead to economic and social instability and may risk the health of others. Effective messaging strategies include: cooperative approaches; social mobilization and building a broader base of support; empowering disadvantaged groups; forming coalitions and networks with business, scientists, and policymakers; engaging the media; involvement in the political process; and taking advantage of windows of opportunity (Shankardass et al., 2012).

*Advocacy for health equity* is defined as "a deliberate attempt to influence decision makers and other stakeholders to support or implement policies that contribute to improving health equity using evidence" (Farrer, Marinetti, Cavaco, & Costongs, 2015, p. 394). The types of data analysis that are useful include: program evaluation data,

---

### THEORY APPLICATION
#### Critical Caring

*Critical caring* is a theory that is linked in the social activism of Nightingale and grounded in Watson's human caring theory and creative health promotion processes, and in feminist theory. Critical caring provides a framework for PHNs to engage in empowered caring (Falk-Rafael & Betker, 2012). Falk-Rafael and Betker interviewed expert Canadian PHNs using a multimodal research design. Their research identified three overarching themes from participants' reports: 1) the moral imperative and difficulty in articulating an ethical framework for practice, 2) pursuing social justice by advocating for health equity, and 3) experiencing barriers to their moral agency (i.e., being unable to do what their moral sense impelled them to do) and moral distress. The premise that "critical caring is a caring ethic through which social justice may be expressed" was supported by Falk-Rafael and Betker's research (p. 110). Caring is also a relational ethic based on the experiential aspects of PHN practice. The critical caring theory supports the importance of creating and maintaining supportive physical, social, economic, and political environments for clients and nurses having a critical role in creating these environments (p. 110).

---

particularly an analysis of cross-sector initiatives that show the impact on health disparities; cost-benefit analysis to assure policymakers that resources are not being wasted; analysis of the differential impact of specific policies to determine expected and unexpected outcomes; and presentation of narratives and stories.

It is important to consider how data is collected and when and where it is presented. Effective data is recent, timely, and local (Farrer et al., 2015). The data collection and evaluation process should include participation of community members. Disadvantaged and vulnerable populations have less voice and less power in shaping public policy. Finding ways to include community members who do not normally have a voice is important. Strategies to include community members are discussed in Chapter 8.

## Advocacy and Empowerment

To foster self-determination, facilitate empowerment, and promote self-advocacy, nurses need to create an atmosphere that supports and respects the rights of the populations they advocate for (Mallik, 1997). Nurses also need to feel and be empowered to take action (Cawley & McNamara, 2011). Table 13.7 outlines an empowerment framework for nurses.

**TABLE 13.7 A Framework for Becoming Empowered and for Empowering Others**

| Definition | Components | Empowerment Strategies |
|---|---|---|
| *Personal power* is the power you acquire and exercise through your informal and formal roles in your family and community. | ▪ Personal roles: family and friends<br>▪ Community roles: neighborhood, volunteer, elected official<br>▪ Cultural and ethnic ties<br>▪ Organizational membership: religious, political, other | ▪ Become involved as a citizen with an issue you are passionate about.<br>▪ Get to know your neighbors and community.<br>▪ Identify yourself to family, friends, neighbors, community members, and stakeholders as a professional who is committed to improving the health of the community.<br>▪ Participate in community or organizational meetings. Share your knowledge about healthcare.<br>▪ Form linkages and networks between different groups and organizations that share common beliefs and goals.<br>▪ Know your elected and appointed officials. |
| *Professional power* is the power you acquire and exercise through your formal role as a professional nurse. | ▪ Legitimacy through licensure<br>▪ Social contract with public<br>▪ Professional expertise and competencies<br>▪ Membership in professional organizations<br>▪ Professional networks | ▪ Find a professional and career mentor.<br>▪ Join a professional nursing organization.<br>▪ Attend conferences and meetings.<br>▪ Embrace the concept of lifelong learning through continuing education, certification, and formal higher education.<br>▪ Strive to provide evidence-based care.<br>▪ Develop strategies for monitoring quality and safety of care.<br>▪ Role-model professional nursing practice.<br>▪ Become a mentor for novice nurses. |
| *Organizational power* is the power you acquire and exercise through your formal and informal roles in your workplace and the healthcare system. | ▪ Position and job description<br>▪ Organizational communication<br>▪ Coordination of care<br>▪ Dispersed power of nursing throughout your organization and society | ▪ Become involved in the work of the organization beyond patient care.<br>▪ Become a member of a practice committee.<br>▪ Collaborate with people in other disciplines, management, and administration.<br>▪ Join an interdisciplinary group whose goal is improvement in patient care or population health.<br>▪ Work with a consumer group to improve healthcare in your community.<br>▪ Be politically active at the local level. Be GLOCAL: Think global, act local. At some point, you may wish to become involved at the state and national levels. |

*Source:* Schoon, Miller, Maloney, & Tazbir, 2012, p. 188

## Advocacy at the Individual/Family Level of Public Health

Nurses advocate for individuals and families by safeguarding their autonomy, acting on their behalf, and championing social justice in the provision of healthcare (Bu & Jezewski, 2006). Advocacy is aimed at building the capacity of individuals or families to manage their own healthcare needs. PHNs recognize the inequalities that exist within social determinants of health and challenge the status quo to change the social environment.

When PHNs advocate for individuals and families, they often do so within trusting relationships (MacDonald, 2006). For example, over time, nurses working with abused children or women often become aware of the abusive situations when they are providing trustworthy care for common physical health conditions. Trusting relationships make it possible for the clients to disclose very personal information

about abuse, and then the nurses can effectively intervene and advocate for safety (Hughes, 2010; Vanderburg, Wright, Boston, & Zimmerman, 2010). Home visiting by itself has been identified as a nursing intervention that reduces health disparities (Abbott & Elliott, 2016). See Chapter 10 for more information on caring relationships.

PHNs are aware that they can take actions to advocate for specific health needs of families that are related to both individual health determinants and social health determinants. They know that individuals and families can only change health determinants that are related to their own biological, behavioral, and life circumstances. They generally cannot change the health determinants that are societal in nature, or the social determinants of health. See Chapter 1 for a discussion of health determinants, protective factors, and risk factors. Table 13.8 illustrates the diverse individual and social determinants of health confronting a young family at risk for elevated blood lead levels at the individual/family, community, and systems levels.

**TABLE 13.8  Erica's Clients: Health Determinant Analysis—Risk for Elevated Blood Lead Levels in Children**

| | Protective Factors | Risk Factors |
|---|---|---|
| **Individual/family health determinants** | ■ Mother exhibits health-seeking behaviors and accepts assistance from the PHN and public health resources.<br>■ Children are healthy except for increased lead levels.<br>■ Apartment owner is concerned about the tenants' health and willing to apply for funding for lead abatement. | ■ Exposure to lead-based paint in home<br>■ Children's developmental stages and ages<br>■ Children's liver and kidneys unable to excrete excess lead<br>■ Family's inability to afford safe housing<br>■ Lack of medical insurance |
| **Social determinants of health—Community level** | ■ Community volunteer resources for transportation<br>■ Faith-based resources<br>■ Community health priorities of child health and environmental health | ■ Older, substandard housing with lead-based paint<br>■ Lack of safe, affordable housing<br>■ High poverty level due to poor economy<br>■ Downsizing of local businesses |
| **Social determinants of health—System level** | ■ Taxpayer funding of public health services<br>■ Public health nursing services available<br>■ Environmental health services available<br>■ Medicaid and CHIP funds for healthcare available for low-income, uninsured families<br>■ Local clinic willing to admit Medical Assistance clients<br>■ Public health clinic able to arrange for blood lead level testing.<br>■ Lead-abatement funding available | ■ Lack of affordable private or public health insurance<br>■ Limited access to affordable healthcare<br>■ Fewer medical clinics accepting Medical Assistance clients |

"*Erica receives a phone call from the mother of the children with suspected high lead levels. She has been able to enroll her children in a state-run healthcare plan and is looking for a medical clinic on a bus line. The clinic she finds is no longer taking patients on government assistance. Erica knows that not many medical clinics are in the mother's neighborhood and cannot think of one on a bus line. She checks the county's database on medical clinics and the metropolitan transportation agency website to investigate bus service routes. She contacts the American Red Cross and faith-based and charitable organizations in the neighborhood for transportation assistance. These searches take an entire afternoon, but Erica is successful in finding a clinic that accepts people on government assistance and a local church that has a volunteer transportation program. Erica tells the mother that she will make a home visit to draw blood from the children to screen them for high lead levels.*

*Erica asks her supervisor how to code these hours on her time sheet, as she is not providing direct nursing care. Her supervisor tells Erica that she is carrying out the nursing interventions of Advocacy and Case Management by finding resources that can help her client become more self-sufficient.*

*Erica returns to the family and draws blood from the children. Environmental Health staff has visited the family's apartment to determine whether the paint and paint chips are lead-based. Two weeks later, Erica, her PHN supervisor, and the Environmental Health staff meet to review their findings. Both children have increased blood lead levels, and a significant amount of lead-based paint has been found throughout the apartment. Erica arranges for the mother and children to be seen in the county public health clinic. Chelation therapy is recommended for the children, but the county does not provide that service. Lead abatement is recommended for the apartment building, but the owner says that he cannot afford it.*

*Erica knows that the human rights of the families in the apartment complex are at risk because of their exposure to lead-based paint and inability to change their living situation because of poverty and lack of affordable and safe housing. She knows that the human rights of the children cannot be met if they do not receive the medical care they need. Realizing that the individual rights of the apartment owner are in conflict with the social justice rights of the apartment residents, Erica tries to find just solutions. Erica refers the family to a social worker to apply for the state Medicaid/Medical Assistance program and Children's Health Insurance Program (CHIP) services. She thinks funding is available for medical treatment for the children through these programs. Erica also refers the apartment owner to a state program that provides financial assistance for lead abatement. The apartment owner is relieved to know that he can get financial assistance for lead abatement to provide a safer environment for his tenants.*

*Erica reflects on the positive health outcome for the two children with increased lead levels and the lead abatement of the apartment building that is scheduled for next month. She remembers that she had been in a hurry on the home visit and was impatient when the mother started talking about her children rather than responding to the questions Erica was asking. Luckily, Erica managed to focus on the mother's concerns rather than her own. She knows that if she had not taken the time to listen carefully, she might have missed the mother's comments about the children's symptoms and might not have noticed the paint chips. Erica renews her commitment to listen to clients telling her what their priorities and needs are. She decides she will be more observant when assessing the homes and neighborhoods of children in her caseload. Erica knows that collecting data and reporting her findings are the first steps in advocating for change.*"

## Advocacy at the Community and Systems Levels of Public Health

To reduce health disparities, PHNs need to be engaged in interventions at both community and systems levels of practice. PHNs spend most of their time working with individuals and families to modify their health determinants (i.e., reduce their risk factors and strengthen their protective factors) and empower them to manage their own healthcare needs. PHNs are interested in reducing health disparities among populations as well. To do this, PHNs must understand the multiple causes or health determinants that influence populations' health statuses. Individuals and families within populations that experience health disparities suffer consequences even if their personal behaviors and biological/genetic factors encourage health. Thus, PHNs must advocate for change in the societal causes of population health disparities by working at the community and systems levels of practice. Working with individuals and families to help them change their own behaviors and risk factors cannot by itself eliminate health disparities at the population level. In a perfect world, health resources would be infinite, and everyone would have access to all the healthcare they need. Unfortunately, this is not the case, and much of the time people cannot even agree on the type of healthcare that is needed. It is important for PHNs to work with other community members to create a sustainable community partnership to work to achieve health equity. Table 13.9 provides

**TABLE 13.9 Public Health Nursing Interventions at the Community and Systems Levels of Practice That Include and Support Advocacy**

*Advocacy:* Florence Nightingale demonstrated advocacy throughout her nursing career. As superintendent of a London hospital for impoverished women, she successfully had the hospital policy changed from admitting only those who belonged to the Church of England to admitting women of all faiths. Her nursing leadership of 38 nurses in Ottoman, Turkey, during the Crimean War was directed primarily at improving the plight of the wounded (Selanders & Crane 2012).

*Community Organizing:* A community action model was used in California to increase the community's capacity to address the social health determinants of tobacco-related health disparities and to develop local policies to eliminate or weaken smoking-related social health determinants (Lavery et al., 2005).

*Collaboration:* PHNs in Alberta, Canada, were concerned about the incidence of postpartum depression. They initiated a demonstration project in which they collaborated with a group of obstetricians and a group of midwives to have pregnant women referred to PHNs for psychosocial screening, health education, referral, and follow-up. Of the 150 women assessed, 37% had a history of postpartum depression, and 33% had a family history of depression. They accessed 93 services. Of the 75 women who participated in the program evaluation, 68% reported that the PHN intervention was helpful. The outcomes were so positive that the collaborative program was continued (Strass & Billay, 2008).

*Policy Development and Policy Enforcement:* Barriers that limit access to healthcare in the uninsured elderly population were explored in a journal article in a special health policy feature. Key barriers were lack of transportation, lack of insurance, complexity of the healthcare system, poverty, lack of family support, culture, communication, and race and ethnicity. Recommendations included improvements to health insurance coverage, use of the case management model of care, outreach services, improvements to transportation, and cultural competency and communication. Many of these recommendations were directed toward needed changes in federal healthcare policy (Horton & Johnson, 2010).

**EVIDENCE EXAMPLE 13.3**
**National Association of School Nurses— Speaking Up for Children**

The National Association of School Nurses (NASN) advocates for child health and the resources needed to promote health and safety among school children. School nurses are aware of the significant number of children coming to school with preventable physical and mental health conditions. School nurses work hard to obtain the needed health and social services for these children, but they know that they cannot solve the problem of inadequate resources by working one nurse to one child at a time. NASN has a history of lobbying for school health resources to meet children's needs. To more effectively lobby at the national level, NASN moved its headquarters to Washington, DC, in 2005. The NASN Annual Conference in 2005 brought hundreds of school nurses to Washington, DC; prepared them for lobbying efforts; and provided opportunities for the nurses to meet with their elected representatives to talk about child and school health issues, explain the role of the school nurse, and discuss the positive impact school nurses have on child health. The NASN 2007 policy agenda, Capital Investment for Children, was an effort to secure a place at the national policymaking table for school nurses so that they could advocate for children with unmet health needs. NASN continues its efforts to work with national, state, and local officials to achieve its goal of achieving a ratio of school nurses to students in each school that can adequately meet their health needs (Denehy, 2007).

examples of how advocacy at the community and systems level can lead to improved population health status.

Lathrop (2013) believes that nurses can take a leadership role in advocating for health equity at the local, national, and global levels of society. The areas targeted for advocacy are: structural change at the national and global levels; living and working conditions at the national and local levels; community interventions such as health fairs at the local levels; and individual and family interventions.

## Determining Public Health Priorities

PHNs need to identify the social justice and human rights issues they encounter in their practice to determine what actions they need to take and what their agencies' priorities should be. Dealing with the issue of health disparities often appears overwhelming. Tools to identify the disparities in specific populations and their causes help PHNs and their partners develop targeted interventions. One example is a Health Equity Assessment Tool (HEAT) developed in New Zealand (Signal, Martin, Cram, & Robson, 2008) that provides a planning and intervention process to identify and reduce health disparities in the Maori population. Table 13.10 provides a list of 10 questions that guides the process from assessment through intervention.

**TABLE 13.10  The Ten HEAT Planning Process Questions to Reduce Health Disparities Among Maori**

1. Which inequalities exist in relation to the health issue under consideration?

2. Who is most advantaged and how?

3. How did the inequities occur? What are the mechanisms by which the inequalities were created, maintained, or increased?

4. Where/how will you intervene to tackle the issue?

5. How will you improve Maori health outcomes and reduce health inequalities experienced by the Maori?

6. How could this intervention affect health inequalities?

7. Who will benefit most?

8. What might the unintended consequences be?

9. What will you do to make sure the intervention does reduce inequalities?

10. How will you know whether inequalities have been reduced?

*Source:* Signal et al., 2008

## Reducing Health Disparities— Downstream Versus Upstream Approach

Evidence has shown that the medical model alone, based on market justice, will not eliminate health disparities. Social determinants of health have been identified as a major cause of health disparities; however, the medical model deals primarily with individual causes of morbidity and mortality, such as genetics, healthcare access and quality, and individual health knowledge and behaviors. When the focus of healthcare is on the individual experiencing disease (secondary and tertiary prevention), this is called the *downstream approach*. Interventions aimed at reducing these causes, although important, will not by themselves alleviate health disparities. Individuals and families do not have equal access to private healthcare systems, governmental supports, or societal resources.

When the focus of healthcare is on modifying the social determinants of health to prevent disease and disability (primary prevention), this is called the *upstream approach*. Beauchamp (2013) argues that collective societal and governmental action based on social justice is necessary to protect the health of the public and that the burdens and benefits of

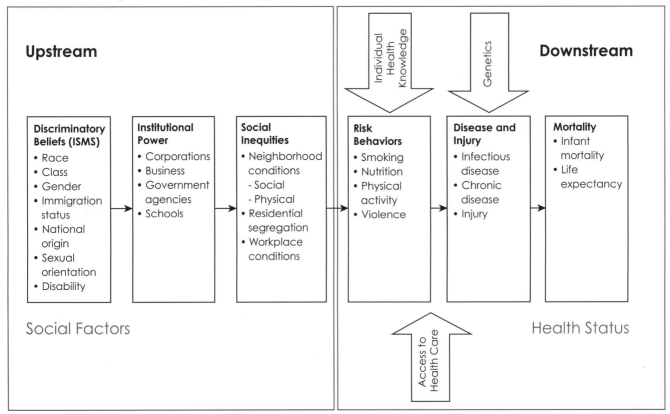

**FIGURE 13.6**  A Framework for Health Equity
*Source:* Alameda County Public Health Department, 2008, p. 4

these efforts should be shared equally except in situations where health disparities exist. However, there is no consensus within U.S. society for this position. Iton (2008) advocates a dual *upstream-downstream* approach (Figure 13.6). The dual approach involves taking an *upstream* approach to prevent disease and improve the health of populations while maintaining the *downstream* approach that treats individuals' diseases and disabilities. Figure 13.6 illustrates the dual *upstream-downstream* approach.

The collective social action that is needed to integrate the *upstream and downstream approaches* and to create inter-sectoral partnerships among governmental and private institutions is a journey that the United States has just begun. However, until there is an integrated system of healthcare that addresses all of the determinants of health, there will be little of the social change required to achieve health equity. A community partnership model that could be implemented at the local, national, and global levels to achieve health equity is presented in Figure 13.7.

## Activity

Read the following story and reflect upon upstream versus downstream thinking:

Two people were walking by a river. Suddenly, they observed babies floating down the river. They ran to the river to pull out as many babies as they could possibly reach. One of the rescuers yelled, "I'm going upstream to find out how these babies are getting into the river." This rescuer climbed the pathway up the side of the river, found where the babies were being thrown into the river, and immediately prevented more babies from being thrown into the water. This is upstream thinking and action in contrast to downstream action. Falk-Rafael (2005b) explains how downstream approaches that are aimed at meeting the needs of individuals and families must be paired with upstream approaches that aim to change power in societal relationships and structures to give voice to those with poor health and social disadvantages.

Think of a health disparity you would like to see decreased in a specific population. How would you use upstream thinking to achieve your goal? Do you think a dual approach of combining upstream and downstream strategies might work? What would you propose?

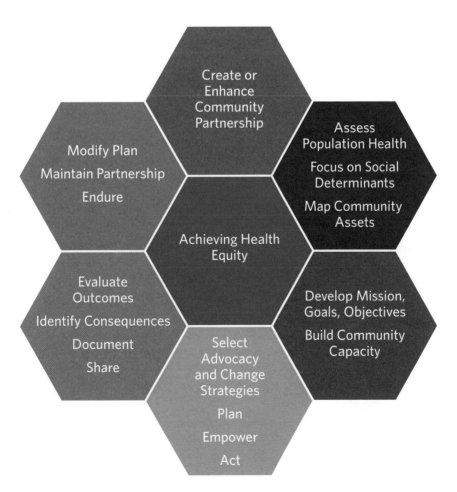

**FIGURE 13.7** Community Partnership Model to Achieve Health Equity

*Source:* Modified from *Phases of a Social Determinants of Health Initiative*, Brennen Ramirez et al., 2008, p. 33

# Civic Engagement as Social Justice Intervention

As advocates for social justice, PHNs by necessity must be involved in the civic life of their communities to have an impact on the social determinants of health. Nurses have both professional and citizenship obligations to the communities in which they work and live as part of the collective responsibility for social action to improve population health. Civic engagement involves working to improve the civic life of communities in partnership with community members. Nursing students who participate in civic engagement develop knowledge, skills, values, and motivations to make a difference (Gehrke, 2008, p. 53–54). Many nursing students are comfortable volunteering in their communities as a form of charity. These actions are commendable, but volunteering is not considered civic engagement. Charity is downstream action—an adaptive response to ameliorate the

outcomes of societal inequities and health disparities. Civic engagement involves more than charity: It is a means to achieve social justice through upstream actions—changing the social structure that creates health disparities. It involves social and political advocacy. Like others, you might tend to prefer to carry out acts of charity and avoid political engagement (Gehrke, 2008; Iton, 2008). However, it is important that you participate in civic engagement at some point in your nursing education and career. Civic engagement may occur at the local, national, and international levels.

# Participating in the Political Process

Professional nurses are expected to advocate for populations experiencing health disparities by using the political process. The role of a political advocate is embedded in the social contract that the profession of nursing has with

**TABLE 13.11 Political Process Activities**

| Stages of the Political Process | Examples of Civic Engagement |
| --- | --- |
| **Electoral process**<br>Candidate selection, endorsement, and support in the primary and general elections. | Work for a candidate by making phone calls, knocking on doors, assembling mailings, putting up yard signs, donating money, and attending rallies and other campaign activities for candidates who support your political health agenda. Participate in candidate screening through your local nurses' association. |
| **Legislative process**<br>Writing, introducing, passing the bill, and enabling legislation for funding. Both houses of Congress (one or two at state level) must pass the bill, and the bill must then be signed by the governor. | Contact your legislators about bills you want legislators to support; write letters and emails or go to the Hill for a face-to-face meeting and attend hearings on the bill. Testify at conference hearings, write letters to the editor of the local newspaper, post blog entries, and call in to radio programs. |
| **Budgeting process**<br>The omnibus reconciliation bill at the end of each legislative session provides funding. A government department is given "budget authority," or the right to implement the legislation and allocate the funding. | Lobby for a bill's funding. Find out which state agency has budget authority to enact and fund the legislation. Provide testimony on the best way to fund programs, and discuss who is going to benefit. |
| **Regulatory process**<br>The department with budget authority holds hearings to determine the rules and regulations that need to accompany the bill. | Attend hearings about the rules and regulations that are going to enable the bill to be implemented and monitored for cost, quality, and access. Ask to be put on an email list to receive notice of meetings and actions taken. |
| **Evaluation process**<br>Legislation that is enacted is usually evaluated at the end of the 2-year budget cycle of the legislature. Every program funded and implemented has to be evaluated and a report sent to the legislative auditor's office. The evaluation of the success of a project is a significant factor in determining whether the program is continued or renewed. | Testify and present reports about the effectiveness and impact of programs. Download a copy of the report and meet with a legislator's staff person or the "budget authority" agency to discuss the evaluation and make recommendations for continuing or modifying the program. |

society (Des Jardin, 2001). Nurses who have personal and professional senses of empowerment are able to work within their communities to improve population health through the political process (Carnegie & Kiger, 2009). PHNs are uniquely suited to participate in the political process, as they are confronted daily with the social determinants of health that often negatively affect their clients' health.

PHNs often participate in the Policy Development and Enforcement process, which requires an understanding of how the political process works and the critical points in moving forward. Taking the time to understand the policy-making process is essential if you want to advocate for vulnerable populations with your elected officials (e.g., legislators, mayor, city council, county commissioners, school board). After you understand how laws, regulations, and ordinances are made, you can be more confident about participating in the process. Your knowledge of healthcare and the health needs of your community makes you an expert in the eyes of elected officials. Developing a trusting relationship with your legislators can help you influence health policy development (Deschaine & Schaffer, 2003).

Nurses need to be involved in the political process from the electoral process to the legislative audit process. However, most citizens, nurses included, have no experience actively participating in the political process. So, it is time to start! Table 13.11 can guide you through the stages of the political process and provide examples of how you can become involved.

The American Public Health Association (APHA, 2018) has identified ten key points of advocacy that might be helpful to you as you think about approaching your legislators (see Table 13.12). Which of these strategies would you feel comfortable using? Think about your authentic leadership style.

## TABLE 13.12  Strategies for Working With Legislators

- Get to know legislators well—their districts and constituencies, voting records, personal schedules, opinions, expertise, and interests. Be sure to have a good understanding of the legislator and his/her concerns, priorities, and perspectives.

- Acquaint yourself with the staff members for the legislators, committees, and resource officials with whom you will be working. These people are essential sources of information and have significant influence in some instances in the development of policy.

- Identify fellow advocates and partners in the public health community to better understand the process, monitor legislation, and assess strengths and weaknesses. Finding common ground on an issue sometimes brings together strange bedfellows but makes for a stronger coalition.

- Identify the groups and other legislators with whom you may need to negotiate for changes in legislation. Do not dismiss anyone because of previous disagreements or because you lack a history of working together. Yesterday's opponent may be today's ally.

- Foster and strengthen relationships with allies and work with legislators who are flexible and tend to keep an open mind. Don't allow anyone to consider you a bitter enemy because you disagree.

- Be honest, straightforward, and realistic when working with legislators and their staff. Don't make promises you cannot keep. Never lie or mislead a legislator about the importance of an issue, the opposition's position or strength, or other matters.

- Be polite, remember names, and thank those who help you—both in the legislature and in the public health advocacy community.

- Learn the legislative process and understand it well. Keep on top of the issues and be aware of controversial and contentious areas.

- Be brief, clear, accurate, persuasive, timely, persistent, grateful, and polite when presenting your position and communicating what you need/want from the legislator or staff member.

- Be sure to follow up with legislators and their staff. If you offer your assistance or promise to provide additional information, do so in a timely and professional manner. Be a reliable resource for them today and in the future.

*Source:* APHA, 2018

*Erica is going to attend a Nurses Day on the Hill event at the state capitol. She wants to talk with her senator and representative about the need for funding programs to rehab older homes to remove lead paint. She asks the mother of the children with lead paint poisoning if it would be okay to share her family's story. She knows that real-life stories are more effective than statistical data. Erica attends Nurses Day on the Hill and talks with her senator and representative. She provides them with a one-page handout on the dangers of lead-based paint to young children. She is surprised at how receptive they are to her and that they treated her as an expert! More than 1,000 nurses are at the event. Erica is surprised that so many nurses took the time to attend. She feels proud to be part of such a large group that advocates for the health needs of the community. She realizes that nursing requires more than just working a shift. Erica knows that if she is going to make a difference as a public health nurse, she needs to advocate for her clients at both the systems and the community levels of practice.*

*Erica has been with the county public health agency for a year. She is committed to social justice and wants to improve her ability to advocate for vulnerable individuals and families. She wants to be able to support agency initiatives to improve population health in her community.*

*Erica has noticed that agency nurses in management positions frequently carry out community-organizing, coalition-building, and policy-development interventions. Sometimes she supported these agency initiatives. Erica makes a list of the opportunities she participated in and the opportunities she missed.*

Table 13.13 lists the opportunities that Erica put together.

## Ethical Application for Social Justice and Nursing Advocacy

PHNs often make ethical decisions related to social justice and human rights. Most of the time these decisions are related to the health status of individuals and families, but sometimes they are clearly related to the health status and health disparities of diverse populations. You need to be able to identify and describe the ethical principles based on social justice and human rights that guide you. It is also important to understand how your ethical beliefs and the ethical beliefs of others affect your capacity to act when confronted with health disparities. You need to have a strong sense of your own ethical beliefs. All PHNs bring personal biases to

**TABLE 13.13 Erica's List of Agency Initiatives**

| Opportunities Taken | Opportunities Missed |
|---|---|
| Brief conversation with a county health board member. Told a client story about a teenage mom who benefitted from the existence of a Healthy Families Collaborative. (Coalition Building) | In the past legislative session during a debate on a ruling regarding preservatives in vaccines, I could have written a personal letter to my legislator. (Policy Development) |
| Articulated several "talking points" from the state department of health policy on vaccines and autism at the early childhood meeting for parents to encourage other parents to have their children vaccinated. (Community Organizing) | Did not attend a meeting organized by city hall regarding hiking and biking trails in my community. I could have been a voice for obesity prevention in my community. (Community Organizing) |
| Led a focus group with Cambodian immigrants on cultural competency in services for the elderly in their community. Provided a summary report to the Cambodian community and service providers. (Collaboration) | Missed an opportunity for PHN team case study discussion to identify unmet health needs among their caseloads. I could have learned how my caseload was similar to or different from other PHNs' caseloads and how this influences our decision-making and priority-setting processes. (Collaboration) |
| Represented the agency on a task force organized by the state health department to develop guidelines on blood lead and healthy housing. (Policy Development) | Missed a meeting with a senior coalition to lobby county commissioners to extend green light walking time to allow seniors to walk across streets safely. I could have learned more about this health risk for the elderly. (Coalition Building) |
| Met with the OB nurse manager, the Newborn Nursery nurse manager, and the Infection Control nurse at the local hospital to discuss Tdap vaccination of staff as a means to prevent pertussis in newborn infants. (Collaboration) | Did not return a survey regarding vending machine policies in the school district. I could have helped with the data-collection process. (Policy Development) |

ethical decision-making, and they have differing abilities and skills to take action. Consider your level of *moral courage,* the ability to confront moral challenges based on steadfast commitment to fundamental ethical principles despite potential risks (Edmonson, 2010; Gallagher, 2011; Lachman, 2010; Murray, 2010). Think about the *ethical environment* that surrounds you, the social environment consistent with principles of human rights and social justice that is supportive of individual or collective actions of moral courage. Do you have the personal and professional resources you need as a student and future nurse to be the advocate you want to be?

## Activity

Reflect on the experiences you and your peers have participated in or observed as part of your community clinical. Were any of these ethical principles demonstrated in PHN practice?

## Activity

Consider the following case study: A PHN making a home visit to a recently paroled inmate of the local jail notes on the referral that the man is PPD positive on repeat testing and needs to start antiviral medications for TB. The man has the medication with him but is not taking it. The PHN considers her options:

- Should she encourage him to resume treatment for latent TB infection?

- Should she notify his physician or his parole agent of his noncompliance?

- What is the ethical problem, and how would you resolve it?

- Review the ethical principles listed in Table 13.14, and use them to resolve the ethical dilemma.

## TABLE 13.14 Ethical Principles and Actions in Advocacy

| Ethical Perspectives | Examples |
| --- | --- |
| Rule ethics (principles) | ▪ Public health resources and services are allocated based on need, so they might be distributed unequally—maximizing utility.<br>▪ Identify individuals, families, populations, and communities who are vulnerable and experiencing health disparities.<br>▪ Provide public health nursing services to those who are most vulnerable, at greatest health risk, and experiencing health disparities and health inequities, focusing on equal access to goods. |
| Virtue ethics (character) | ▪ Make ethical decisions based on social justice and human rights.<br>▪ Focus on fair procedures rather than outcomes.<br>▪ Provide support for individuals, families, populations, and communities who advocate for themselves.<br>▪ Be caring and compassionate.<br>▪ Select advocacy goals and actions that are culturally congruent with the racial and ethnic diversity of individuals, families, and populations within the community. |
| Feminist ethics (reducing oppression) | ▪ Advocate for the health and well-being of individuals, families, populations, and communities.<br>▪ Include and partner with clients in priority setting, goal setting, and advocacy actions.<br>▪ Empower clients to manage their own healthcare needs.<br>▪ Increase capacity of individuals, families, populations, and communities to manage their healthcare needs.<br>▪ Take actions to address social injustice at all levels of public health nursing practice.<br>▪ Focus on ensuring equal access to resources.<br>▪ Focus on traditions and practices in a community. |

*Sources:* Table based on work by Racher, 2007, and Volbrecht, 2002

## ! KEY POINTS

1. Social justice and human rights serve as the foundation for public health nursing advocacy.

2. Public health priorities and actions are directed at vulnerable populations experiencing health disparities and health inequities.

3. To reduce health disparities at the local, national, and global levels, it is necessary to eradicate the social determinants of health that create negative health outcomes.

4. PHNs advocate for health equity and justice for individuals, families, populations, and communities at all three levels of practice—individual/family, community, and systems.

5. PHNs bear professional accountability to advocate for vulnerable individuals, families, populations, and communities experiencing health disparities.

6. It is important for students and PHNs to become involved in civic engagement and the political process to help create social and structural change for health equity.

## REFLECTIVE PRACTICE

It is difficult to think about the bigger picture on a daily basis when providing nursing care to vulnerable individuals and families. The annual review period is a good time to compare your professional goals with actual practice to determine the congruence between goals and practice and to identify future opportunities for professional growth and development.

Think about your experiences in your public health nursing clinical and the advocacy competencies you developed during it:

■ Which vulnerable populations have you worked with as a student nurse?

■ How did you know whether an individual, family, or population was experiencing a health disparity?

■ Which health disparities did you identify in your community?

■ How did you explore the causes of health disparities in your community?

■ Which unmet health needs did you identify in your community?

■ Which clients did you advocate for as part of your public health clinical?

■ Which advocacy actions did you observe or participate in during your public health nursing clinical?

■ What worked and what did not? What would you do differently?

■ If you were going to develop an intervention at the community or systems level of practice for an unmet health need, what would it be? How would you start?

Refer to the Cornerstones of Public Health in Chapter 1. Which of these cornerstones support the social justice approach of achieving health equity through community partnerships? Does this cornerstone also support social justice as a foundation of public health nursing?

*Erica is preparing for her annual review with her supervisor. She decides that one of her goals for the following year will be to develop her advocacy skills at the community and systems levels of practice. She believes that her values and perspectives are consistent with social justice and the mission and goals of the county public health agency. She believes that she has been effective in advocating for individuals and families, such as the family whose children had increased blood lead levels. She now understands that she has to intervene at all three levels of practice to create change sufficient to improve population health. Erica is ready to work on her ACTIONS!*

## APPLICATION OF EVIDENCE

Think about how Erica developed and demonstrated public health nursing advocacy competencies as she worked with the two young children with increased blood lead levels and their mother, analyzed her own practice, and set the goal of developing additional advocacy competencies. Discuss the following questions with your classmates:

1. Which values and perspectives motivated Erica to act in a socially just manner?

2. Which aspects of the situation required Erica to take actions for this family?

3. Which ethical conflict between social justice and individual human rights did Erica have to resolve? How did she resolve it?

4. Why was it important for Erica to include others and work as part of a team?

5. Which health determinants required Erica to take actions at the systems level of practice?

6. Which advocacy actions did Erica take to help the family and owner of the building?

7. What were the health outcomes of her actions and the team's actions?

8. Which future civic engagement or community engagement actions might Erica participate in to protect children from environmental hazards?

## References

Abbott, L. S., & Elliott, L. T. (2016). Eliminating health disparities through action on the social determinants of health: A systematic review of home visiting in the United States, 2005–2015. *Public Health Nursing, 34*(1), 2–30. doi:10.1111/phn.12268

Alameda County Public Health Department. (2008). *Life and death from unnatural causes—Health and social inequity in Alameda County.* Oakland, CA: Author. Retrieved from http://www.acphd.org/media/53628/unnatcs2008.pdf

American Nurses Association. (2013). *Public health nursing: Scope and standards of practice.* Silver Springs, MD: Author.

American Nurses Association. (2015). *Code of ethics for nurses with interpretive statements.* Washington, DC: Author. Retrieved from https://www.nursingworld.org/nurses-books/code-of-ethics-for-nurses/

American Nurses Association. (2016). *The nurse's role in ethics and human rights: Protecting and promoting individual worth, dignity, and human rights in practice settings* [Position statement]. Silver Springs, MD: Author. Retrieved from https://www.nursingworld.org/~4af078/globalassets/docs/ana/ethics/ethics-and-human-rights-protecting-and-promoting-final-formatted-20161130.pdf

American Public Health Association. (2018). Ten top rules of advocacy. Retrieved from https://www.apha.org/policies-and-advocacy/advocacy-for-public-health/coming-to-dc/top-ten-rules-of-advocacy

Association of State and Territorial Health Officials. (2016). Triple aim: Implementing a 'health in all policies' approach with health equity as the goal. Retrieved from http://www.astho.org/Health-Equity/2016-Challenge/Implementing-a-health-in-all-policies-approach-with-health-equity-as-the-goal/

Baum, N., Gollust, S., Goold, S., & Jacobson, P. (2007). Looking ahead: Addressing ethical challenges in public health practice. *Journal of Law, Medicine, and Ethics, 35*(4), 657–667.

Beauchamp, D. E. (2013). Public health as social justice. In M. T. Donohoe (Ed.), *Public health and social justice* (pp. 11–19). San Francisco, CA: Jossey-Bass/John Wiley & Sons, Inc.

Blodern, A., O'Brien, L. T., Cheryan, S., & Vick, S. B. (2016). Understanding perceptions of racism in the aftermath of Hurricane Katrina: The roles of system and group justification. *Social Justice Research, 29,* 139–158. doi:10.1007/s11211-016-0259-9

Brenan, M. (2017). Nurses keep healthy lead as most honest, ethical profession. Gallup. Retrieved from http://news.gallup.com/poll/224639/nurses-keep-healthy-lead-honest-ethical-profession.aspx

Brennen Ramirez, I. K., Baker, E. A., & Metzler, M. (2008). *Promoting health equity: A resource to help communities address social determinants of health.* Atlanta, GA: U.S. Department of Health and Human Services, Centers for Disease Control and Prevention.

Bu, X., & Jezewski, M. A. (2006). Developing a mid-range theory of patient advocacy through competency analysis. *Journal of Advanced Nursing, 57*(1), 101–110.

Budetti, P. (2008). Market justice and U.S. healthcare. *Journal of the American Medical Association, 299*(1), 92–94.

California Newsreel. (2008). Backgrounders from the unnatural causes health equity database. *Unnatural Causes.* Retrieved from http://www.unnaturalcauses.org/assets/uploads/file/primers.pdf

Carnegie, E., & Kiger, A. (2009). Being and doing politics: An outdated model or 21st century reality? *Journal of Advanced Nursing, 65*(9), 1976–1984. doi:10.1111/j.1365-2648.2009.05084.x

Cawley, T., & McNamara, P. M. (2011). Public health nurse perceptions of empowerment and advocacy in child health surveillance in West Ireland. *Public Health Nursing, 28*(2), 150–158. doi:10.1111/j.1525-1446.2010.00921.x

Centers for Disease Control and Prevention. (2016). Native diabetes wellness program. Retrieved from https://www.cdc.gov/diabetes/ndwp/about-us/index.html

Central Intelligence Agency. (2017). *The world factbook*. Retrieved from https://www.cia.gov/library/publications/the-world-factbook/rankorder/2091rank.html

Cloos, P. (2015). The racialization of U.S. public health: A paradox of the modern state. *Cultural Studies ← → Critical Methodologies, 15*(5), 379–386. doi:10.1177/1532708615611719

Curtin, L. (1979). The nurse as advocate: A philosophical foundation for nursing. *Advances in Nursing Science, 1*(3), 1–10.

Denehy, J. (2007). National Association of School Nurses: Speaking up for children. *Journal of School Nursing, 23*(3), 125–127.

Deschaine, J. E., & Schaffer, M. A. (2003). Strengthening the role of the public health nurse leaders in policy development. *Policy, Politics, & Nursing Practice, 4*, 266–274. doi:10.1177/1527154403258308

Des Jardin, K. E. (2001). Political involvement in nursing—Education and empowerment. *AORN Journal, 74*(4), 481–482.

Doede, M. S. (2015). Black jobs matter: Racial inequalities in conditions of employment and subsequent health outcomes. *Public Health Nursing, 33*(2), 151–158. doi:10.1111/phn.12241

Edmonson, C. (2010). Moral courage and the nurse leader. *Online Journal of Issues in Nursing, 15*(3). doi:10.3912/OJIN.Vol15No03Man05

Falk-Rafael, A. (2005a). Advancing nursing theory through theory-guided practice—The emergence of a critical caring perspective. *Advances in Nursing Science, 28*(1), 38–49.

Falk-Rafael, A. (2005b). Speaking truth to power: Nursing's legacy and moral imperative. *Advances in Nursing Science, 28*(3), 212–223.

Falk-Rafael, A., & Betker, C. (2012). Witnessing social injustice downstream and advocating for health equity upstream: "The Trombone Slide" of Nursing. *Advances in Nursing Science, 35*(2), 98–112. doi:10.1097/ANS.0b013e31824fe70f

Farrer, L., Marinetti, C., Cavaco, Y. K., & Costongs, C. (2015). Advocating for health equity: A synthesis review. *The Milbank Quarterly, 93*(2), 392–437.

Feagin, J., & Bennefield, Z. (2014). Systemic racism and U.S. health care. *Social Science & Medicine, 103*, 7–14. Retrieved from http://dx.doi.org/10.1016/j.socscimed.2013.09.006

Feeding America. (2017). Food insecurity in the United States. Retrieved from http://map.feedingamerica.org/

Ford, C. L., & Harawa, N. T. (2010). A new conceptualization of ethnicity for social and epidemiologic and health equity research. *Social Science & Medicine, 71*(2010), 251–258. doi:10.1016/j.socscimed.2010.04.008

Fowler, M. (2015). *Guide to nursing's social policy statement: Understanding the profession from social contract to social covenant* (3rd ed.). Silver Springs, MD: American Nurses Association.

Frank, R. (2008). Functional or futile?: The (in)utility of methodological critiques of genetic research on racial disparities in health. A commentary on Kaufman's "Epidemiologic analysis of racial/ethnic disparities: Some fundamental issues and a cautionary example." *Social Science & Medicine, 66*(2008), 1670–1674. doi:10.1016/j.socscimed.2007.11.047

Gadow, S. (1999). Relational narrative: The postmodern turn in nursing ethics. *Scholarly Inquiry for Nursing Practice: An International Journal, 13*(1), 57–70.

Gallagher, A. (2011). Moral distress and moral courage in everyday nursing practice. *Online Journal of Issues in Nursing, 16*(2). doi:10.3912/OJIN.Vol16No02PPT03

Garcia, M. C., Faul, M., Massetti, G., Thomas, C. C., Hong, Y., Bauer, U. E., & Iademarco, M. F. (2017). Reducing potentially excess deaths from the five leading causes of death in the rural United States. *Surveillance Summaries, 66*(2), 1–7. doi:http://dx.doi.org/10.15585/mmwr.ss6602a1. Retrieved from https://www.cdc.gov/mmwr/volumes/66/ss/ss6602a1.htm

Gehrke, P. M. (2008). Civic engagement and nursing education. *Advances in Nursing Science, 31*(1), 52–66. doi:10.1097/01.ANS.0000311529.73564.ca

Gordon-Burns, D., & Walker, H. P. (2015). Institutional racism in the public health system. *New Zealand Journal of Occupational Therapy, 62*(2), 43–47.

Gruskin, S., & Daniels, N. (2008). Justice and human rights: Priority setting and fair deliberative process. *American Journal of Public Health, 98*(9), 1573–1577.

HealthyPeople.gov. (n.d.). Social determinants of health. Retrieved from https://www.healthypeople.gov/2020/topics-objectives/topic/social-determinants-of-health

Henry Street Consortium. (2017). *Entry-level population-based public health nursing competencies*. St. Paul, MN: Author. Retrieved from www.henrystreetconsortium.org

Horning, M. L., & Fulkerson, J. A. (2014). A systematic review on the affordability of a healthful diet for families in the United States. *Public Health Nursing, 32*(1), 68–80. doi:10.1111/phn.12145

Horton, S., & Johnson, R. J. (2010). Improving access to health care for uninsured elderly patients. *Public Health Nursing, 27*(4), 362–370.

Hughes, J. (2010). Putting the pieces together: How public health nurses in rural and remote Canadian communities respond to intimate partner violence. *Online Journal of Rural Nursing and Health Care, 10*(1), 34–47.

International Council of Nurses. (2011). *Nurses and human rights* [Position statement]. Geneva, CH: Author. Retrieved from http://www.icn.ch/images/stories/documents/publications/position_statements/E10_Nurses_Human_Rights.pdf

Isaacs, K. P., & Choudhury, S. (2015). *The growing gap in life expectancy by income: Recent evidence and implications for the Social Security retirement age*. Congressional Research Service. Retrieved from https://fas.org/sgp/crs/misc/R44846.pdf

Iton, A. B. (2008). The ethics of the medical model in addressing the root causes of health disparities in local public health practice. *Journal of Public Health Management Practice, 14*(4), 335–339.

Jaja, C., Gibson, R., & Quaries, S. (2013). Advancing genomic research and reducing health disparities: What can nurse scholars do? *Journal of Nursing Scholarship, 45*(2), 202–209. doi:10.1111/j.1547-5069.2012.01482.x

Kleinfehn-Wald, N. (2010). Social justice and human rights issues identified by practicing public health nurses [Unpublished research].

Kochanek, K. D., Arias, E., & Anderson, R. N. (2015). *Leading causes of death contributing to decrease in life expectancy gap between black and white populations: United States, 1999–2013.* National Center for Health Statistics Data Brief 218. Centers for Disease Control and Prevention.

Lachman, V. D. (2010). Strategies necessary for moral courage. *Online Journal of Issues in Nursing, 15*(3). doi:10.3912/OJIN.Vol15No03Man03

Lathrop, B. (2013). Nursing leadership in addressing the social determinants of health. *Policy, Politics, and Nursing Practice, 14*(1), 41–47. doi:10.1177/1527154413489887

Lavery, S. H., Smith, M. L., Esparza, A. A., Hrushow, A., Moore, M., & Reed, D. F. (2005). The community action model: A community-driven model designed to address disparities in health. *American Journal of Public Health, 95*(4), 611–616.

Lee, C. (2009). "Race" and "ethnicity" in biomedical research: How do scientists construct and explain differences in health? *Social Science & Medicine, 68*(2009), 1183–1190. doi:10.1016/j.socscimed.2008.12.036

Ludwick, R., & Silva, M. C. (2000). Ethics: Nursing around the world: Cultural values and ethical conflicts. *Online Journal of Issues in Nursing, 5*(3). Retrieved from http://ojin.nursingworld.org/mainmenucategories/anamarketplace/anaperiodicals/ojin/columns/ethics/culturalvaluesandethicalconflicts.html

MacDonald, H. (2006). Relational ethics and advocacy in nursing: Literature review. *Journal of Advanced Nursing, 57*(2), 119–126.

Mallik, M. (1997). Advocacy in nursing—A review of the literature. *Journal of Advanced Nursing, 25*(1), 130–138.

Matthews, T. J., & Driscoll, A. K. (2017). *Trends in infant mortality in the United States 2005–2014.* NCHS Data Brief 279. Retrieved from https://www.cdc.gov/nchs/data/databriefs/db279.pdf

Matwick, A. L., & Woodgate, R. L. (2016). Social justice: A concept analysis. *Public Health Nursing, 34*(2), 176–184. doi:10.1111/phn.12288

Minnesota Department of Health. (2001). *Public health interventions: Application for public health nursing practice.* St. Paul, MN: Author. Retrieved from http://www.health.state.mn.us/divs/opi/cd/phn/docs/0301wheel_manual.pdf

Minnesota Department of Health. (2014). *Advancing health equity in Minnesota—Report to the legislature.* St. Paul, MN: Author. Retrieved from http://www.health.state.mn.us/divs/chs/healthequity/ahe_leg_report_020414.pdf

Murray, J. S. (2010). Moral courage in healthcare: Acting ethically even in presence of risk. *Online Journal of Issues in Nursing, 15*(3), Manuscript 2. doi:10.3912/OJIN.Vol15No03Man02

National Academies of Sciences, Engineering, and Medicine. (2017). *Communities in action: Pathways to health equity.* Washington, DC: National Academies Press. doi:10.17226/24624.

National Vital Statistics System. (2016). Table 18: Years of potential life lost before age 75 for selected causes of death, by sex, race, and Hispanic origin: United States, selected years 1980–2015. National Center for Health Statistics. Retrieved from https://www.cdc.gov/nchs/data/hus/2016/018.pdf

Office of the High Commissioner for Human Rights, United Nations Human Rights. (n.d.). Your human rights. Retrieved from http://www.ohchr.org/EN/Issues/Pages/WhatareHumanRights.aspx?Pages/WhatareHumanRights.aspx

Public Health Leadership Society. (2002). *Principles of the ethical practice of public health* (Version 2.2). Retrieved from https://www.apha.org/~/media/files/pdf/membergroups/ethics_brochure.ashx

Racher, F. E. (2007). The evolution of ethics for community practice. *Journal of Community Health Nursing, 24*(1), 65–76.

Ramaswamy, M., & Kelly, P. J. (2015). Institutionalized racism as a critical social determinant of health. *Public Health Nursing, 32*(4), 285–286. doi:10.1111/phn.12212

Reutter, L., & Kushner, K. E. (2010). "Health equity through action on the social determinants of health": Taking up the challenge in nursing. *Nursing Inquiry, 17*(3), 269–280.

Robinson, L. R., Bitsko, R. H., Thompson, R. A., Dworkin, P. H., McCabe, M. A., Peacock, G., & Thorpe, P. G. (2017). CDC Grand Rounds: Addressing health disparities in early childhood. *Morbidity and Mortality Weekly Report, 66*(29), 769–772.

Salm Ward, T. C., Mazul, M., Ngui, E. M., Bridgewater, F. D., & Harley, A. E. (2013). "You learn to go last": Perceptions of prenatal care experiences among African-American women with limited incomes. *Journal of Maternal Child Health, 17,* 1753–1759. doi:10.1007/s10995-012-1194-5

Schoon, P. M., Miller, T. W., Maloney, P., & Tazbir, J. (2012). Power and politics. In P. Kelly & J. Tazbir (Eds.), *Essentials of leadership and management* (pp. 186–208). Clifton Park, NJ: Delmar/Centage.

Selanders, L. C., & Crane, P. C. (2012). The voice of Florence Nightingale on advocacy. *Online Journal of Issues in Nursing, 17*(1), 1–10. doi:10.3912/OJIN.Vol17No01Man01

Shankardass, K., Lofters, A., Kirst, M., & Quinonez, C. (2012). Public awareness of income-related health inequalities in Ontario, Canada. *International Journal of Equity Health, 11*(26). Retrieved from https://equityhealthj.biomedcentral.com/track/pdf/10.1186/1475-9276-11-26?site=equityhealthj.biomedcentral.com

Signal, L., Martin, J., Cram, F., & Robson, B. (2008). *The Health Equity Assessment Tool: A user's guide.* Wellington, NZ: Ministry of Health.

Singh, G. K., Siahpush, M., & Kogan, M. D. (2010). Rising social inequalities in U.S. childhood obesity, 2003–2007. *Annals of Epidemiology, 20*(1), 40–52. Retrieved from http://www.sciencedirect.com/science/article/pii/S104727970900324X

Smedley, A., & Smedley, B. D. (2005). Race as biology is fiction, racism as a social problem is real. *American Psychologist, 60*(1), 16–20. doi:10.1037/0003-066X.60.1.16

Strass, P., & Billay, E. (2008). A public health nursing initiative to promote antenatal health. *Canadian Nurse, 104*(2), 29–33.

United Nations. (1948). *Universal declaration of human rights.* Geneva, CH: Author. Retrieved from http://www.un.org/en/documents/udhr/

United Nations. (2015). *Transforming our world: The 2030 agenda for sustainable development.* Sustainable development knowledge platform. Retrieved from https://sustainabledevelopment.un.org/post2015/transformingourworld

Vanderburg, S., Wright, L., Boston, S., & Zimmerman, G. (2010). Maternal child home visiting program improves nursing practice for screening of woman abuse. *Public Health Nursing, 27*(4), 347–352.

Volbrecht, R. M. (2002). *Nursing ethics: Communities in dialogue.* Upper Saddle River, NJ: Pearson Prentice Hall.

Williams, D. R., Costa, M. V., Oduniami, A. O., & Mohammed, S. A. (2008). Moving upstream: How interventions that address social determinants of health can improve health and reduce disparities. *Journal of Public Health Management Practice, 14*(Suppl.), S8–S17. doi:10.1097/01.PHH.0000338382.36695.42

World Health Organization. (n.d.). About social determinants of health. Retrieved from http://www.who.int/social_determinants/sdh_definition/en/

World Health Organization. (2015). *Human rights and health* [Fact sheet]. Retrieved from http://www.who.int/mediacentre/factsheets/fs323/en/

# COMPETENCY #12

## Demonstrates Leadership in Public Health Nursing With Communities, Systems, Individuals, and Families

■ **Patricia M. Schoon**

*with Bonnie Brueshoff, Erin Karsten, and Marjorie A. Schaffer*

> " *José is with the Elders at Home Program for his public health nursing clinical. He is assigned to Mr. and Mrs. Santos, a couple in their 70s struggling to manage their healthcare needs and stay in their home in an older inner-city neighborhood. Mrs. Santos provides primary assistance for her husband, who has advanced chronic obstructive pulmonary disease (COPD). After a recent hospitalization, Mr. Santos received home care services from a home care nurse, respiratory therapist, occupational therapist, and home health aide. These services were reimbursed by Medicare because Mr. Santos met the criteria of potential for rehabilitation and progress toward independent living. All went well. Then a 60-day health assessment resulted in a determination that Mr. Santos was no longer eligible for home care services. He was referred to the county public health Elders at Home Program but has been resisting a home visit. José wonders, "I am just a student nurse. What can I do?" He sighs, "Well, it looks like my preceptor has handed me a challenge I can't avoid. Isn't there a chapter we are supposed to read on leadership in public health nursing?"* "

---

### JOSÉ'S NOTEBOOK

**COMPETENCY #12** Demonstrates Leadership in Public Health Nursing with Communities, Systems, Individuals, and Families

A. Seeks learning opportunities when working with peers, organizations, and communities

B. Demonstrates ability to be flexible, adapt to change, and tolerate ambiguity while working in an unstructured environment

C. Seeks from and provides consultation and support to peers and community partners

D. Responds to population health needs in collaboration with systems and communities

E. Contributes to team efforts to improve the quality of care provided to client populations

F. Prioritizes and organizes workload, time, materials, and resources to maximize benefits to clients and stakeholders

G. Participates in the political process to advocate for changes in health and social policies that affect population health, workforce health, and public health services delivery

*Source: Henry Street Consortium, 2017*

*(continues)*

## JOSÉ'S NOTEBOOK (continued)

### USEFUL DEFINITIONS

**Advocacy-Based Leadership:** Advocacy-based leaders are motivated by the needs of others to take actions to improve others' health and well-being.

**Authentic Leadership:** Authentic leaders are reflective practitioners whose actions are consistent with their values, ethical standards, and convictions (Murphy, 2012; Wong, Spence Laschinger, & Cummings, 2010).

**Leadership:** Leadership is the process and art of influencing, motivating, and leading others to achieve shared goals.

**Leadership Journey:** The leadership journey is a lifelong process of self-discovery, self-efficacy, and goal-directed actions.

**Shared Leadership:** Shared leadership refers to the concept of being an effective team member (Avolio, Walumbwa, & Weber, 2009).

## Leadership in Public Health Nursing Practice

Leadership is often taught as a separate course in the nursing curriculum. So, you may be asking, why is leadership content included in this book? Why is there a separate leadership competency? Isn't leadership the same no matter where it is practiced?

Leadership theories are certainly applicable to all forms of nursing practice. However, there are two aspects of public health nursing practice that are unique. Public health nurses (PHNs) are often alone in community settings and required to take immediate actions independently. Sometimes PHNs are the only healthcare provider available in a community setting. PHNs must be comfortable making decisions and taking actions independently and know how to access consultation and support by phone and Internet. They need to be risk takers, able to advocate for their clients in situations where they may be alone and in situations that may not always be comfortable. It is important for PHNs to be comfortable in community settings where there is minimal structure and maximum uncertainty. PHNs must be comfortable providing mentorship and being mentored. Leadership skills are essential.

PHNs spend their daily lives in the community and deal with social determinants of health and the impact of these determinants on health outcomes with individuals, families, populations, and communities. They know that they often must go outside the healthcare system to promote and protect their clients' health. Effective use of leadership skills is crucial to the success of their efforts. PHNs carry out leadership at the individual/family, community, and systems levels; in the home; in interprofessional public health and community teams; and in diverse community systems, such as government, healthcare organizations, schools, home-care agencies, prisons, faith-based communities, and homeless shelters. PHNs employ many strategies including persuasion, influencing, role-modeling, networking, and collective social action. Interventions often used are collaboration, community organizing, coalition-building, social marketing, surveillance, and policy development and enforcement. PHNs who work in governmental agencies are responsible for carrying out the core functions and essential services of public health (see Chapter 7). Leadership skills are essential to the success of these services.

> Public health nurses practice at that intersection where societal attitudes, government policies, and people's lives meet. Such privilege creates a moral imperative not only to attend to the health needs of the public but also, like Nightingale, to work to change the societal conditions contributing to poor health (Falk-Rafael, 2005, p. 219).

PHNs are expected to have a passionate commitment to advocate for the health of the clients they serve and the health of their community.

## The Leadership Journey

Nurses are presented with leadership challenges throughout their careers. *Leadership challenges* are events or situations that require nurses to use critical thinking and ethical problem-solving to arrive at equitable and effective solutions. These situations propel nurses along their leadership journey. The *leadership journey* is a lifelong process of self-discovery, self-efficacy, and goal-directed actions. Nursing students and professional nurses are on a lifelong journey as they develop their leadership potential, explore their authentic leadership styles, and identify their personal and professional reasons and motivations for taking leadership actions. Students and nurses entering public health have their own unique leadership journey.

Nursing leadership begins with the nurse-patient relationship in clinical practice. You started your leadership journey as a nursing student the moment you identified an unmet patient need and advocated for your patient by working to influence other members of the care team to take actions to meet your patient's needs. In other words, you began to *lead* when you identified an unmet client need and took the lead in advocating for your client with others. In doing so, you demonstrated *advocacy-based nursing leadership.* The actions you took were based on your beliefs and values and reflected your own personal and professional way of being, the beginning of *authentic leadership* practice. When you move beyond the nurse-client relationship and advocate within the healthcare system or community for changes in attitudes, beliefs, knowledge, actions, and resources that will help meet your client's needs, you are practicing *leadership.* You do not have to be in a formal position of authority, such as a supervisor or manager,

to be a leader. Staff nurses usually work within healthcare teams and share the workload. Knowing how to work effectively within the healthcare team and with groups within the community is referred to as *shared leadership.* These three forms of leadership are consistently practiced in public health nursing.

## Authentic Leadership

Choosing to lead is a conscious choice to take action. The authentic leader moves from concerns about self to concerns about the other. Leadership is a journey from the "I" to the "We" (George & Sims, 2007). Leadership consciousness starts with an awareness and understanding of one's own values, beliefs, and convictions. Self-awareness or consciousness leads nurses to develop their own personal and professional leadership competencies. This consciousness then leads them to an awareness of the needs of others, thus creating a moral challenge and a call to action. When nurses respond to this call for action, they develop authentic personal and professional leadership styles and competencies. Figure 14.1 demonstrates how you move along your leadership journey throughout your nursing career as you respond to transitional moments in your nursing practice.

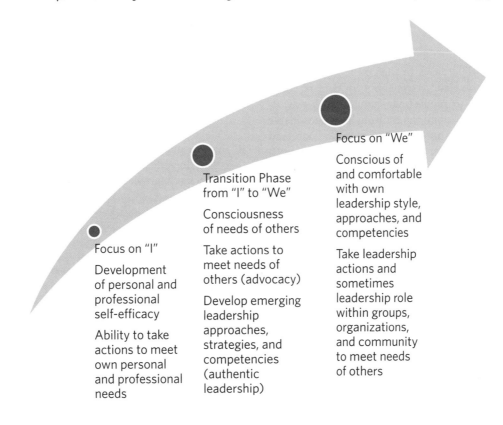

**FIGURE 14.1** The Leadership Journey—Ongoing Leadership Challenges
*Source:* Based on concepts from George & Sims, 2007

You have already developed some beginning leadership skills and practices in your previous nursing clinicals. These skills and practices are consistent with the situational challenges you have faced and your authentic sense of self. You may further develop your leadership style and skills as you progress through your public health clinical. This chapter provides guidance to help you consider the public health nursing leadership styles and skills that fit your authentic self. Which transitional moments in your leadership journey do you think you might encounter during your public health nursing clinical experiences?

## The Leadership Journey: Reflections of a Public Health Nurse Leader

As you progress along your leadership journey, you may want to reflect on the situations, personal decisions, and role models or supporters who helped you develop your authentic leadership style and skills. In the following interview, a PHN leader describes her leadership journey and what she learned along the way (Brueshoff, personal communication, 2013):

*Tell a story about how your early experiences in public health nursing and the leadership challenges you confronted helped you along your leadership journey.*

My first job as a nurse was working in a PHN position in northern Minnesota. I had a generalized caseload of young families and elderly clients. One of my specific roles in the department was to provide follow-up for the Sudden Infant Death Syndrome (SIDS) cases in the county. As a novice PHN, I found my knowledge base about SIDS to be inadequate, which led me to request additional training available at the state level. Through the training, I made valuable connections with the Minnesota SIDS Center and accessed expertise from SIDS Center staff that provided me with resources for families and much-needed emotional support. Needless to say, I became better prepared to provide the support and assistance that benefited SIDS families during subsequent home visits. This experience early on in my career reinforced the importance of ongoing education and reaching out to access resources and expertise from other professionals. Later in my career, my experience working with SIDS families helped me mentor other PHNs who were working with SIDS cases and was a factor in my leadership journey as I was hired in a position as an apnea home monitoring coordinator.

*Who were your role models and guides along the way?*

I was extremely fortunate to have the support and guidance from two public health directors who offered me opportunities for growth and challenged me to take on leadership roles. I consider both directors to be my role models and mentors. I also looked to the Minnesota Department of Health (MDH) PHN nurse consultants for guidance with my PHN practice and took every opportunity I could to volunteer for state work groups and committees. Through the

encouragement that was given to me, I gained confidence and was motivated to advance my knowledge and skills. For example, I received the support to apply to serve on the MDH Maternal and Child Health (MCH) State Advisory Task Force. I was appointed to be a member of this task force, which gave me leadership experience in dealing with statewide policy and programs and expanded my professional network. I was given support to pursue the Robert Wood Johnson (RWJ) Executive Nurse Fellowship program that I completed.

*What inspires you and keeps you fresh in your leadership vision and strategies?*

Both my practice experiences and professional development activities have kept me inspired including (1) experiencing the impact that public health has in helping us all be healthy, because the focus of public health is on prevention; (2) being able to be innovative in trying new approaches and using evidence-based practice; (3) reading leadership literature and articles; (4) networking with my colleagues; (5) mentoring new PHN staff; and (6) working to influence policies and decision-making on all levels—local, state, and national.

*What are your three most important "lessons learned" about leadership in your public health nursing practice?*

- To lead, you have to be willing to take risks and know it is OK to fail and learn from your mistakes—to learn how to "fail forward."

- Networking and lifelong learning are key. You can do more with others than by being solo. Join professional organizations and stretch yourself. Get involved. Never stop. Learning self-awareness is very important and will help you immensely! Ask for honest feedback from others so you can build on your strengths.

- Become politically savvy. Learn about policies and processes that affect public health. The ability to influence policy has a far-reaching influence on nursing!

–Bonnie Brueshoff, DNP, RN, PHN, Public Health Director and Robert Wood Johnson Executive Nurse Fellow (2006–2009), Dakota County Public Health

## Leading Through Relationships

PHNs work with their clients, team members, interprofessional colleagues, and various members of the community in striving to meet their goals of improving population health. Public health nursing leadership requires influencing others to achieve public health goals (Morrison, Jones, & Fuller, 1997). You are starting your public health nursing leadership journey at the individual/family level of practice, which is where entry-level PHNs often begin to develop their skills and understanding of their role. Table 14.1 outlines leadership styles that are often used in public health nursing practice and provides examples of how students may develop skill in using these styles.

## TABLE 14.1 Nursing Leadership Styles in Public Health Nursing

| Leadership Style | Student Leadership Learning Examples |
| --- | --- |
| *Advocacy-based leadership:* Advocacy-based leaders are motivated by the needs of others to take actions to improve their health and well-being. Advocacy-based leadership is based on the ethical principles of social justice. Advocacy-based leaders are risk takers who act with moral purpose and demonstrate moral courage when faced with perceived or actual opposition. (Refer to a discussion of advocacy and moral courage in Chapter 13.) | ■ Students meet with county commissioners to advocate for additional funding for low-cost or free dental services to Medicaid clients.<br>■ Students work with local grocery stores to form a coalition to provide food items to stock a school-based backpack program where students take home backpacks filled with food on Fridays so that they have food over the weekend. |
| *Authentic leadership:* Authentic leaders are reflective practitioners whose actions are consistent with their values, ethical standards, and convictions. They are true to themselves and know why they do what they do. Authentic leaders objectively consider all available information and the opinions of others, clearly and openly share their perspectives, are open and honest in their communication, and have an awareness of their own strengths and weaknesses. They are considered trustworthy and reliable (Murphy, 2012; Wong et al., 2010). | ■ Students visit a community center hosted by a recent immigrant group to learn how to communicate and develop respectful, trusting relationships in a culturally sensitive manner.<br>■ Students have a post-clinical debrief with their PHN preceptors to reflect on the communication strategies they used in working with developmentally delayed adults in a sheltered living setting. |
| *Shared leadership:* Shared leadership refers to the concept of being an effective team member: sharing responsibilities, mutually organizing the team's work, maintaining team communication, taking the initiative to try a new approach if something is not working, supporting team members, providing positive feedback, and allocating resources equitably (Avolio et al., 2009). When leadership is shared, PHNs have more time and energy to care for their clients. | ■ Students plan for and staff a hearing and vision screening program at a local elementary school. Each group of students has a lead student who is the primary liaison with the school nurse and takes the lead in organizing a team of fellow students to provide the screening.<br>■ Students work with a PHN team to reach out to families who are eligible for PHN services but have not accessed them. |

Think about the leadership journey you have been on since starting your public health nursing clinical. Are you able to identify when you began to focus more on your clients and the community than yourself? Can you identify a transformative moment when you realized that it was morally necessary for you to advocate for the unmet health needs of a vulnerable population by enlisting the help of others?

*José has just completed his first visit to Mr. and Mrs. Santos. Mrs. Santos is experiencing caregiver stress, and Mr. Santos is becoming less and less active. He loves to smoke even though he has a portable oxygen tank in his bedroom. Mr. and Mrs. Santos do not want nurses and social workers coming in and telling them what to do. They are afraid of strangers. José tells them he will make a joint visit with the social worker and introduce them to her. He is going to take the initiative to find the resources Mr. and Mrs. Santos need to live independently in their own home.*

Which public health nursing leadership competencies has José demonstrated? Which leadership styles is he using in working with Mr. and Mrs. Santo?

## Advocacy-Based Leadership

Advocacy-based leadership is foundational to public health nursing. Advocating for clients—whether those clients are individuals, families, populations, or communities—is part of the social justice mission of public health nursing. Although all nurses advocate for the unmet needs of their individual clients, PHNs have a responsibility to advocate for the health of the public, to care about what is causing the health disparities in their communities, and to take action to improve the health status of the affected individuals, families, populations, and communities. This means that PHNs need to be aware of emerging health needs and connect the patterns of health disparities they observe among their individual clients. Sometimes advocacy-based leadership is an unconscious response to an unmet healthcare need. Sometimes it is a conscious choice triggered by an ethical or moral call to action. Evidence Example 14.1 illustrates advocacy-based leadership taken by a public health nursing student from a school of nursing in the Henry Street Consortium.

## EVIDENCE EXAMPLE 14.1
### PHN Student Initiative Demonstrates Leadership and Improves Population Health

A student nurse completed her leadership clinical in an inner-city school with a 95% poverty rate among its students. She developed a dental screening program for third-graders as her leadership project. After screening all the children, she found that almost all of them had dental disease, such as decay, bleeding gums, abscesses, and missing or broken teeth. Almost none of them had received dental care in the last year, and few owned a toothbrush. Each child was given a toothbrush and toothpaste and taught how to brush his or her teeth. The PHN student then attempted to screen all the children in the elementary school, managing to screen about 90%. She prepared a report showing the need for dental care in almost all the children screened, sent home referrals to all the parents, and included information on local dental clinics that provided care for low-income patients. The principal used the report to obtain a grant to put a dental clinic in the school. Within a few years, dental clinics were established in elementary schools located in high-poverty neighborhoods throughout the school district.

—Senior Student Nurse

## THEORY APPLICATION
### Caring Leadership Model

The McDowell-Williams Caring Leadership Model combines Watson's Human Caring Theory (2008) and Kouzes and Posner leadership theory (2007). This model was developed for and implemented in an acute care setting. However, it is applicable to any clinical setting. The model is based on six core values (Williams, McDowell, & Kautz, 2011, p. 33):

- **A**lways lead with kindness, compassion, and equality.
- **G**enerate hope and faith through co-creation.
- **A**ctively innovate with insight, reflection, and wisdom.
- **P**urposely create protected space founded upon mutual respect and caring.
- **E**mbody an environment of caring-helping-trusting for self and others.

The acronym AGAPE is defined historically as brotherly love and charity, which fits with the social justice and equity precepts of public health nursing.

"*José returns to visit with Mr. and Mrs. Santos. Mrs. Santos is crying and wringing her hands. José asks Mrs. Santos whether she would be willing to see a mental health case worker. She refuses. He remembers that the local Latino Catholic church has a pastoral ministry home visiting program. He wonders whether Mrs. Santos would allow the pastoral minister to visit her. Mrs. Santos agrees to let José contact the church. José is pleased that he is developing his advocacy-based leadership skills. He is really stretching himself to try to find ways to help Mr. and Mrs. Santos and be an effective advocate.*

*Margaret, José's public health nursing preceptor, says to him, "I hope you like a challenge, because this couple has lots of them. You are going to have to think outside the box to keep Mr. and Mrs. Santos in their own home. You really are going to have to use all your communication, advocacy, and leadership skills to work successfully with this family."*

*José wonders and then reflects, "Do I have any leadership skills? I thought those came later, after 5 to 10 years of practice. Hmm. Well, maybe I was practicing advocacy-based leadership."*

*Margaret agrees, "Yes, you certainly took the lead in advocating for Mr. and Mrs. Santos.*"

### Using Public Health Interventions as Part of the Leadership Journey

You might have noticed that José is practicing many of the public health nursing interventions described in Chapter 2 in his role as Mr. and Mrs. Santos's PHN. Leadership is integrated into many of the activities that PHNs and student nurses carry out. Table 14.2 has examples of leadership activities utilizing the Public Health Intervention Wheel (Minnesota Department of Health [MDH], 2001). The intervention examples are suggested student learning activities.

## What Are Leadership Expectations for Entry-Level Public Health Nurses?

The expectation of what leadership roles and responsibilities PHNs take on are dependent of the needs of specific organizations and the community. Individual nurses also bring different leadership abilities to their work. Diverse styles of leadership are necessary to accomplish the work of public health nursing. PHNs select leadership strategies and interventions based on what is most effective. Characteristics such as flexibility, a willingness and openness to develop new leadership skills, and the courage to practice them in the public arena are the key to successful PHN leadership. Consider what a public health nursing director has to say about leadership and PHNs who are just starting out:

Based on the PHN population-based practice focus in public health, a new PHN needs to demonstrate clinical leadership for the work with individuals and families as well as at the community level. This leadership role might be as a participant or a lead position on various committees such as an interagency collaborative, an early childhood intervention, or a school health team. The PHN must also be a leader in engaging community members in efforts to improve health and address health inequities. The PHN needs to utilize communication and collaboration skills to lead groups, coalitions, and committees to achieve the goals of improving the health of the population.

–Bonnie Brueshoff, DNP, RN, PHN, Public Health Director and Robert Wood Johnson Executive Nurse Fellow (2006–2009), Dakota County Public Health, 2017

## What Are Essential Leadership Skills for Becoming a Public Health Nursing Leader?

PHNs are often confronted with the need to use their leadership skills in advocating for their clients. As someone new to public health nursing, you might find thinking about the skills needed for leadership in this field daunting. Remember that all good nursing leaders start at the beginning by becoming competent in their practice specialties; as they develop confidence as expert practitioners, they build a repertoire of leadership skills.

Nursing leadership can be formal or informal. PHNs demonstrate leadership at all levels of nursing practice from novice to expert and as staff nurses, clinical experts,

### TABLE 14.2 Taking the Lead in Using Public Health Interventions

| PHN Intervention | Example |
|---|---|
| Advocacy | ▪ Observing/participating in a town meeting designed to address or change a determinant of health<br>▪ Advocating for parenting classes at a conference center in an apartment complex (community level) |
| Policy development | ▪ Working with schools/work sites to change vending and fundraiser policies to include healthy food choices (systems level) |
| Policy enforcement | ▪ Responding to concerns/complaints about smoking in restricted areas based on the Freedom to Breathe Act (community level) |
| Surveillance | ▪ Attending or participating in immunization registry meetings (systems level)<br>▪ Locating unlicensed daycare providers and providing teaching on home safety (individual level) |
| Coalition building | ▪ Recruiting and inviting family daycare providers to join the childhood-obesity prevention committee (community level) |
| Community organizing | ▪ Participating in/helping plan youth programs, such as smoking or alcohol-use prevention (community level)<br>▪ Helping/coordinating a bioterrorism tabletop exercise (systems level) |
| Disease and health event investigation | ▪ Following up on reports of pertussis cases; communicating with the state health department, clinics, and area schools about the outbreak and doing case investigation (individual and systems levels)<br>▪ Meeting with clinics and hospitals regarding prenatal hepatitis B program (systems level)<br>▪ Working with veterinarians, meat packers, and hunting associations on chronic wasting disease (systems level) |
| Case management | ▪ Participating in a Student Attendance Review Board (SARB) meeting within a school (systems level) |
| Collaboration | ▪ Participating in meetings to observe the collaborative process, decision-making, and problem-solving in groups (e.g., children's mental health, early childhood family education) (systems level) |
| Consultation | ▪ Working with child daycare centers, adult daycare centers, and battered women's shelters to establish standards and criteria for prevention of infectious disease (systems level) |
| Social marketing | ▪ Designing messages and materials on "how to make a healthy home" that PHNs can use on home visits to help families deal with asthma (systems level) |

*Sources:* Dakota County Public Health, 2004; Henry Street Consortium, 2004; MDH, 2001

nursing specialists, supervisors, managers, educators, or administrators. Leadership is a process, not a role. Much of the research on leadership in the literature looks at the leadership roles of managers; however, all nurses can utilize leadership styles and strategies. Leadership is an expected competency for PHNs, regardless of their position (American Nurses Association [ANA], 2013; Quad Council of Public Health Nursing Organizations, 2011).

New PHNs need to be able to carry out entry-level leadership competencies. Initially, their leadership opportunities are tied to their daily clinical practice with individuals and families. However, depending on the size and nature of the agency, they might soon become involved in leadership activities at the community and systems levels of practice. Some public health agencies include leadership development in their annual performance appraisals (Kalb et al., 2006). You might be expected to demonstrate the leadership skills you have developed after you have been in public health nursing for a year or so. The Henry Street Consortium has generated a set of leadership skills that beginning PHNs need to develop and strengthen to practice effective PHN leadership (see Table 14.3).

## TABLE 14.3 Essential Leadership Skills for Public Health Nurses

| Skill | Strategies and Considerations | Your Leadership Action |
|---|---|---|
| Seeks learning opportunities | ▪ Determine goals for professional development.<br>▪ Strive to see the "big picture" by attending to community and systems processes. | Match your interests and goals to learning opportunities. |
| Works independently; is autonomous in practice | ▪ PHNs make many independent decisions based on established programs or protocols.<br>▪ PHNs make decisions based on their own expertise within the framework of ethical and professional standards or practices. | Attend a PHN team meeting to observe how PHNs share experiences. Seek suggestions about evidence-based practice and tools to use for complex family situations. |
| Willing to work in an unstructured environment; tolerates ambiguity | ▪ PHNs practice in settings where people live, learn, and work—the priorities in these settings are often not health or healthcare.<br>▪ Sometimes the goals of others are not clear or consistent with the goals of PHNs.<br>▪ PHNs learn to be in ambiguous situations while working to determine individual, family, and community goals.<br>▪ PHNs suggest health-oriented goals but ultimately work within the structure of each setting to accomplish goals that are mutually determined or sometimes rejected. | Talk with your preceptors about the challenges they have confronted. |
| Seeks consultation and support | ▪ It is essential to seek consultation and support in a practice area where role models are often not physically present.<br>▪ PHNs use technology to access resources and expertise when additional information is needed. | By reflecting on your experiences with expert practitioners, you can validate your thinking and actions and learn about more effective approaches to your work. |
| Takes initiative; is a self-starter | ▪ PHNs are responsible for organizing their own schedules.<br>▪ Many activities in public health nursing involve long-term planning, especially when building partnerships and coalitions that focus on community and systems changes. | As you are learning the skills needed for public health nursing practice, you can be proactive in identifying ways to prepare for clinical experiences. Do you need to do background reading? Do you need to identify specific objectives to guide your preparation? Which questions do you need to ask? |

| Skill | Strategies and Considerations | Your Leadership Action |
|---|---|---|
| Adapts to change | ■ The settings where people live, work, and learn undergo constant changes.<br><br>■ Adapting to change is a constant in public health nursing practice. | As someone new to public health nursing, you need to change your frame of thinking to a public health model in contrast to the medical model (see Chapter 7). |
| Is willing and able to respond to population needs | ■ Healthy People 2020 priorities are based on the most recently identified health goals for the United States (U.S. Department of Health and Human Services [U.S. DHHS], n.d.).<br><br>■ PHNs and local health departments must adapt to these changes if they are to be relevant in the interventions selected to improve population health. | Review the health data and health disparities data for your community. Ask your preceptor how the public health or community agency is responding to those needs. Identify a priority that you would like to work on as a student or volunteer in your community. |
| Demonstrates flexibility | ■ Flexibility is required in situations where families or coworkers oppose change.<br><br>■ Sometimes being flexible means being patient and waiting while encouraging others to make a change. | Compare your plan for the day and reflect on what actually occurred. Analyze how you were flexible in adapting to changes in your plan. |
| Contributes to team efforts | ■ PHNs need to cultivate skills that make them effective team leaders and team players.<br><br>■ Listening, being open, valuing the contributions of others, and identifying a common vision and goals are important when bringing others together to improve public health. | Many public health learning experiences include collaborating with your peers on a health promotion project for the community. Use this experience to work on your team-building skills. Take time to learn more about team members and different styles of working together. |
| Prioritizes and organizes workload, time, materials, and resources | ■ Public health nursing can be overwhelming because so many areas exist in which nurses could spend time and energy for improving population health.<br><br>■ PHNs use technology (e.g., cellphones, digital calendars) to organize their workloads and manage their time. | Learning time-management skills at the beginning of your public health nursing experience can serve you well. Make a plan for what you need to do, gather the information you need, work on prioritization, and seek needed resources. You can always modify your plan as you evaluate how well it is working. You can also share your plan with your preceptor or mentor, who can help you reflect on your organization and preparation for your learning experiences. |

The day-to-day work of the public health or community health agency needs to be accomplished. This means two things: carrying out the organization's mission and goals, and carrying out the organization's priority work. For staff nurses, that means managing their caseload of clients on a daily basis, setting priorities based on the changing needs of their clients, and being willing to take on tasks that need to be done. As you work with preceptors and expert nurses in the community, notice their leadership approaches and styles that meet the health needs of their clients as well as the needs of the organization.

## Activity

Review the activities, strategies, and actions in Table 14.3.

■ What skills do you consider your strengths? Choose two strengths and decide what strategies you might use to help you succeed in your public health nursing clinical.

■ Consider which nursing skills and strategies you might use to help achieve the mission and work of the public health/community health agency in which you are working.

■ What skills do you think you could strengthen during your clinical? Choose one skill to strengthen. What strategies might you use to help you do this?

# Challenges of Working in the Community

Working in the community is challenging because of the diversity, uncertainty, and constant change you experience in an environment that is not within your control. As one student said, "The patients aren't lined up nicely in their beds all in a row down the hall." In home settings, children are running around, animals abound, and the sounds of the television and people coming and going are often disconcerting. Older or disabled adults might like their slippery throw rugs on the floor and might want to have their favorite snacks available even though they are not on their prescribed diets. You might find homes without heat in the winter and homes without refrigerators in the summer. Some people live alone, and others live with myriad relatives and friends. You never know what to expect when you knock on the door. But you need to be ready for both the expected and the unexpected. The following student example demonstrates several leadership skills:

> During a home visit, a student was in the process of changing a catheter for a paraplegic man when the man's cat jumped on the bed. What was the student to do? Her sterile field was about to be compromised. She was wearing her only pair of sterile gloves, and her equipment was laid out on the bed. She thought for a moment. Then, very calmly, she asked the man whether he would hold his cat while she changed his catheter.

## Activity

- What leadership skills did this student nurse demonstrate?
- If you were the student in this situation, what might you do?
- What leadership skills would you use in this situation?

As you develop the ability to practice nursing in the community, whether in a home, school, clinic, faith-based organization, or other type of community agency, you are developing your leadership skill set.

# Achieving the Work of the Organization—Systems Level of Practice

The primary work of a public health organization is to improve the health status of the population. PHNs in formal leadership roles (e.g., team leaders, supervisors, managers, administrators) are responsible for achieving the work of the organization. Much of this work is done at a systems

level of public health practice. The aims of this work are to ensure a high level of care, to create supportive practice environments for nurses, and to build strong partnerships that achieve community health outcomes (Giddens, 2013). Staff nurses use their leadership skills as part of the team to achieve the work of the organization.

## Organizational Culture and Leadership

The leadership and culture of the organization in which the PHN works determine the support available for effective PHN practice. The culture of support for achieving public health nursing practice goals must permeate the entire organization, as demonstrated in Figure 14.2. Nurses at all levels within the organization must take responsibility for carrying out the work of public health nursing practice. Figure 14.2 illustrates who needs to provide leadership to shape and maintain a supportive organizational culture at all levels within a public health nursing agency. Evidence Example 14.2 identifies the organizational attributes that support public health nursing leadership and practice.

> *José makes a joint visit to Mr. and Mrs. Santos with the social worker. Margaret, his PHN preceptor, tells him that the directors of Public Health Nursing and Human Resources have made a renewed commitment for public health nursing and social work staff to work together in the Elders at Home Program. Joint visiting is encouraged. In preparation for that shared visit, José reviews the job description of the social worker and considers how his role as a public health nursing student is both similar to and different from the role of the social worker. He phones the social worker in advance of the visit to discuss how they might work together. During the visit, José and the social worker spend time evaluating the home environment of Mr. and Mrs. Santos and talking with the couple about their goals to live in place. Mr. and Mrs. Santos are committed to living in this home that they have worked so hard to purchase and maintain. It is obvious that home maintenance is poor. Stacks of old papers litter the house, they lack working smoke detectors, and they have minimal food stored in the cupboards or refrigerator. The kitchen sink is not draining properly, and the washer and dryer are not working. The social worker offers to help the couple apply for assistance for home repairs and for Meals on Wheels. José is glad he can share the care needs with the social worker. He believes they will be more effective in helping Mr. and Mrs. Santos by working as a team. After the visit, he asks his preceptor for feedback about the leadership skills he demonstrated as a member of the care team.*

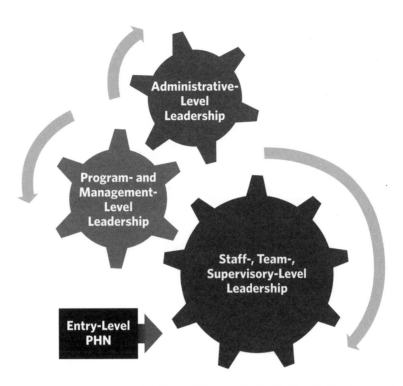

**FIGURE 14.2** Organizational Culture of Support for Public Health Nursing Practice

## EVIDENCE EXAMPLE 14.2

### Organizational Attributes That Support Public Health Nursing Practice

A Canadian study (Meagher-Stewart et al., 2010; Underwood et al., 2009) identified effective leadership as an organizational attribute that supports public health nursing practice. The study analyzed survey data from more than 13,000 community nurses across Canada and data from 23 focus groups of PHNs and policymakers. The organizational factors that were identified as requisite for effective public health nursing practice included government policy that supports public health, supportive organizational culture, and good management practices. Visionary and empowering leadership that permeated the organization facilitated the PHNs' ability to practice their full scope of competencies. These organizational attributes and leadership qualities empowered and motivated staff to be effective in their roles. Researchers concluded that it was essential for leadership to respect, trust, and value public health for PHNs to be effective.

Students can take the initiative to create their own leadership opportunities and share leadership with their peers. Evidence Example 14.3 on the next page demonstrates that when students worked together to plan and organize their nursing care, their shared leadership actions enhanced their ability to provide patient-centered care.

*José makes another joint visit with the social worker. They talk with Mr. and Mrs. Santos about their healthcare needs. Mr. Santos is on oxygen therapy. Mrs. Santos states that she knows her husband should stop smoking and that she turns off his oxygen when he does smoke. Mr. Santos cannot care for his personal needs. Mrs. Santos says that she is uncomfortable assisting him with hygiene and that he has not had a good bath or shower for several weeks. Mrs. Santos is becoming stressed and showing signs of depression. No one has contacted Mr. and Mrs. Santos about home maintenance. José decides he needs to prioritize their health needs. The social worker starts the application process for a home health aide to assist Mrs. Santos with Mr. Santos's personal needs. José is going to follow up on the home-maintenance referral and work with Mr. Santos on a safe smoking program. He will focus on Mrs. Santos's stress and possible depression on the next visit. José is excited to share with his fellow students what he has learned about his own leadership abilities and how he has been able to work with Mr. and Mrs. Santos and the social worker to help the Santoses stay independent in their own home.*

### EVIDENCE EXAMPLE 14.3

#### Shared Leadership Enhances Nursing Care in a Homeless Center

An example of how nursing students effectively practiced leadership occurred during a clinical at a homeless shelter. Public health nursing students conducted a monthly foot-care clinic from September through May. During a 3-hour clinic, six to eight students provided foot care to 20 to 45 clients. The instructor and homeless shelter staff oriented the students to the shelter and the foot-care clinic. Then the instructor turned the clinic over to the students to manage. The students determined how to arrange the clinic space, how to allocate the foot-care supplies, and who would carry out the different clinic roles (recruitment and registration of the clients; assigning the clients to students for their foot care; keeping each workspace stocked with supplies; providing hospitality; documenting client assessments and services provided; and following up with clients after they received care to make sure all their priority health needs were met). The instructor noticed that when she turned over the management of the clinic to the students, they were much more engaged and took more responsibility for the clinic and their clients. Every group of students organized its clinic a little differently. Each month, the shared responsibility, freedom to be creative and practice autonomously, and mutual contributions to team efforts led to a successful clinic. Because of their ability to prioritize what needed to be done and organize their workload effectively, students managed to take the time to provide a therapeutic encounter with each client who visited the clinic. As one man said, after he spent an hour with one of the students who listened patiently to his story, "This has been the best day of my life."

## Workload and Resource Management

To move the organization toward its vision, a PHN leader must effectively manage workloads and resources. Public health organizations rely on formal leaders to manage budgets, supplies, and performance. In a business sense, public health organizations require a variety of management activities to operate effectively (Baker & Baker, 2014). Because the business of a public health organization is service to its population, public health nursing leaders must make thoughtful, responsible decisions as they plan and direct various aspects of the organization's work. Figure 14.3 illustrates how the day-to-day work of formal PHN leaders impacts quality and ensures efficiency.

Although their duties differ from those of a formal leader, informal PHN leaders are just as vital to an organization's success. Staff and entry-level PHNs can use their leadership skills to effectively manage their workload and achieve the goals of the team. PHN leaders set the standard and role model for their peers of what it looks like to take initiative and to be proactive. They understand how their daily work impacts the mission of the organization and the overall health of the community that they serve. PHN leaders are skilled at time management, problem solving, communication, and relationship building. They regularly share their ideas and volunteer for collaborative projects outside of their regular job duties. These leaders bring a positive energy to the team, which contributes to a high level of morale.

> Each of us has a spark of life inside us and our highest endeavor ought to be to set off that spark in one another.
>
> –Florence Nightingale

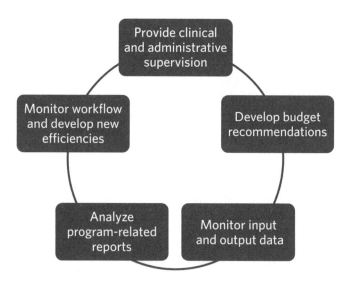

**FIGURE 14.3** Workload and Resource Management Responsibilities

## Measuring Outcomes of Population-Based Practice

The core public health function of assurance requires those working in governmental public health to evaluate the outcomes of programs and interventions (see Chapter 7). PHN leaders rely on meaningful data to demonstrate the positive outcomes of their interventions for individuals/families and communities. The Omaha System is a valuable tool for public health nursing practice to capture the correlation between PHN interventions and client outcomes (see Chapter 3). The Omaha System helps to create meaningful concepts for public health practice. Public health nursing leaders use knowledge-behavior-status (KBS) ratings to evaluate client and program outcomes. This is evidence that the PHN leader can use to leverage population health data (U.S. DHHS, 2016). By evaluating which interventions and targets caused the most effective changes for certain problems, PHN leaders can decide how to adjust practice to meet the anticipated outcomes. Use of the data also supports leveraging funding and policy support.

Reports that demonstrate the effectiveness of public health nursing interventions provide a rationale for continued or increased funding for public health nursing services.

## Strategies for Improving Quality in PHN Interventions

Ongoing evaluation and improvement of services provided by public health and other community agencies is carried out as part of the core public health function of assurance. Public health nursing staff and managers use the quality improvement process to meet this challenge. *Quality improvement* is defined as "the use of a deliberate and defined improvement process and the continuous ongoing effort to achieve measurable improvement in the efficiency, effectiveness, performance, accountability, outcomes, and other indicators of quality that improve the health of the community" (MDH, 2017a, para. 1).

Along with continuous program assessment and staff supervision, public health nursing leaders use this process to improve quality in PHN interventions. Evidence Example 14.5 describes how a local public health nursing agency utilizes the quality improvement processes.

---

### EVIDENCE EXAMPLE 14.4
**Health Literacy Outcomes**

A study of health literacy outcomes (Monsen et al., 2012) used Omaha System data to examine knowledge scores across problems over time. Monsen's team collected pre-intervention and post-intervention KBS (knowledge-behavior-status) scores by traditional racial categories. Their findings showed significant inequities across race categories in pre-intervention knowledge ratings. However, the post-intervention KBS ratings improved for all race categories and, in fact, their ratings began to parallel one another. Racial disparities decreased post-intervention, and all races saw a marked increase in their KBS outcomes. The targeted intervention worked to increase KBS outcomes and promoted health equity.

---

### EVIDENCE EXAMPLE 14.5
**Dakota County Family Health Practice Advisory Committee**

The Family Health Practice Advisory Committee is a quality assurance committee for the family health unit at the Dakota County Public Health Department. The committee is composed of PHNs with varying levels of experience and is facilitated by the unit coordinator. The main responsibility of the committee is to ensure the implementation of evidence-based practice in family home visiting. The committee utilizes the nursing process and a continuous quality improvement approach for projects, literature reviews, case consultation, chart audits, and continuing education for PHNs. PHNs on this committee act as evidence champions when changes to practice are implemented. This advisory committee ensures that the unit is in compliance with targeted state and federal benchmarks for family home visiting programs. The work of this committee has resulted in improved quality in PHN interventions.

One project this committee worked on was the implementation of a Sexually Transmitted Infection (STI) assessment for the Family Home Visiting program. For this project, the identified problem was that the PHNs did not currently have a standardized STI assessment form, although they were working with a population known to be at-risk for STIs. The committee used evidence from the Minnesota Department of Health and the Centers for Disease Control and Prevention to develop and implement a standardized assessment and teaching kit. The assessment included basic screening questions to ask clients as a part of the nursing assessment, and the kit included information on low-cost testing clinics, a laminated sexual health exposure chart, educational pamphlets, and STI testing recommendations. The committee held an in-person training for all staff prior to implementation, which included presentations by a local epidemiologist and a nurse practitioner. Each PHN received an assessment kit at the training. The initial evaluation of this project showed that 90% of the clients who were screened using the new assessment form had at least one risk factor, indicating that they were at-risk and required follow-up testing for STIs. The Family Home Visiting program continues to use the assessment and evaluate the data.

*Source:* Karsten, 2017

# Maximizing Benefits to Clients and Stakeholders

Public health organizations are the guardians of available community health resources. Both fiscal and human resources are finite. It is important to manage resources in a way that benefits the public as a whole while not disadvantaging those who are most in need of assistance. Public health organizations rely on nursing leaders to develop and implement creative approaches that maximize benefits to clients and stakeholders and ensure health equity for all (U.S. DHHS, 2016). Recipients, or customers, of PHN interventions include direct clients, as well as stakeholders in the community. Public health organizations are continually challenged to respond to the question, *what do our customers need from us?* Population health models suggest that investments in prevention efforts are highly likely to have a substantial impact on improving a community's health. Increased spending on traditional medical services does not appear to have the same level of impact on overall population health. Rather, interventions that have a broad reach across populations have the potential to improve quality of life for community residents (National Home Visiting Resource Center [NHVRC], 2017).

# Shared Leadership Through Collaboration

Today's healthcare system requires nurses to work with others to meet the goal of improving population health. The definition of public health, what nurses do *together* as a society to ensure the conditions in which everyone can be healthy, reinforces the importance of PHNs working collaboratively

---

### EVIDENCE EXAMPLE 14.6

**Family Home Visiting Return on Investment**

Public health programs such as home visiting have yielded a strong return on investment over the years. Numerous studies have shown that the cost-effectiveness of home visiting yields $3.75 on average for every dollar invested (NHVRC, 2017). Outcomes of home visiting programs include a reduction in the number of childhood emergency room visits, early identification of developmental and social-emotional delays in children, higher employment rates and tax revenues, and reduced dependence on welfare programs. These improvements in child health and well-being and parental self-sufficiency demonstrate how public health services maximize benefits not only to individuals, but to entire communities.

---

(see Chapter 8) to achieve the goals of public health (Committee on Assuring the Health of the Public, 2003; Institute of Medicine, 1988). Creative, cost-saving solutions to population health concerns can result from interprofessional collaboration (Giddens, 2013). This collaboration is especially important in public health nursing practice. PHNs work regularly with their clients, team members, interprofessional colleagues, and various members of the community. This collaborative practice is a form of shared leadership.

Collaboration also occurs between the PHN and the client at the individual/family level of practice. This form of collaboration is part of case management, in which the PHN works to optimize the self-care capacities of the client and empower the client to make positive, healthy decisions (MDH, 2001). The PHN must be flexible and comfortable working in the unstructured environment of the client's home to share leadership and collaborate with the client in making decisions.

> *José makes another visit to Mr. and Mrs. Santos. He notices that Mr. Santos is still smoking in the same room as his oxygen tank. José is concerned about the safety issues and the possible neglect of a vulnerable adult. He wants to honor the couple's independence and wishes but understands that his professional responsibility requires him to report the potential for harm to this vulnerable adult. José consults with Margaret, his preceptor. She says she will make a joint visit with José the next day to determine whether there is anything else they can do. During the visit the next day, José observes Margaret's approach to Mr. Santos. Margaret and Mr. and Mrs. Santos set up a smoking schedule for Mr. Santos that allows him to smoke while on the front porch. Mr. Santos will use his oxygen before and after each smoking session but not during it. José is impressed with Margaret's skill in working with Mr. Santos. He is going to use her technique during his next visit.*

Collaboration at the systems and community levels of practice occurs through strategic partnerships between two or more parties that use a structured approach to pursue agreed-upon goals. As PHNs work with the community both as client and partner, they share data collection, problem solving, planning, and evaluation in carrying out community assessment, setting priorities, and developing programs (see Chapters 3 and 8). The ability to develop and work in strategic partnerships has become more important in public health nursing practice. A growing expectation of public health practice and PHN leadership is the ability to influence others to achieve the public health goal of health equity (see Chapter 13). A 2016 Public Health 3.0 initiative speaks to this expectation (U.S. DHHS, 2016).

## EVIDENCE EXAMPLE 14.7

### Public Health 3.0

Public Health 3.0 (PH 3.0) refers to "a new era of enhanced and broadened public health practice that goes beyond traditional public department functions and programs" (U.S. DHHS, 2016, p. 11). Led by the U.S. Department of Health and Human Services, PH 3.0 emphasizes collaboration across public and private sectors in an effort to advance health equity. This initiative requires businesses, lawmakers, community leaders, and federal policymakers to incorporate health into all areas within their span of control. Collaboration with community partners and the involvement of multiple sectors is essential to the vision of PH 3.0, which is aimed at improving the social determinants of health. Strong public health leadership is necessary to develop and maintain cross-sector relationships because this interprofessional collaboration is the foundation for policy approaches that have the potential to affect large populations (U.S. DHHS, 2016). Throughout 2016, a series of regional listening sessions brought community leaders from the private and public sectors together to learn more about opportunities to improve and modernize public health. In October 2016, the Office of the Assistant Secretary for Health (OASH) issued a white paper titled *Public Health 3.0: A Call to Action to Create a 21st Century Public Health Infrastructure*. This white paper provides recommendations for advancing Public Health 3.0 (see Table 14.4).

**TABLE 14.4  Five Critical Leadership Dimensions in Enhanced Scope of Public Health Practice**

| Dimension | Scope |
|---|---|
| Strong leadership and workforce | ■ Think outside of the box to leverage data in communications within and outside the traditional health sector<br>■ Partner with educational institutions to build a strong public health workforce pipeline<br>■ Create opportunities for growth within the organization to maintain strong public health professionals already working in the field |
| Strategic partnerships | ■ Cultivate relationships and identify collective goals<br>■ Develop sustainable partnerships |
| Flexible and sustainable funding | ■ Advocate for flexible funding models that allow leaders to respond more rapidly to emerging community needs<br>■ Capture and document cost-savings attributable to public health efforts<br>■ Engage funders in shared goals and values |
| Timely and locally relevant data, metrics, and analytics | ■ Explore new types of data, including healthcare utilization trends, that paint a more complete picture of the community's strengths and challenges<br>■ Address data gaps and challenges by advocating for timely, sub-county, de-identified data that will quickly move evidence into action |
| Foundational infrastructure | ■ Develop a clear mission and values statement that guides the organization's strategic plan<br>■ Document processes for decision-making<br>■ Build interdisciplinary teams within the organization<br>■ Focus on equity and cultural competence |

*Source:* Based on U.S. DHHS, 2016

# Leadership at the Community Level of Practice

As leaders, PHNs aim to be change agents to reduce the social conditions that contribute to poor health (health disparities and inequity). Power to influence key stakeholders and decision-makers is gained through developing alliances (coalition building) with individuals and groups who have influential power. The PHN's ability to engage with communities and develop effective partnerships to address the priorities in the community is critical. Nurses have a long history of advocacy and coalition-building to improve the health of populations. Florence Nightingale made alliances with politicians, journalists, philosophers, scientists, and influential thinkers and writers who contributed to her understanding of the public health issues of her time, but also helped her bring about change for improving the health

of populations (Falk-Rafael, 2005). PHNs need to move from behind the scenes to put forward strategies that can make a difference for the health of populations. This means increasing their knowledge and skills to transform the environments where they live, learn, work, and play into settings that foster good health through public health interventions and public policy (French, 2009).

Taking the initiative to improve health by reducing risk factors that contribute to chronic disease demonstrates nursing leadership. Evidence Example 14.8 in the school environment outlines leadership interventions that PHNs can use to create good health by decreasing obesity rates and reducing tobacco use and exposure, both major contributing factors to chronic diseases and rising healthcare costs (MDH, 2017b).

PHNs can bring about change through initiating public discussion and building awareness of proven strategies to promote healthy eating and physical activity. Actions include putting chronic disease prevention on the agenda of professional organizations and using the media to increase awareness. PHNs can use the data from their monitoring activities to inform other professionals, organizations, and the public about how the lack of access to healthy food and physical activity contributes to health disparities and inequities. Partnership skills for collective action (see Chapter 8) are essential in bringing about change through advocacy action.

Although PHNs can identify and study the impact of health determinants, they cannot solve such problems as poverty, housing, unemployment, and unsafe environments. PHNs can, however, call attention to these problems and get them on the policy agenda and into the public discourse. PHNs can also study the causes and results of these health determinants and examine the effectiveness of social and collective responses to these problems. They can help mobilize public will and coordinate actions of the public and private healthcare, education, and business sectors. Leading successful change in communities involves many different strategies (Hill, 2008; Nissen, Merrigan, & Kraft, 2005). Examples of such strategies are outlined in Table 14.5.

## EVIDENCE EXAMPLE 14.8

### Statewide Health Improvement Partnership (SHIP) in Action Working to Create Good Health

The SHIP program uses evidence-based strategies based on the latest science, compiled by the Minnesota Department of Health (MDH) in collaboration with local public health (MDH, 2017b). Local public health staff, including PHNs, are involved in working with communities to choose strategies that address local needs. The community-led improvements have resulted in healthy eating, physical activity, and reduced commercial tobacco use. One successful component of SHIP in Dakota County, Minnesota, has been working with schools to create healthier food environments (Dakota County Public Health, 2017). This partnership, called Smart Choices, has engaged schools with the highest rates of students receiving free and reduced-price lunch (a measure of poverty). Currently, 32 schools across 6 districts are involved in Smart Choices. Public health provided startup funds to schools to support projects that are sustainable and impact school policies or practices. Changes to systems or policies are important to reach all children regardless of race, income, or other factors. Partner school districts have made multiple successful changes to their food environments. For example, during a visit to a school, public health staff observed that most students in the lunch room had water bottles. A senior at the school commented that they could remember when the food and drink options weren't nearly as healthy, and they were glad that incoming freshman would never know a time when the water wasn't the norm. Other successes include establishing district-wide farm-to-school infrastructure, including salad bars, water-only vending options, and district-wide treat-free classroom birthday celebration policies (MDH, 2017b).

 **Healthy People** **2020** **healthypeople.gov** Immunization rates across the life span are highlighted in Healthy People 2020 Topics and Objectives (https://www.healthypeople. gov/2020/topics-objectives). Click the National Snapshots tab under the topic "Immunization and Infectious Diseases" to find the proportion of children in your state who have been immunized for measles, mumps, rubella, hepatitis B, and pneumonia. Which vaccination rate is of most concern to you? Click the Interventions & Resources tab to find evidence-based information and recommendations for best practices for immunizations. Which intervention would you like to see implemented in your community to increase immunization rates? Which leadership strategies might you use to convince elected officials to fund this intervention to increase the immunization rate in your community?

The leadership skill of being willing and able to respond to population needs is extremely important. PHNs often refer to this as having a passion for public health. Taking the initiative to advocate for and to participate in the process of social change to improve the health status of vulnerable populations requires a passionate commitment to the health of the public. Evidence Example 14.9 illustrates the complex mix of leadership skills required to improve the health status of vulnerable populations.

PHNs can bring about social change through initiating public discussion on the effects of poverty and the contribution of policy decisions to reduce poverty. Actions include putting poverty on the agenda of professional organizations and using the media to increase awareness. Working with the community as your client, just as working with individuals and families, requires a mutual egalitarian approach as you share data collection, problem solving, planning, and evaluation with community members. See Chapter 8 for examples of PHNs collaborating with communities, and note in Chapter 3 how they work with community members in carrying out a community assessment. Taking leadership in working toward social change involves skills in shared leadership strategies.

## TABLE 14.5 Leadership Strategies for Successful Community Change

- Define the roles and responsibilities for stakeholders involved in leading the change.
- Seek input from all who will experience the change.
- Be present "at the table." As Hill says, "Interpersonal and political skills and personal presence are essential during periods of change" (Hill, 2008, p. 460).
- Look for traditional as well as nontraditional partners, including funding sources.
- Consider the big picture.
- Collaborate with others to create a positive vision of the future, and choose strategies to work toward that vision.
- Remember that leadership is about relationships every day.
- Engage in self-examination and self-correction.
- Consistently integrate evidence-based approaches.
- Be hopeful but realistic when planning change.

*Sources:* Hill, 2008; Nissen et al., 2005

## EVIDENCE EXAMPLE 14.9
### Bringing About Social Change to Reduce Child Poverty

Cohen and Reutter (2007) reviewed literature from Canada, the United States, and the United Kingdom as well as the professional standards and competencies for nursing practice in Canada. Based on their review, the authors recommend using Blackburn's (1992) framework for working with families living in poverty. Blackburn conceptualizes three broad roles, which can be carried out at all levels of practice:

- **Monitoring:** Collecting and analyzing information to determine the impact of poverty on families
- **Alleviating and preventing:** Helping families avoid, reduce, and counteract the impact of poverty
- **Bringing about social change:** Working with organizations and the government to create policies that reduce or eliminate poverty

---

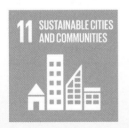 **SUSTAINABLE DEVELOPMENT GOALS**

**Public-Private Partnership in the Health Sector**

**GOAL 11** At the global level, private public partnerships (PPP) have been encouraged to achieve specific national healthcare goals in countries where there is a mismatch between demand for and supply of healthcare services. The Chiranjeevi Yojana Scheme in Gujarat, India, was initiated in 2005 when the government realized it did not have the resources to provide necessary emergency and routine obstetrical care to its population due to lack of medical providers and emergency hospital care. Its goals were to: reduce the maternal mortality ratio from 389/100,000 to 100/100,000 live births, reduce total fertility rate from 3.0 to 2.1, and reduce the infant mortality rate from 53/1,000 to 30/1,000 live births by 2010. The assumption for the PPP is that the private sector has experience and resources to provide quality and cost-effective services. The government operationalized this scheme to provide obstetrical care to nontaxpaying families, families below the poverty line, and tribal families. The District Health Service enrolled trust hospitals and private gynecologists and obstetricians to provide maternity services. The Maternal Mortality Rate in 2010 was 200/100,000 live births, so although that goal was not achieved, significant progress was made. Problems identified were lack of enrolled physicians providing care, high cost of care provided by private providers and hospitals, poor quality of care with some providers, and tendency to refer complex cases to the public hospitals. Several PPP models currently in use are working to balance existing resources, skills, and expertise and to reduce disparities between rich and poor by expanding access.

*Source:* Thadani, 2014

## Collaborative Leadership at the Community Level of Practice

Public health nurses are skilled at adapting to change and responding with flexibility and creativity when working with groups in the community. PHNs work collaboratively as leaders in two different ways (Work Group for Community Health and Development, University of Kansas, 2016):

■ *Collaborative leadership*: Leadership of a collaborative effort, such as a coalition or inter-agency task force, in which the leader guides and coordinates the group to solve a problem, create something new, or lead an initiative

■ *Leading collaboratively*: Leadership as a collaborative effort within a community organization in which leadership shifts to take advantage of different talents or abilities, or leadership is permanently shared by the entire group or members of the group

### Finding Common Ground

One of the most difficult challenges public health professionals experience is to build consensus in a community with groups who have diverse histories, values, and beliefs. A barrier to consensus-building or finding common ground is *dissensus,* which is demonstrated by community controversy, disagreement, and conflict. However, enduring change seldom occurs without the consensus of disparate groups. So PHNs take on the challenge by working within communities to form coalitions to achieve a common purpose. The process of consensus-building takes both commitment and persistence, as illustrated in Figure 14.4.

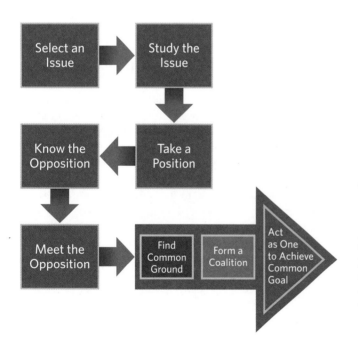

**FIGURE 14.4** Consensus-Building to Achieve a Common Goal

> *José has almost completed his public health nursing clinical. He is feeling like he has taken on leadership in working with Mr. and Mrs. Santos. He has a meeting with Margaret, his PHN preceptor, to review his leadership journey throughout the clinical experience. Margaret tells him that in her evaluation of his leadership competencies, he has shown initiative in taking on challenges and responsibilities and has become more flexible in accepting Mr. and Mrs. Santos's independence in deciding on their own healthcare and lifestyle. She tells him that he has demonstrated collaborative leadership in working with her and the social worker. Margaret asks José if he wants to go to a community meeting where a group of PHNs, social workers, faith community leaders, and members of the business community are considering forming a coalition to influence legislators to fund more living-in-place programs for older adults. She would like him to support Mr. and Mrs. Santos in telling their story at the meeting. Margaret believes that storytelling will help the different members of the group find the common ground needed to form the coalition. José agrees. He is ready to work on strengthening his advocacy-based leadership.*

### Coalition Formation as Community and Civic Engagement

PHNs work in community and interprofessional coalitions to build capacity to meet the health and social needs of diverse community groups. These coalitions are part of community engagement. When public health nursing leaders work in coalitions to influence elected and appointed officials and key community decision-makers, they are participating in civic engagement or the political process. See Chapter 13 for a discussion of civic engagement. Evidence Example 14.10 demonstrates the long-term commitment of a public health department and collaborative leadership to work with partners at a state-wide level to influence policy development, a core function of public health.

### Ethical Considerations

In addition to considering the impact of decisions on the health of individuals, families, communities, and systems, public health nursing leaders must consider how decisions affect PHNs and other public health staff. Nursing leaders can apply ethical perspectives to guide decisions that affect their teamwork and leadership activities (see Table 14.6).

## EVIDENCE EXAMPLE 14.10
### Tobacco Prevention Program

Haley Thorson, the PHN Tobacco Prevention Coordinator, recounted the activities of the Grand Forks Public Health Department in Grand Forks, North Dakota, as a statewide leader in tobacco prevention since the early 1990s.

The public health nurses have led the tobacco prevention efforts in Grand Forks for nearly three decades. The nurses working in the Tobacco Prevention Program have focused primarily on evidence-based policy changes recommended by the Centers for Disease Control (CDC, 2014) to shift the social and cultural norms related to tobacco use. When this norm changes, it is realized in reductions of tobacco use rates among youth and adults within the community. Specifically, in 2010, the tobacco prevention nursing staff led a local coalition who collaborated with key partners in the community to strengthen the local smoke-free law, removing exemptions that left several pockets of the workforce unprotected from exposure to secondhand smoke. In the months prior, the nurses utilized relationship-building skills to cultivate both a champion on the city council and a well-known champion within the medical community. With past tobacco-related policy initiatives taking controversial tones, the nurses decided that a community-wide assessment of attitudes, awareness, and perceptions surrounding the policy change would be important.

A collaboration with the University of North Dakota's research department led to the conduction of the Grand Forks Secondhand Smoke Study (Social Science Research Institute-University of North Dakota, 2010), which validated the community support for a secondhand smoke policy. The nurses' connectedness and respect in the community led to relationships with unconventional partners such as the Convention and Visitor's Bureau and the Chamber of Commerce. These connections were instrumental in sharing messages to calm unsubstantiated financial fears related to the policy change within the business community. These newfound partnerships in combination with focused, on-point health messaging led to the successful passage of the proposed changes to the local smoke-free law. In an effort to evaluate the effectiveness of the new law, the public health nurses collaborated on several key pieces of research, including an indoor air quality study (Travers & Vogl, 2011), a community impact study (Social Science Research Institute-University of North Dakota, 2012), and a study on the economic impact of the policy change (Goenner, 2013). These data were instrumental in building the evidence base to assist additional communities across the state in passing similar policies and eventually a comprehensive statewide law in 2012.

*Source:* Thorson, 2017

## TABLE 14.6  Ethical Action in Public Health Nursing Leadership

| Ethical Perspective | Application |
|---|---|
| Rule ethics (principles) | ▪ Make leadership decisions that promote good and prevent harm to families, communities, organizations, and public health workers.<br>▪ Consider which leadership actions promote social justice in the community and among public health staff members.<br>▪ Use advocacy-based leadership to improve population health at the individual/family and community levels of practice. |
| Virtue ethics (character) | ▪ Be conscious of the needs of others, moving from the "I" to the "we" perspective.<br>▪ Use your authentic leadership styles based on your beliefs, values, ethical standards, and convictions.<br>▪ Be a leader who establishes caring relationships as a foundation for leadership actions.<br>▪ Be a leader who values both the success of the organization and the well-being of public health staff members.<br>▪ Value the contributions of all team members. |
| Feminist ethics (reducing oppression) | ▪ Identify the moral and ethical leadership challenges related to population health and health disparities.<br>▪ Be inclusive in the decision-making process within the community. Include all population groups that will receive services.<br>▪ Use a team approach versus a hierarchical approach to prioritizing public health strategies.<br>▪ Use a shared leadership approach to be an effective team member within the interprofessional public health team and within the community.<br>▪ Use an advocacy-based leadership approach to empower communities to take charge of and manage their own healthcare needs. |

Table based on work by Racher, 2007 and Volbrecht, 2002

## KEY POINTS

- Providing leadership at all three levels of public health nursing practice—individual/family, community, and system—is a professional expectation of nurses who work in public health.

- Students and professional nurses are on leadership journeys that will continue throughout their nursing careers. Leadership approaches that are particularly relevant to public health nursing practice include advocacy-based leadership, authentic leadership, and shared leadership.

- Students and new graduates demonstrate entry-level leadership skills in public health by their ability to seek learning opportunities; work independently and autonomously; work in unstructured environments and tolerate ambiguity; contribute to team efforts; prioritize,

organize, and complete assigned workloads; seek consultation and support; take initiative and be self-starters; be flexible and adapt to change; and respond to population needs.

- PHNs use many of the interventions from the Public Health Intervention Wheel (see Chapter 2) to carry out leadership activities.

- PHNs are able to be effective leaders when they are supported by a shared leadership culture that permeates all levels of the organization.

- PHNs are expected to advocate for improvement in population health and to reduce health disparities by working collaboratively with interprofessional and community groups.

## REFLECTIVE PRACTICE

Think about the imperative that PHNs are expected to provide leadership to improve the health status of individuals, families, and communities. Think about how you might respond to an unexpected situation that might prompt you to take the *lead* in resolving a healthcare concern in the community. How might you respond to the leadership challenge in the following scenario?

During a staff meeting, several PHNs in a health department shared their concerns about new moms dealing with postpartum depression and the lack of a postpartum depression support group in the county. Working with their supervisor, the PHNs discovered that a hospital bordering the county did have an active postpartum support group/program. Through several meetings and discussion of the needs that could be met and roles that each could provide, a partnership was established. The hospital agreed to provide staff with the expertise to facilitate the support group at no cost,

and the PHNs were able to make space and childcare available at no cost, as well as do outreach and advertise this new program. Through these PHNs' leadership, the postpartum support group was established and continues to be successful in reaching many new moms who benefit from the encouragement and support provided during the group meetings.

Consider the following questions:

- What was the leadership challenge in this situation?
- Which ethical principles might be used to resolve this leadership challenge?
- How did the PHNs demonstrate advocacy-based and authentic leadership?
- Which leadership skills did the PHNs demonstrate?
- Which levels of practice did PHNs use in planning and implementing nursing interventions?

## APPLICATION OF EVIDENCE

1. Which examples of public health nursing leadership have you observed at the individual, community, and systems levels when working with PHNs during your clinical experience?

2. Identify three leadership skills you have read about in this chapter that you have observed during your public health clinical.

3. Give an example of how a PHN has used advocacy-based leadership to improve the health of an individual/family or community during your public health nursing clinical.

4. Give an example of a PHN who has used authentic leadership to carry out the mission and the work of the public health agency.

# References

American Nurses Association. (2013). *Public health nursing: Scope and standards of practice.* Silver Springs, MD: Author.

Avolio, B. J., Walumbwa, F. O., & Weber, T. J. (2009). Leadership: Current theories, research, and future directions. *Annual Review of Psychology, 60,* 421–449.

Baker, J. J., & Baker, R. W. (2014). *Health care finance: Basic tools for nonfinancial managers* (4th ed.). Burlington, MA: Jones & Bartlett Learning.

Blackburn, C. (1992). *Improving health and welfare work with families in poverty: A handbook.* Buckingham, UK: Open University Press.

Centers for Disease Control and Prevention. (2014). *Best practices for comprehensive tobacco prevention and control programs.* Atlanta, GA: U.S. Department of Health and Human Services, Centers for Disease Control and Prevention, National Center for Chronic Disease Prevention and Health Promotion, Office on Smoking and Health.

Cohen, B. E., & Reutter, L. (2007). Development of the role of public health nurses in addressing child and family poverty: A framework for action. *Journal of Advanced Nursing, 60*(1), 96–107.

Committee on Assuring the Health of the Public. (2003). *The future of the public's health in the 21st century.* Institute of Medicine. Washington, DC: National Academies Press. Retrieved from https://www.nap.edu/read/10548/chapter/1

Dakota County Public Health. (2004). *Dakota County clinical menu, modified from Henry Street Consortium clinical menu.* West St. Paul, MN: Author.

Dakota County Public Health. (2017). *Building a healthier Dakota County – SHIP progress report, January 2017.* West St. Paul, MN: Author.

Falk-Rafael, A. (2005). Speaking truth to power: Nursing's legacy and moral imperative. *Advances in Nursing Science, 28*(3), 212–223.

French, M. (April 2009). *Shifting the course of our nation's health: Prevention and wellness as national policy.* American Public Health Association issue brief. Retrieved from https://www.apha.org/~/media/files/pdf/factsheets/finalpreventionpolicy.ashx

George, B., & Sims, P. (2007). *True north—Discover your authentic leadership.* Hoboken, NJ: Jossey-Bass/Wiley.

Giddens, J. F. (2013). *Concepts for nursing practice.* St. Louis, MO: Mosby.

Goenner, C. F. (2013). *The impact of tobacco legislation on economic activity in the city of Grand Forks, North Dakota.* University of North Dakota Business and Public Administration. Retrieved from http://ndeconomist.com/papers/misc/Goenner_Tobacco_2012.pdf

Henry Street Consortium. (2004). *The Henry Street Consortium clinical menu.* St. Paul, MN: Author. Retrieved from http://www.health.state.mn.us/divs/opi/cd/phn/docs/0405henryst_clinicalmenu.pdf

Henry Street Consortium. (2017). *Entry-level population-based public health nursing competencies.* St. Paul, MN: Author. Retrieved from www.henrystreetconsortium.org

Hill, K. S. (2008). Leading change: The creativity of a public health nurse leader. *Journal of Nursing Administration, 38*(11), 459–460.

Institute of Medicine. (1988). *The future of public health.* Washington, DC: National Academies Press.

Kalb, K. B., Cherry, N. M., Kauzloric, J., Brender, A., Green, K., Miyagawa, L., … Shinoda-Mettler, A. (2006). A competency-based approach to public health nursing performance appraisal. *Public Health Nursing, 29*(3), 115–138.

Karsten, E. (2017). *Case study: Dakota County Family Health Practice Advisory Committee.* Unpublished manuscript. Apple Valley, MN: Dakota County Public Health.

Kouzes, J. M., & Posner, B. Z. (2007). *The leadership challenge* (4th ed.). San Francisco, CA: Jossey Bass/John Wiley & Sons.

Meagher-Stewart, D., Underwood, J., MacDonald, M., Schoenfeld, B., Blythe, J., Knibbs, K., … Crea, M. (2010). Organizational attributes that assure optimal utilization of public health nurses. *Public Health Nursing, 27*(5), 433–441.

Minnesota Department of Health. (2001). *Public health interventions: Applications for nursing practice.* St. Paul, MN: Author. Retrieved from http://www.health.state.mn.us/divs/opi/cd/phn/wheel.html

Minnesota Department of Health. (2017a). Quality improvement and performance management. St. Paul, MN: Author. Retrieved from http://www.health.state.mn.us/qi/

Minnesota Department of Health. (2017b). *Statewide Health Improvement Partnership fact sheet.* Office of Statewide Health Improvement Initiatives. St. Paul, MN: Author. Retrieved from https://www.co.dakota.mn.us/Government/publiccommittees/SHIP

Monsen, K. A., Areba, E. M., Radosevich, D. M., Brandt, J. K., Lytton, A. B., Kerr, M. J., … Martin, K. S. (2012). Evaluating effects of public health nurse home visiting on health literacy for immigrants and refugees using standardized nursing terminology data. In P. Abbott & C. Hullin (Eds.), *NI 2012: Advancing global health through informatics. Proceedings of the 11th International Congress on Nursing Informatics.*

Morrison, R. S., Jones, L., & Fuller, B. (1997). The relation between leadership style and empowerment on job satisfaction of nurses. *Journal of Nursing Administration, 27*(5), 27–34.

Murphy, L. G. (2012). Authentic leadership—Becoming and remaining an authentic nurse leader. *Journal of Nursing Administration, 42*(11), 507–512.

National Home Visiting Resource Center. (2017). *2017 home visiting yearbook.* Retrieved from https://www.nhvrc.org/wp-content/uploads/NHVRC_Yearbook_2017_Final.pdf

Nissen, L. B., Merrigan, D. M., & Kraft, M. K. (2005). Moving mountains together: Strategic community leadership and systems change. *Child Welfare, 84*(2), 123–140.

Quad Council of Public Health Nursing Organizations. (2011). *The Quad Council competencies for public health nurses.* Retrieved from http://www.achne.org/files/Quad%20Council/QuadCouncilCompetenciesforPublicHealthNurses.pdf

Racher, F. (2007). The evolution of ethics for community practice. *Journal of Community Health Nursing, 24*(1), 65–76.

Social Science Research Institute-University of North Dakota. (2010). *Grand Forks secondhand smoke study.* Grand Forks, ND: Author.

Social Science Research Institute-University of North Dakota. (2012). *Comprehensive smoke-free ordinance community impact study.* Grand Forks, ND: Author.

Thadani, K. B. (2014). Public private partnership in the health sector: Boon or bane. *Procedia – Social and Behavioral Sciences, 157,* 307–316. Retrieved from https://ac.els-cdn.com/S1877042814058534/1-s2.0-S1877042814058534-main.pdf?_tid=420af4be-bf8e-11e7-b480-00000aacb361&acdnat=1509600517_16b4a026ae2ae1b08ce163757d3eabde

Thorson, H. (2017). *Tobacco prevention program.* Unpublished manuscript. Grand Forks, ND: Grand Forks Public Health Department.

Travers, M. J., & Vogl, L. (2011). *Grand Forks, North Dakota air quality monitoring study.* Buffalo, NY: Roswell Park Cancer Institute.

Underwood, J. M., Mowat, D. L., Meagher-Stewart, D. M., Deber, R. B., Baumann, A. O., MacDonald, M. B., … Munroe, V. J. (2009). Building community and public health nursing capacity: A synthesis report of the national community health nursing study. *Canadian Journal of Public Health, 100*(5), I-1–I-11.

U.S. Department of Health and Human Services. (n.d.). Healthy People 2020—About Healthy People. Retrieved from https://www.healthypeople.gov/2020/About-Healthy-People

U.S. Department of Health and Human Services. (2016). *Public health 3.0: A call to action to create a 21st century public health infrastructure.* Retrieved from https://www.healthypeople.gov/sites/default/files/Public-Health-3.0-White-Paper.pdf

Volbrecht, R. M. (2002). *Nursing ethics: Communities in dialogue.* Upper Saddle River, NJ: Pearson Prentice Hall.

Watson, J. (2008). *Nursing: The philosophy and science of caring* (Rev. ed.). Boulder, CO: University Press of Colorado.

Williams, R. L., McDowell, J. B., & Kautz, D. D. (2011). A caring leadership model for nursing's future. *International Journal of Human Caring, 15*(1), 31–35.

Wong, C. A., Spence Laschinger, H. K., & Cummings, G. G. (2010). Authentic leadership and nurses' voice behavior and perceptions of care equity. *Journal of Nursing Management, 18,* 889–900.

Work Group for Community Health and Development, University of Kansas. (2016). *Chapter 13: Section 11. Collaborative leadership.* Community Tool Box. Retrieved from http://ctb.ku.edu/en/table-of-contents/leadership/leadership-ideas/collaborative-leadership/main

# Putting It All Together: What It Means to Be a Public Health Nurse

■ **Marjorie A. Schaffer**
*with Patricia M. Schoon*

This is the beginning of your story as a public health nurse (PHN). The chapters in this book have given you a foundation in the Henry Street Consortium entry-level population-based public health nursing competencies, which emphasize the knowledge, skills, and attitudes needed to be an effective PHN. What are your next steps for developing your expertise in public health nursing?

## What Do You Need to Know?

When PHNs and educators created the Henry Street Consortium competencies, they also generated a basic public health nursing knowledge base to serve as a foundation for public health nursing practice. In smaller local health departments, PHNs need a broader knowledge base so that they are competent to provide services in many areas of public health. In larger public health agencies, PHNs might need more in-depth knowledge and expertise in specific areas of public health, such as following up on a population with drug-resistant tuberculosis or working with schools and community agencies to prevent teen pregnancy. Keep in mind that PHNs also work in many organizations other than official public health agencies, such as home-visiting nurse associations, schools, corporations that include occupational health positions, and nonprofit organizations that value and need the expertise of PHNs. Following is a list of basic public health nursing knowledge areas for population-based practice:

- Antepartum/postpartum
- Chemical health issues and behaviors
- Chronic disease prevention and management
- Death and dying
- Disaster and bioterrorism response
- Disease prevention and control
- Environmental health and safety
- Family development
- Family planning
- Health determinants
- Health informatics
- Health promotion for all ages
- Human growth and development
- Human sexuality
- Immunizations across the life span
- Injury prevention
- Medication administration/management
- Mental health
- Nutrition
- Parenting
- Social and market justice
- Technical nursing skills
- Violence prevention

Many nursing students worry about being knowledgeable in medication administration and technical nursing skills as they seek their first employment as a nurse. Nurses new to public health nursing might feel similarly less prepared in public health knowledge areas that are essential to successful public health nursing practice. Look carefully at your position description to determine whether you have an adequate knowledge base and skill set to perform the job responsibilities. Seek a mentor and establish a plan for strengthening your knowledge base and skill set. Consider volunteering for community-based health-related activities, such as the Medical Reserve Corps, to increase your exposure to public health and the needs of the community.

## Preparing for Population Health Practice

PHNs have provided public health nursing services for populations since Lillian Wald focused on the needs of the population surrounding the Henry Street Settlement in New York City in the 1890s (Kub, Kulbok, Miner, & Merrill, 2017). In 2014, the National Advisory Council on Nurse Education and Practice (NACNEP) Annual Report to Congress addressed new roles for nurses in population health management (2016). The report's Executive Summary states, "Healthcare organizations need nurses capable of gathering and analyzing population-level data, promoting wellness and disease prevention in the community, adopting and disseminating best practices for population health, and identifying patients who may benefit from greater outreach efforts to promote health screening and related primary care services" (p. 5).

In 2017, the Robert Wood Johnson Foundation published "Catalysts for Change: Harnessing the Power of Nurses to Build Population Health in the 21st Century," which summarized recommended population-focused competencies (Storfjell, Winslow, & Saunders, 2017). The competencies, recommended for all registered nurses, are based on a compilation of the literature; expert researchers, practitioners, and thought leaders; regional meetings on models of care, research findings, and policy implications; and a national consensus conference. The Henry Street Entry Level Population-Based Public Health Nursing Competencies are consistent with these recommended competencies (Table 15.1).

**Activity**

In the study by Schaffer, Keller, and Reckinger (2015), PHNs were asked what would be the greatest impact on their community if there were no public health nursing services. See Table 15.2 for examples of PHN comments.

Based on PHN comments, discuss how the health of populations would be affected if counties or cities reduced or eliminated public health nursing services.

PHNs are essential contributors to community health and well-being. They must continue to provide evidence about the outcomes of their work and become "visible" to policymakers who make decisions about public health funding. This means PHNs must advocate for themselves and their accomplishments as well as for services for the populations they serve.

Public health nurses have contributed to population health, well-being, and equity for over a century. Robert Wood Johnson Foundation Public Health Nurse Leaders (2017) identified 10 ways that PHNs improve health. Consider how PHNs impact populations in the following summary of how PHNs improve health through population health practice (see Table 15.3).

**TABLE 15.1 Recommendations for Key Population-Focused Nursing Competencies: Consistency With Henry Street Competencies**

| Population-Focused Nursing Competency | Henry Street Model Competency |
|---|---|
| Wholeness (whole-person & whole-community care) | Incorporates mental, physical, emotional, social, and spiritual aspects of health into assessment, planning, implementation, and evaluation |
| Coordination | Works within the responsibility and authority of the governmental public health system |
| Collaboration (teamwork/partnering) | Utilizes collaboration to achieve public health goals |
| Advocacy | Shows evidence of commitment to social justice, the greater good, and the public health principles |
| Communication | Effectively communicates with communities, systems, individuals, families, and colleagues |
| Assessment/Analysis | Applies the public health nursing process to communities, systems, individuals and families |
| Cultural competency/Diversity | Demonstrates nonjudgmental/unconditional acceptance of people different from self |
| Attention to determinants of health | Applies the public health nursing process to communities, systems, individuals, and families |
| Relationship-building | Establishes and maintains caring relationships with communities, systems, individuals, and families |
| Leadership | Demonstrates leadership in public health nursing with communities, systems, individuals, and families |

*Source:* Storfjell et al., 2017

**TABLE 15.2  PHNs' Perceptions of the Impact of No Public Health Nursing Services on the Community**

| Category | PHN Comments |
|---|---|
| Occurrence of disease and health problems | "I believe more children would be placed in increasingly violent or dangerous environments." |
| Lack of prevention accompanied by declining health in the community | "The biggest impact on the health of the community would be a much less healthy society." |
| Less care for vulnerable populations | "The most vulnerable among us would suffer immeasurably."<br><br>"The poor and vulnerable would go without primary/preventive care and would flood our emergency departments."<br><br>"Mentally ill and disabled clients that do not have health insurance would be wandering with nowhere to be treated." |
| Negative effects on public health infrastructure | "The high-risk individuals that are uninsured or underinsured would fall through the cracks of the system and would not have any resources for healthcare on any level, with the exception of the already overused and misused emergency room, for their healthcare." |
| Negative effects on local health department programs | "The impact would be devastating. While all aspects of public health are important, it is the nurse who pulls all the little pieces together. It is the nurse who looks at the big picture to ensure services are being received." |

*Source:* Schaffer et al., 2015

**TABLE 15.3  Ten Ways Public Health Nurses (PHNs) Improve Health**

| Strategy | Example |
|---|---|
| Prevent | PHNs work inside and outside clinic walls to prevent conditions such as obesity, diabetes, injuries, school absenteeism, infant mortality, and spread of communicable disease. |
| Educate | PHNs educate individuals, families, communities, and stakeholders about health behaviors, environments, and policies that make the healthy choice the easy choice. |
| Coordinate | PHNs coordinate and integrate care and services across the life span to improve individual and population health outcomes, improve health equity, and reduce costs. |
| Protect | PHNs protect people by educating about environmental hazards, preparing for emergencies, and mobilizing during disasters. |
| Lead | PHNs lead evidence-based quality practice and policy changes. They lead cross-sector and transdisciplinary collaborations that impact communities. |
| Promote | PHNs promote health equity and health as a shared value through individual and community engagement and inclusion. |
| Advocate | PHNs advocate for community assets that lead to healthier people such as safe and affordable housing, healthy school meals, tobacco prevention policies, safe places to walk and bike, access to healthy foods, appropriate behavioral health treatment services, violence prevention, and trauma-informed care. |
| Care | PHNs care for people, families, and communities. They understand the importance of culture, language, literacy, and how these shape health, well-being, and equity. |
| Integrate | PHNs recognize that health is a function of physical, mental, emotional, and spiritual well-being. They assist individuals and communities in integrating a variety of needed services through collaborating, mobilizing, and leading interdisciplinary teams, partners, and consumers. |
| Research | PHNs use research to inform their practice and do research to improve the health of individuals, families, and communities. |

*Source:* Robert Wood Johnson Foundation Public Health Nurse Leaders, 2017

## Who Do You Need to Be?

Henry Street Consortium members identified personal characteristics that contribute to effective public health nursing practice. The following characteristics are virtues that can enhance your ability to be successful and committed to public health nursing (Henry Street Consortium, 2017):

- Adaptability
- Caring
- Compassion
- Confidence
- Courage
- Creativity
- Flexibility
- Hard work
- Humor

- Independence
- Leadership qualities
- Lifelong-learning attitude
- Passion
- Persistence
- Positive attitude
- Resourcefulness
- Risk-taking
- Self-care

### Activity

Consider the following questions as you review the personal characteristics/virtues that enhance your public health nursing practice.

- Why are these characteristics important for effective public health nursing practice?
- Which of these characteristics have you observed in practicing PHNs? Give a specific example of how you see the characteristic exemplified in the practice of the expert PHN.
- How do you see these characteristics contributing to the accomplishment of the population-focused competencies identified in Table 15.1?
- How do you think your personal characteristics/virtues match with the kind of PHN you would like to be?

## What Can You Learn from the Stories of Nursing Students?

You can also learn about public health nursing strategies from the following stories of nursing students. The student stories represent the process and experiences encountered in becoming a PHN.

As you reflect on the meaning of the stories, think about how you are learning to be a PHN. Use the following questions to guide your reflections about the three student stories:

1. Which competencies is the student working on developing?

2. Which public health interventions are the student and preceptor using in this story?

3. Which Cornerstones of Public Health Nursing (see Chapter 1) is the student expressing?

4. What are the implications for population health practice for each story?

5. Which personal characteristics would it be helpful to have or develop to carry out this public health nursing practice example?

### Student Story #1

School children are a population at high risk for infection and transmitting infectious organisms. In terms of epidemiology, the "chain of infection" is the process by which pathogens are transmitted from the environment to a host, invade the host, and cause infection. Breaking the chain of infection at any point prevents the spread of infection. Hand-washing is the most effective mechanism to break the chain and prevent the spread of infection. With two of my classmates, I taught three sessions on hand-washing to first graders. A curriculum and resource program had provided us with a hand-washing kit that consisted of a 3-minute video of a young boy explaining and demonstrating how to correctly wash one's hands to remove as many germs as possible, several bottles of "GloGerm Potion" that makes invisible germs glow a bright white under a black light, a black light, and a bunch of "Germbusters!" stickers.

As each session began, we did a few minutes' worth of very basic health teaching about how germs can cause illness; are everywhere, especially on our hands; and by washing our hands well and often, we can prevent the spread of germs and stay healthy. After our short presentation, we helped the children practice correct hand-washing techniques with the GloGerm product. This gave me a nice chance to do some one-on-one teaching and interact with a few children who were somewhat timid or shy and see them respond positively and come out of their shell. The kids absolutely loved the presentation and our "magic potion"!

This experience shows growth in my ability to communicate effectively and work with others to complete a task. Good communication and organization were required between me and my classmates to work out our own teaching time to learn about the hand-washing kit, pick up and return the kit, and put together a good presentation. It was also necessary to communicate with first-graders and to understand child development to teach health concepts at their developmental level and not speak over their heads. I believe any one of us could have done the job alone, but it was much more enjoyable to share the work and be a part of a team than to do it alone. Being a team player is something I, a loner by nature, need to work on. I learned that I am likable and competent, work well with others, and really enjoy it, and I showed that I am responsible by carrying my share of this clinical assignment. This teaching experience was FUN and gave me more confidence in my nursing knowledge and teaching skills. In looking back, I see that I have become more spontaneous and flexible and can laugh more as I spend more time in real-world settings as opposed to the nursing lab or classroom. This experience of working with others and the necessity of good communication were most useful to me and will help me continue improving in those areas. This teaching experience will serve as a positive example in times when I feel less confident in my abilities.

*Source:* Senior Nursing Student

## Student Story #2

My preceptor and I went out to a home to carry out a developmental assessment on a two-year-old suspected of being developmentally delayed. My preceptor had a very friendly, informal, yet professional demeanor, which I believe is a very beneficial and important asset to have and develop; she explained what the assessment consisted of and the actions that would ensue following the assessment as well as the other areas of specialty services that might be involved. During the assessment, my preceptor was very warm and casual, but one could see that she was observing our young client very carefully. She observed him in a way that was not distressing to the mother. Afterward, my preceptor and I discussed the results and the process she uses when collecting and processing data within the realm of public health nursing. She stated that working within public health really exposes one in a community. For example, it is not uncommon to run into clients at the grocery store or in various other establishments around the area, and one has to face the questions, "Do I say hello? Do I ask how things are going? Do they recognize me?" I asked her how she deals with these simple, yet complex questions. She remarked that a nurse needs to be very sensitive and prepared for these issues: "We are in their lives and homes and must be respectful." She stated that she leaves it up to the clients to make the initial contact and allows them to lead the direction of the conversation. She also made it clear how important confidentiality is, because at times a PHN visits one family member and the other members are unaware, so even confidentiality within families is instituted and mandated by HIPAA [Health Insurance Portability and Accountability Act].

I became more aware of the importance of having guidelines, such as the Nurse Practice Act, to help us provide effective and competent care. My preceptor was an excellent example and resource to whom I can look back and reflect when I begin my career as a nurse. The Nurse Practice Act encompasses nurses in all fields; however, the means by which it is carried out is customized to each specialty field. For example, independent nursing functions, in reference to public health nursing, differ from delegated medical functions that nurses carry out in hospitals. Independent functions consist of educating, teaching, and providing information to clients and not performing skilled nursing care, such as caring for wounds or giving injections that would be done in the hospital. Also, boundaries are harder to manage in public health nursing than within the hospital. It is the client who "runs the show" and is in charge, not the nurse; one must be extra cautious when exchanging information in the field. I feel I will be more adequately prepared and aware of when and how to set boundaries and how to deal with a situation where I might not want to reveal as much to clients as they might want or expect.

*Source:* Senior Nursing Student

## Student Story #3

I worked with my preceptor in a breast and cervical cancer screening program. Part of the screening consisted of checking total (fasting) cholesterol and blood glucose levels. I did a finger stick to draw up a drop of blood into a little plastic case that fit into a machine that would give us the cholesterol and glucose results in about 5 minutes. After we had the results, I entered the data into a computer program created by the Centers for Disease Control and Prevention (CDC) that analyzes and creates a bar graph and written description of the results that are very easy for the average nonmedical person to understand and learn from. It also generates a "Diagnostic Referral" form if any test result is too high. This form can then be faxed to a healthcare provider immediately, with no other data needing to be added. When I had printed out the report, I went over it in great detail with my client, asking her to stop me if she needed additional clarification or had any other questions. She was able to verbalize a general understanding of her results. The computer program had created a referral form for her to be evaluated by a physician because of high cholesterol, and she requested that my preceptor set up an appointment for her. My preceptor will follow up with the woman in two weeks to find out whether she has kept the doctor appointment and whether she wants to participate in the lifestyle interventions and counseling services that are also offered at the clinic.

I learned how to use new-to-me technology in both the blood testing and data entry experiences, and I learned so much about the community resources available for this (my) age group. More important to my nursing practice was the review of cholesterol and glucose normal values and the opportunity to do some teaching with my client, in which I had to use good communication and listening skills to facilitate her learning. I noticed afterward that I had picked up some of my preceptor's mannerisms in talking with clients—nonverbal communication skills, such as leaning forward toward the client. I also learned that I often get in a rush when I am talking about something I understand but the person I am talking to does not and that I need to slow down. I have become more aware of my interpersonal behaviors, and this will help make me a better nurse in the future.

*Source:* Senior Nursing Student

**TABLE 15.4  Telling Your Story**

| Focus | Questions |
|-------|-----------|
| Who? | Who are the people in the story? What are their environments? What does each person want? |
| Ouch! | What are the obstacles that stand in the way of accomplishing the want or goal? What are the internal and external factors that cause difficulty, distress, or concern? |
| What? | What is the truth about the situation/experience that impacts relationships and connections to resources, needed services, and actions? |
| Why? | Why is each person in the story making the choices he or she is making? Why are the obstacles making it difficult to accomplish the goal? |
| So? | What is the emotional effect on people in the story and the reader? What is the meaning? Why should we care? |

*Source: Adapted from Klein, 2016, pp. 46–47*

### Activity

From your clinical learning experiences in public health nursing, select an experience and write your own story. Reflect on the competencies, public health nursing interventions, and Cornerstones of Public Health Nursing (see Chapter 1) represented in your story. Identify additional knowledge areas and skills that you will need to develop as you work toward expertise in public health nursing.

Table 15.4 provides questions you can use to develop your story. The story does not need to follow the order of the questions. The questions will help you to think about key features of your story and what is important about your story.

## Transition From Student to Public Health Nursing Practice

You may feel overwhelmed by how much there is to know about public health nursing. How can a new graduate be a successful PHN? When Molly Hoff was new to public health nursing practice, she reflected on her experience of becoming a PHN in writing:

*What support helped you to make a transition to your new position?*

The biggest support I had transitioning to PHN practice was other nurses and social workers in my orientation. Some of them were more experienced than me, and it was great to draw on that knowledge. With little experience, it was nice to be able to relate and lean on them for support.

*What knowledge areas and skills did you find you needed for public health nursing practice?*

Far and above, you need to have great critical thinking skills—before anything else, you need that. I was taught this very well in school, but it got rusty in some of my clinical practice, which was less autonomous than this position. You need to be able to think through, around, and over a myriad of issues that are constantly coming up with our clients. Another skill needed is active listening/motivational interviewing—this is the crux of our contact with the clients and unless they feel supported and that they are not being judged, we will not be able to do our jobs. Having a base in holistic treatment doesn't hurt either, knowing how to look at the person as a complete being and not the sum of their diagnoses.

*What is especially rewarding to you about public health nursing practice?*

Public health practice is great because it is helping people live their lives to the fullest possible degree. Going into the hospital is an event; what we do is everything after and before that—the person's everyday life.

*What advice do you have for a new PHN?*

Learn as much as possible about health and wellness, because you never know what will come in handy or help you in your job.

*Source: Molly Hoff (personal communication, September 2013)*

## Reflections on Being a Public Health Nurse

Expert PHNs explained why they practice public health nursing and what they find rewarding in practice. Their comments capture the essence of what is important to PHNs and what inspires them to do their work:

> "Being a public health nurse is an honor and a privilege. You are constantly doing work important to the public 'common good.' You constantly give back each and every day. It is an amazing privilege to be allowed such an important place in others' lives."
> –Karen

> "Being a public health nurse fits best with my philosophy—giving people the resources and supports they need to make good decisions that maximize their health, safety, and independence."
> –Chris

> "Being a public health nurse includes looking beyond the obvious and looking for what is happening in the client situation that we do not yet know. Making genuine connections and building

caring relationships undergirds public health. A public health nurse is both a nurse investigator and caregiver, blending holistic inquiry with thoughtful interventions that can make a real difference in people's everyday lives by impacting health and imparting hope."

–Renee

"Public health nursing involves healthcare of an entire community. I personally thrive in a work environment where all aspects of nursing care might be required on any given day. A public health nurse needs to be flexible in the work day, because priorities can be continually changing."

–BJ

"Public health nursing is rewarding when I help improve the health of the community while assisting individuals with taking action to optimize their own health."

–Bruce

"I enjoy working with different cultures—learning about their traditions, beliefs, and how frequently there is a commonality to all people, regardless of which country they were born in or their economic status."

–Mary

"I know that each family I visit will find their path a little easier and more focused because of me. As a public health nurse, I need to be flexible, nonjudgmental, caring, and empathetic, but I also need to keep myself distanced enough to see the big picture and to help my clients look at options and goals for their health and their lives. I am a public health nurse because I want to make a difference."

–Barb

"Being in the community is so rewarding—I work with people of all ages and backgrounds and establish partnerships to carry out the public health mission to reach those in need. Being a public health nurse means being a voice for prevention and early intervention, being a voice for making healthy choices, and being an advocate to help people to be healthy. For me, public health nursing is fulfilling, rewarding, challenging, and is my passion. It is a true calling and a blessing to be a public health nurse."

–Bonnie

## References

Henry Street Consortium. (2017). *Henry Street Consortium entry-level competencies (long form)*. Retrieved from http://www.henrystreetconsortium.org/uploads/1/1/1/9/11196081/henry_street_competencies_long_form.pdf

Klein, C. B. (2016). *The magic world: Writing great books for children and young adults*. New York, NY: W. W. Norton & Company.

Kub, J. E., Kulbok, P. A., Miner, S., & Merrill, J. A. (2017). Increasing the capacity of public health nursing to strengthen the public health infrastructure and to promote and protect the health of communities and populations. *Nursing Outlook, 65*(5), 661–664. Retrieved from http://dx.doi.org/10.1016/j.outlook.2017.08.009

National Advisory Council on Nurse Education and Practice. (2016). *Preparing nurses for new roles in population management*. Retrieved from https://www.hrsa.gov/advisorycommittees/bhpradvisory/nacnep/Reports/fourteenthreport.pdf

Robert Wood Johnson Foundation Public Health Nurse Leaders. (2017, August). 10 ways public health nurses (PHNs) improve health. Retrieved from https://health.wyo.gov/wp-content/uploads/2017/11/10-Ways-PHNLs-Improve-Health-09.14.17.pdf

Schaffer, M. A., Keller, L. O., & Reckinger, D. (2015). Public health activities: Visible or invisible? *Public Health Nursing, 32*(6), 711–720. doi:10.1111/phn.1291

Storfjell, J. L., Winslow, B. W., & Saunders, J. S. D. (2017, September 1). Catalysts for change: Harnessing the power of nurses to build population health in the 21st century. Robert Wood Johnson Foundation. Retrieved from https://www.rwjf.org/en/library/research/2017/09/catalysts-for-change--harnessing-the-power-of-nurses-to-build-population-health.html

# PART III

# Appendixes

# Entry-Level, Population-Based Public Health Nursing (PHN) Competencies for the New Graduate or Novice Public Health Nurse

## PHN KNOWLEDGE AND SKILLS

### CORNERSTONE

Public health nursing practice focuses on entire populations and reflects community priorities and needs.

1. **Applies the public health nursing process to communities, systems, individuals, and families**
   A. Identifies the population(s) for which the PHN is accountable
   B. Assesses the health status of communities, systems, individuals, and families
      1) Uses a health and social determinants framework to determine risk factors and protective factors that lead to health and illness in communities, systems, individuals, and families
      2) Identifies relevant and appropriate data and information sources for the populations to which the PHN is accountable
         a. Familiar with data used in the health department
         b. Familiar with data in the programs in which the PHN works
      3) Works in partnership with communities, systems, individuals, or families to attach meaning to collected quantitative and qualitative data
      4) Works in partnership with communities, systems, individuals, and families to establish priorities
   C. Creates public health strength, risk, and asset-based diagnoses for communities, systems, individuals, and families
   D. In partnership with communities, systems, individuals, and families, develops a plan based on priorities (including nursing care plans for individuals/families)
      1) Selects desired outcomes that are measurable, meaningful, and manageable
      2) Selects public health interventions that
         a. Are supported by current literature as evidence-based
         b. Reduce health determinant risk factors and strengthen health determinant protective factors
         c. Have the greatest potential for improving the health of the population
         d. Respect and are consistent with the culture and ethnic beliefs of the community
         e. Are consistent with professional standards, the Nurse Practice Act, existing laws, ordinances, and policies
      3) Selects level(s) of intervention (community, systems, individuals, and families)
      4) Selects level(s) of prevention (primary, secondary, tertiary)
   E. Implements the plan with communities, systems, individuals, and families
      1) Works in partnership with communities, systems, individuals, and families to implement public health interventions
      2) Utilizes best practices when implementing the public health nursing intervention

F. Evaluates
   1) Measures outcomes of public health nursing interventions using evidence-based methods and tools
   2) Documents the public health nursing process by completing forms, records, and charts for communities, systems, individuals, and families
   3) Uses information technology to collect, document, analyze, store, and retrieve the health status of communities, systems, individuals, and families

## CORNERSTONE

Public health nursing practice promotes health through strategies driven by epidemiological evidence.

2. **Utilizes basic epidemiological (the incidence, distribution, and control of disease in a population) principles in public health nursing practice**
   A. Understands the relationship between community assessment and health promotion/disease prevention programs, especially the populations and programs with which the PHN works
   B. Understands the relationships between risk/protective factors and health issues
   C. Obtains and interprets information regarding risks and benefits to the community
   D. Applies an epidemiological framework when assessing and intervening with communities, systems, individuals, and families

3. **Utilizes the principles and science of environmental health to promote safe and sustainable environments for individuals/families, systems, and communities**
   A. Promotes environments that facilitate holistic well-being and health, healing, and healthy lifestyles for individuals/families, systems, and communities
      1) Assesses environmental risk factors and protective factors for individuals/families, systems, and communities
      2) Engages in actions to reduce environmental risk factors and strengthens protective factors for individuals/families, systems, and communities
      3) Takes actions to reduce and manage harmful waste products from individuals/families, systems, and communities
      4) Evaluates the outcomes of actions to promote healthy environments
   B. Seeks to protect individuals/families, systems, and communities from environmental hazards
      1) Educates individuals, families, systems, and communities about environmental hazards and harmful lifestyle factors
      2) Recommends modifications in home, neighborhood, workplace, and community environments to increase safety for individuals and families across the life span
      3) Supports right-to-know legislation and regulations that protect and inform the public about hazardous products
   C. Considers the diverse values, beliefs, cultures, and circumstances of individuals/families and populations when recommending and implementing healthy environmental interventions
      1) Is attentive to diverse lifestyle factors and assesses potential health and safety risks related to them
      2) Accepts and supports diversity in environmental lifestyle factors
      3) Makes referrals when appropriate to governmental agencies when harmful environmental lifestyle factors place children and vulnerable adults at risk
   D. Promotes stewardship of the environment at local, national, and international levels
      1) Advocates for sustainable natural and built environments
      2) Advocates for environmental justice for vulnerable and under-represented populations
      3) Supports policies that promote safe and sustainable natural and built environments and water and food systems

## CORNERSTONE

The authority for the independent practice of public health nursing emanates from the Nurse Practice Act.

4. **Practices within the auspices of the Nurse Practice Act**
    A. Understands the scope of nursing practice (independent nursing functions and delegated medical functions)
    B. Establishes appropriate professional boundaries
    C. Maintains confidentiality
    D. Demonstrates ethical, legal, and professional accountability
    E. Delegates and supervises other personnel
    F. Understands the role of a public health nurse as described under public health nursing registration
    G. Considers how to practice public health nursing in a variety of public and private healthcare settings

## CORNERSTONE

Public health nursing practice collaborates with community resources to achieve those strategies but can and will work alone if necessary.

5. **Works within the responsibility and authority of the governmental public health system**
    A. Describes the relationship among the federal, state, and local levels of public health system
    B. Identifies the individual's and organization's responsibilities within the context of the Essential Public Health Services and Core Functions
    C. Understands practice implications for laws, regulations, and rules relevant to public health
    D. Adheres to legal mandates such as data privacy and mandated reporting
    E. Differentiates the public health model from the medical model
    F. Understands the independent public health nursing role as described in the Scope and Standards of Public Health Nursing
    G. Describes the role of government in the delivery of community health services
    H. Identifies components of the healthcare system
        1) Funding streams such as Medicare, Medicaid, Prepaid Medical Assistance Plan (PMAP), categorical grants
        2) Programs utilized by state and local health departments, such as the Women, Infants, and Children (WIC) program, home visiting, and school health
        3) Community resources

6. **Utilizes collaboration to achieve public health goals**
    A. Demonstrates effective participation on interprofessional teams
    B. Develops relationships and builds partnerships with communities, systems, individuals, and families
    C. Utilizes community assets and community engagement to empower communities, systems, individuals, and families

7. **Effectively communicates with communities, systems, individuals, families, and colleagues**
    A. Interacts respectfully, sensitively, and effectively with everyone
    B. Utilizes sound teaching/learning strategies that tailor communication to target individual, family, community, organizational, or system audiences
    C. Selects appropriate communication methods to reach target audience(s)
    D. Presents accurate demographic, statistical, programmatic, and scientific information

## CORNERSTONE

Public health nursing practice establishes caring relationships with the communities, systems, individuals, and families that comprise the populations PHNs serve.

8. **Establishes and maintains caring relationships with communities, systems, individuals, and families**
   A. Demonstrates trust, respect, empathy
   B. Follows through with commitments
   C. Maintains appropriate boundaries
   D. Demonstrates tact and diplomacy
   E. Seeks assistance when needed in managing relationships
   F. Interacts with others in a culturally sensitive manner

## CORNERSTONE

Public health nursing practice encompasses the mental, physical, emotional, social, spiritual, and environmental aspects of health.

9. **Incorporates mental, physical, emotional, social, and spiritual aspects of health into assessment, planning, implementation, and evaluation**
   A. Assesses mental, physical, emotional, social, and spiritual health
   B. Develops and implements holistic public health interventions that meet the needs of individuals, families, communities, and systems
   C. Evaluates the impact of public health nursing interventions on the mental, physical, emotional, social, spiritual, and environmental health of individuals, families, communities, and systems

## CORNERSTONE

Public health nursing practice is grounded in social justice, compassion, sensitivity to diversity, and respect for the worth of all people, especially the vulnerable.

10. **Demonstrates nonjudgmental/unconditional acceptance of people different from self**
    A. Listens to others in an unbiased, respectful manner
    B. Promotes the expression of diverse opinions and perspectives
    C. Identifies the role of diverse factors when selecting or designing public health interventions tailored to specific individuals, communities, or systems
    D. Interacts respectfully, sensitively, and effectively with individuals, families, and communities

11. **Shows evidence of commitment to social justice, the greater good, and the public health principles**
    A. Applies principles of social justice to promote and maintain the health and well-being of populations
    B. Understands the impact of the social determinants of health on vulnerable and at-risk populations
    C. Advocates for the disadvantaged and underserved
    D. Participates in collaborative social actions to reduce health disparities and inequities

## ALL CORNERSTONES

12. **Demonstrates leadership in public health nursing with communities, systems, individuals, and families**
    A. Seeks learning opportunities when working with peers, organizations, and communities
    B. Demonstrates ability to be flexible, adapt to change, and tolerate ambiguity while working in an unstructured environment
    C. Seeks and provides consultation and support to peers and community partners
    D. Responds to population health needs in collaboration with systems and communities
    E. Contributes to team efforts to improve the quality of care provided to client populations
    F. Prioritizes and organizes workload, time, materials, and resources to maximize benefits to clients and stakeholders
    G. Participates in the political process to advocate for changes in health and social policies that affect population health, workforce health, and public health services delivery

## Personal Characteristics That Contribute to Effective Practice

1. Passion
2. Creativity
3. Courage
4. Confidence
5. Adaptability
6. Humor
7. Persistence
8. Independence
9. Positive attitude
10. Lifelong learner
11. Risk taker
12. Hard worker
13. Leader
14. Resourceful
15. Flexibility
16. Caring
17. Compassion
18. Self-care

## Basic Public Health Nursing Knowledge Base

1. Human growth and development across the life span: prenatal, infancy, preschool, school-age, adolescent, adult, elderly
2. Human sexuality
3. Family planning
4. Family development
5. Antepartum/postpartum
6. Parenting
7. Death and dying; grief and loss
8. Health and social determinants
9. Social and market justice
10. Health promotion: infant, preschool, school-age, adolescent, women, men, elderly
11. Nutrition
12. Disease prevention and control, including universal precautions
13. Immunizations across the life span
14. Chronic disease prevention and management
15. Chemical health issues and/or behaviors
16. Mental health
17. Injury prevention
18. Violence prevention
19. Disaster and bioterrorism response
20. Environmental health and safety
21. Medication administration/management
22. Technical nursing skills

Original Publication: March 2003
Henry Street Consortium
Linking Public Health Nursing Practice
  and Education to Promote Population Health
Center for Public Health Nursing
Minnesota Department of Health

Revised June 2017
Henry Street Consortium
www.henrystreetconsortium.org

# Omaha System

---

## BOX B.1
### Domains and Problems of the Omaha System Problem Classification Scheme

### Environmental Domain

Material resources and physical surroundings both inside and outside the living area, neighborhood, and broader community:

- Income
- Sanitation
- Residence
- Neighborhood/workplace safety

### Psychosocial Domain

Patterns of behavior, emotion, communication, relationships, and development:

- Communication with community resources
- Social contact
- Role change
- Interpersonal relationship
- Spirituality
- Grief
- Mental health
- Sexuality
- Caretaking/parenting
- Neglect
- Abuse
- Growth and development

### Physiological Domain

Functions and processes that maintain life:

- Hearing
- Vision
- Speech and language
- Oral health
- Cognition
- Pain
- Consciousness
- Skin
- Neuromusculoskeletal function
- Respiration
- Circulation
- Digestion-hydration
- Bowel function
- Urinary function
- Reproductive function
- Pregnancy
- Postpartum
- Communicable/infectious condition

### Health-Related Behaviors Domain

Patterns of activity that maintain or promote wellness, promote recovery, and decrease the risk of disease:

- Nutrition
- Sleep and rest patterns
- Physical activity
- Personal care
- Substance use
- Family planning
- Healthcare supervision
- Medication regimen

From: Martin, K. S. (2005). *The Omaha System: A key to practice, documentation, and information management* (Reprinted 2nd ed.). Omaha, NE: Health Connections Press.

## BOX B.2

### Categories of the Omaha System Intervention Scheme

**Teaching, Guidance, and Counseling**

Activities designed to provide information and materials, encourage action and responsibility for self-care and coping, and assist the individual, family, or community to make decisions and solve problems.

**Treatments and Procedures**

Technical activities such as wound care, specimen collection, resistive exercises, and medication prescriptions that are designed to prevent, decrease, or alleviate signs and symptoms for the individual, family, or community.

**Case Management**

Activities such as coordination, advocacy, and referral that facilitate service delivery; promote assertiveness; guide the individual, family, or community toward use of appropriate community resources; and improve communication among health and human service providers.

**Surveillance**

Activities such as detection, measurement, critical analysis, and monitoring intended to identify the individual, family, or community's status in relation to a given condition or phenomenon.

From: Martin, K. S. (2005). *The Omaha System: A key to practice, documentation, and information management* (Reprinted 2nd ed.). Omaha, NE: Health Connections Press.

## BOX B.3

### Targets of the Omaha System Intervention Scheme

- anatomy/physiology
- anger management
- behavior modification
- bladder care
- bonding/attachment
- bowel care
- cardiac care
- caretaking/parenting skills
- cast care
- communication
- community outreach worker services
- continuity of care
- coping skills
- day care/respite
- dietary management
- discipline
- dressing change/wound care
- durable medical equipment
- education
- employment
- end-of-life care
- environment
- exercises
- family planning care
- feeding procedures
- finances
- gait training
- genetics
- growth/development care
- home
- homemaking/housekeeping
- infection precautions
- interaction
- interpreter/translator services
- laboratory findings
- legal system
- medical/dental care
- medication action/side effects
- medication administration
- medication coordination/ordering
- medication prescription
- medication setup
- mobility/transfers
- nursing care
- nutritionist care
- occupational therapy care
- ostomy care
- other community resources
- paraprofessional/aide care
- personal hygiene
- physical therapy care
- positioning
- recreational therapy care
- relaxation/breathing techniques
- respiratory care
- respiratory therapy care
- rest/sleep
- safety
- screening procedures
- sickness/injury care
- signs/symptoms-mental/emotional
- signs/symptoms-physical
- skin care
- social work/counseling care
- specimen collection
- speech and language pathology care
- spiritual care
- stimulation/nurturance
- stress management
- substance use cessation
- supplies
- support group
- support system
- transportation
- wellness
- other

From: Martin, K. S. (2005). *The Omaha System: A key to practice, documentation, and information management* (Reprinted 2nd ed.). Omaha, NE: Health Connections Press.

**TABLE B.1** Omaha System Problem Rating Scale for Outcomes

| Concept | 1 | 2 | 3 | 4 | 5 |
| --- | --- | --- | --- | --- | --- |
| **Knowledge:** Ability of client to remember and interpret information | No knowledge | Minimal knowledge | Basic knowledge | Adequate knowledge | Superior knowledge |
| **Behavior:** Observable responses, actions, or activities of client fitting occasion or purpose | Not appropriate behavior | Rarely appropriate behavior | Inconsistently appropriate behavior | Usually appropriate behavior | Consistently appropriate behavior |
| **Status:** Condition of client in relation to objective and subjective defining characteristics | Extreme signs/symptoms | Severe signs/symptoms | Moderate signs/symptoms | Minimal signs/symptoms | No signs/symptoms |

From: Martin, K. S. (2005). *The Omaha System: A key to practice, documentation, and information management* (Reprinted 2nd ed.). Omaha, NE: Health Connections Press.